HANDBOOK OF FRACTURES

Second Edition

EDITORS

Clayton R. Perry, M.D.

Assistant Clinical Professor
Department of Orthopaedic Surgery
St. Louis University School of Medicine
St. Louis, Missouri
U.S. Center for Sports Medicine
St. Louis, Missouri

John A. Elstrom, M.D.

Clinical Assistant Professor
University of Illinois
Chicago, Illinois
Department of Surgery
Northern Illinois Medical Center
McHenry, Illinois

D0002393

McGRAW-HILL, INC.
Health Professions Division
New York   St. Louis   San Francisco   Auckland   Bogotá
Caracas   Lisbon   London   Madrid   Mexico City   Milan
Montreal   New Delhi   San Juan   Singapore
Sydney   Tokyo   Toronto

McGraw-Hill

*A Division of The **McGraw·Hill** Companies*

HANDBOOK OF FRACTURES, SECOND EDITION

Copyright @2000, 1995 by The **McGraw-Hill Companies,** Inc. All rights reserved. Printed in the United States of America. Except as permitted under the United States Copyright Act of 1976, no part of this publication may be reproduced or distributed in any form or by any means, or stored in a data base or retrieval system, without the prior written permission of the publisher.

1 2 3 4 5 6 7 8 9 0 DOC DOC 9 9

This book was set in Times Roman by the PRD Group, Inc.
The editors were Darlene Cooke, Susan Noujaim, and Nicky Panton.
The production supervisor was Richard Ruzycka.
The cover designer was Pehrsson Design.
The index was prepared by Geraldine Beckford.
R.R. Donnelley and Sons was printer and binder.

This book is printed on acid-free paper.

Library of Congress Cataloging-in-Publication Data

Handbook of fractures/editors, Clayton R. Perry, John A. Elstrom. —
   2nd ed.
     p.   cm.
   Includes bibliographical references and index.
   ISBN 0-07-048624-7
   1. Fractures Handbooks, manuals, etc. 2. Orthopedics Handbooks,
manuals, etc. I. Perry, Clayton. II. Elstrom, John A.
   [DNLM: 1. Fractures—therapy Handbooks. 2. Orthopedics—
methods Handbooks. WE 39 H236 2000]
RD101.H24   2000
617.1′5—dc21
DNLM/DLC
for Library of Congress   99-38946
                                             CIP

This book is dedicated to Monica,
without whose help it would not have been possible,
and to my sons, Clay and Kevin
CRP

This book is dedicated to my wife, Quyen,
Quos amor verus tenuit, tenebit
-Seneca
JAE

Contents

Contributors

EDWARD R. ABRAHAM, M.D.
Chairman, Department of
  Orthopaedic Surgery
Abraham Lincoln School of
  Medicine
University of Illinois
Chicago, Illinois [10]

KEITH H. BRIDWELL, M.D.
Professor
Department of Orthopaedic
  Surgery
Washington University School
  of Medicine
St. Louis, Missouri [15]

**C.M. COURT-BROWN,
  M.D., FRCS Ed. (Orth)**
Consultant Orthopaedic
  Surgeon
The Royal Infirmary of
  Edinburgh
Edinburgh, Scotland [21]

**KENNETH A.
  DAVENPORT, M.D.**
Attending Physician
Marquette General Hospital
Marquette, Michigan [19]

JOHN A. ELSTROM, M.D.
Clinical Assistant Professor
University of Illinois
Chicago, Illinois

Department of Surgery
Northern Illinois Medical
  Center
McHenry, Illinois [3, 5, 7, 8, 9,
  and 11]

MARK GONZALEZ
Professor
Department of Orthopaedic
  Surgery
Abraham Lincoln School of
  Medicine
University of Illinois
Chicago, Illinois
Chairman, Department of
  Orthopaedic Surgery
Cook County Hospital
Chicago, Illinois [10 and 14]

MICHAEL E. JOYCE, M.D.
Assistant Clinical Professor
Department of Orthopaedic
  Surgery
University of Connecticut
  School of Medicine
Willimantic, Connecticut [6]

The numbers in brackets show the chapter numbers of each contributor.

ENES KANLIC, M.D., Ph.D.
Associate Professor
TTUHSC for Health Science
Center–El Paso
Orthopaedic Surgery
Department
El Paso, Texas [18 and 23]

**LAWRENCE G. LENKE,
M.D.**
Associate Professor
Department of Orthopaedic
Surgery
Washington University School
of Medicine
St. Louis, Missouri [15]

CARL H. NIELSEN, M.D.
Associate Professor
Department of Anesthesiology
Washington University School
of Medicine
St. Louis, Missouri [4]

**MICHAEL F. O'BRIEN,
M.D.**
Assistant Clinical Professor
Department of Orthopaedic
Surgery
University of Colorado
Denver, Colorado

Instructor
Spine Fellowship Program
University of Colorado
Denver, Colorado

Woodridge Orthopaedic and
Spine Center
Wheatridge, Colorado [15]

CLAYTON R. PERRY, M.D.
Associate Clinical Professor
Department of Orthopaedic
Surgery
St. Louis University School of
Medicine
St. Louis, Missouri

U.S. Center for Sports
Medicine
St. Louis, Missouri [1, 2, 6, 7,
10, 11, 17, 18, 20, 22, and
23]

DONALD L. PRUITT, M.D.
Private Practice
St. Louis Orthopaedic Institute
St. Louis, Missouri [12 and 13]

D. KEVIN SCHEID, M.D.
Director of Orthopaedic
Education
Methodist Hospital
Indianapolis, Indiana

Clinical Instructor
Department of Orthopaedic
Surgery
Indiana University School of
Medicine
Indianapolis, Indiana [16]

**ROBERT SCHENCK, Jr.,
M.D.**
Associate Professor, Deputy
Chairman
Department of Orthopaedics
University of Texas Health
Sciences Center
San Antonio, Texas [20]

Preface

Fracture management is fundamental to orthopaedic practice. In developing this book, we wanted a portable handy reference written for the practicing orthopaedic surgeon. It is not always convenient to refer to the large published tomes for quick management decisions. Our aim has been to create a concise, organized, and readily accessible reference for fracture management. In order to fulfill our objectives, it has been necessary to publish a pocket-size book that can be readily carried.

We have attempted to bring together the basic elements that the reader must know in order to diagnose, classify, and manage specific fractures. Despite the small trim size of the book, we have maximized the use of illustrations to avoid excess use of words in the text and to better present a balanced overview of fracture management; it is not our intention to discuss some of the more controversial issues that can be read elsewhere. Despite this, the author's philosophy of management may be evident, and we encourage the reader to also review other literature for specific technical procedures. In keeping with this scope, we decided to omit references within the text, but to include a more practical list of reading material entitled, "Selected Readings."

The organization of this book is simple. Initially, there are general chapters that cover clinical evaluation, methods of fixation, nonoperative techniques, anesthetic techniques, and fracture healing and bone grafting. Thereafter, each chapter specifically examines fractures organized by anatomy, starting with the glenohumeral joint and working down to the foot. For ease of accessibility, we have divided each chapter into identical sections: anatomy, fracture classification, diagnosis and initial management, radiographic examination, and associated injuries. Bolding of key words within the text is designed to help the reader quickly identify relevant material. The glossary at the end of the book defines terms that are not defined within the text itself, thus, it can be used as a quick reference.

This book is a collaborative effort, representing the method of fracture management from a small group of active orthopaedic trauma surgeons. The editors would like to acknowledge the expertise provided by a select group of contributing authors. We hope that we have fulfilled our goal in providing a practical, accessible guide for all persons involved in the care of fracture management.

Acknowledgments

I would like to acknowledge my indebtedness to the following persons: Lisa Tracy, for her untiring efforts in preparing the manuscript. Dr. Arsen Pankovich, my friend and teacher for his support, criticism, and advice; and Dr. Robert F. Hall, Jr., for his willingness to read over many of the chapters and suggest changes, and for his demonstration of some of the surgical techniques that contributed immeasurably to the section on the upper extremity.

John A. Elstrom, M.D.

HANDBOOK
OF
FRACTURES

Clinical Evaluation/Initial Management of Patients with Multiple Injuries

Clayton R. Perry

A history and physical examination are obtained from all patients who have sustained a fracture or dislocation. Unlike patients with complex medical problems, the diagnosis of a fracture or dislocation is relatively obvious. The key is not to miss an associated injury.

The elements of a **history** are where, when, and how the injury has occurred. A **past medical history** is obtained to determine whether there are preexisting conditions that alter the choice of management (e.g., a recent myocardial infarction mitigates for closed management of a fracture, or a prior injury may have already compromised function of the extremity). Hand dominance and occupation are documented. A **social history** regarding the use of alcohol, tobacco, and drugs is obtained.

A complete **physical examination** of cardiovascular, respiratory, gastrointestinal, genitourinary, and neurologic systems is performed. The examination then focuses on the area of the injury, distal to the injury, and one joint proximal to the injury. The patient is asked to localize the pain. The area is inspected for open wounds and deformity and is then gently palpated to pinpoint the painful area and to determine the position of underlying bones and joints. Active and passive range of motion of surrounding joints is assessed. The circulatory status is determined by palpating pulses, looking for capillary refill in the nail beds, and assessing the color of the skin (blue, pink, or white). The neurologic system is evaluated by determining whether sensation, voluntary movement, and deep tendon reflexes are present and intact.

A specific, detailed pattern of examination of the musculoskeletal, vascular, and neurologic systems of the upper and lower extremities follows.

UPPER EXTREMITY

Musculoskeletal System

Flexion of distal interphalangeal joints of the fingers and thumb indicates intact flexor profundus and flexor pollicis longus. Flexion of the proximal interphalangeal joints of an individual finger while the remaining digits are held in extension indicates an intact flexor superficialis. Interphalangeal extension indicates intact interossei and extensor hood; metacarpal phalangeal extension, an intact extensor digitorum; and wrist dorsiflexion and palmar flexion, intact flexor carpi radialis, ulnaris and extensor carpi radialis longus, and radialis brevis and ulnaris. Radial or ulnar deviation indicates that the contralateral flexor or extensor is not functioning (e.g., radial deviation with extension of the wrist indicates that the extensor carpi ulnaris is not functioning). The ability to pronate the forearm indicates an intact pronator teres (which functions when the elbow is extended) and intact pronator quadratus (which functions when the elbow is flexed). Supination indicates intact supinator and biceps; elbow flexion, intact brachialis and biceps; and elbow extension, intact triceps. Initiation of glenohumeral abduction and the ability to maintain the humerus abducted 60° indicate an intact rotator cuff. The deltoid, pectoralis major, and trapezius are palpated as they contract. The phalanges, metacarpals, radius, ulna, and humerus are gently palpated along their lengths. The examiner looks for a palpable "step off" indicative of a fracture to determine the exact location of the patient's pain. Range of motion of the joints is measured. By convention, full extension is 0° and hyperextension is expressed as negative degrees. Wrist motion is expressed as degrees of dorsiflexion and palmar flexion, with neutral being 0°; forearm rotation is expressed as degrees of supination and pronation, with neutral being 0°. Glenohumeral motion is measured while stabilizing the scapula with one hand to estimate the contribution of scapula-thoracic motion. Bringing the elbow forward is glenohumeral flexion, posteriorly is extension.

Vascular System

Pulses are palpable in the axilla (axillary artery), the antecubital fossae medial to the biceps tendon (brachial artery), and radial to the flexor carpi radialis tendon at the wrist (radial artery); a palpable radial pulse indicates a systolic pressure of at least 80 mmHg. The Allen test determines whether the ulnar artery is intact. Using the thumb and index finger, the examiner compresses and occludes the patient's radial and ulnar arteries at the wrist after the patient has made a fist. The patient then opens the hand. As pressure is taken off the ulnar artery, the hand becomes pink if the ulnar artery is intact. The hand will remain white if the ulnar artery is not contributing to the blood supply of the hand. Capillary refill is assessed by compressing the nail beds and observing the return of oxygenated blood. Brisk, or immediate, capillary refill indicates that oxygenated blood is reaching the extremity. The presence or absence of capillary refill is especially important in two clinical situations. First, when the hand or fingers are injured, pulses cannot be reliably palpated. The presence of brisk capillary refill indicates that the arterial supply is adequate to sustain the viability of the fingers and hand. Second, when there is a known arterial injury proximal to the wrist, the presence of brisk capillary refill indicates that collateral vessels are supplying the extremity distal to the injury.

Neurologic System

Sensory function is assessed by determining the ability to differentiate sharp from dull. Intact sensation on the sides of a digit indicates an intact digital nerve; on the dorsum of the first web space, an intact radial nerve;

on the palmar aspect of the distal index finger, an intact median nerve; on the ulnar aspect of the fifth finger, an intact ulnar nerve; on the dorsum of the forearm, an intact musculocutaneous nerve; and in the "policeman's badge" distribution over the deltoid, an intact axillary nerve. The **motor component of the neurologic system** is assessed by determining the ability to contract a given muscle actively. Abduction of the fingers indicates an intact ulnar nerve; palmar abduction of the thumb, an intact median nerve; thumb and wrist extension, an intact radial nerve; and deltoid contraction, an intact axillary nerve. An intact deep tendon reflex indicates that the arc consists of an efferent nerve from the tendon, the spinal cord at the level of the motor neurons supplying the muscle, and an intact afferent nerve to the muscle. When peripheral nerves are intact, deep tendon reflexes are the best way to assess nerve root function. Presence of the biceps reflex indicates an intact musculocutaneous nerve and C5 root, and that of the brachioradialis and triceps reflex indicates radial nerve and C6 and C7 roots, respectively.

LOWER EXTREMITY

Musculoskeletal System

Foot eversion indicates intact peroneal longus and brevis. The anterior tibialis dorsiflexes the ankle and is palpable at its insertion on the navicular. Ankle plantar flexion indicates triceps surae; knee extension, an intact quadriceps femoris; knee flexion, intact hamstrings; hip extension, intact gluteus maximus; and hip abduction, an intact gluteus medius. The bones of the foot, tibia, patella, and the femoral condyles are palpated. Range of motion of the joints is measured. Subtalar motion is determined by inverting and everting the heel, with the ankle held at a neutral position. Ankle motion is documented as degrees of dorsiflexion and plantar flexion, with neutral being 0°. Knee motion is documented, with full extension being 0°. Hip motion is measured while stabilizing the pelvis with one hand to minimize lumbosacral and sacroiliac motion. Evaluation of the ankle ligaments is described in "Fractures and Dislocations of the Ankle" (Chap. 22). Evaluation of the knee ligaments is described in "Injuries About the Knee" (Chap. 20).

Vascular System

Pulses are palpable lateral to the base of the first metatarsal (dorsalis pedis), behind the medial malleolus (posterior tibial), in the popliteal fossae (popliteal artery), and in the femoral triangle (femoral artery). Capillary refill is observed in the nail beds.

Neurologic System

Intact sensation on either side of a digit indicates an intact digital nerve; in the first web space, an intact deep peroneal nerve; on lateral side of the foot, intact sural and superficial peroneal nerves; and on medial dorsum of the foot, an intact saphenous nerve. **Motor system:** Contraction of the anterior tibial, peroneus longus, and brevis muscle indicates an intact common peroneal nerve; of the triceps surae, an intact tibial nerve; of the quadriceps femoris, an intact femoral nerve; and of the hamstrings, an intact sciatic nerve. Intact deep tendon reflexes of the triceps surae indicates an intact S1 nerve root, and of the patellar tendon, an intact L4 nerve root.

Two extremity injuries which bear special mention are open fractures and compartment syndromes. **Open fractures** are graded 1-3, with 3 being the most severe, and having the highest incidence of complications (i.e., osteomyelitis and nonunion). **Grade 1** open fractures have wounds less than 1 cm in length, **grade 2** wounds are more than 1 cm in length, but clean without devitalization of tissue; **grade 3** wounds are greater than 10 cm in length, or grossly contaminated, have devitalized tissue (e.g., avulsion or crush injuries), or associated with comminuted fractures and vascular injury. Grade 3 fractures are further divided into three groups. **3A** fractures are characterized by the absence of periosteal stripping, and do not have an associated vascular injury. **3B** fractures have periosteal stripping, and soft tissue loss. In general 3B injuries cannot be closed primarily, and require a soft tissue transfer for coverage. **3C** fractures are characterized by the presence of an associated limb threatening vascular injury, or significant nerve injury.

Compartment syndromes are caused by elevated hydrostatic pressure in a closed fascial space, or compartment. There are many causes of elevated pressure including contusion of muscle, a bleed into the compartment, or occlusion of venous outflow from the compartment. As the pressure increases, the capillary beds and arterioles collapse, shunting blood through the compartment via larger arteries without supplying the structures within the compartment. This action results in more ischemia, increased swelling, and higher pressure. The physical signs of compartment syndrome are increased **pain** (for this sign to apply, the patient must be conscious and the extremity involved must have normal sensation), **pain with passive stretch** of involved muscles (this is distinguished from pain due to an associated fracture in that very slight, gentle, motion elicits severe pain in the involved compartment), **paresthesias of nerves** traversing the compartment (this sign is most valuable in the anterior compartment of the leg, with decreased sensation in the first web space, indicating the deep peroneal nerve), **hard tense compartments** (the most equivocal sign), and **elevated pressures** when measured with a manometer (the most objective sign and used to confirm compartment syndrome when the clinical signs are equivocal). Pulselessness and pallor, signs of arterial occlusion, are not necessarily present; in fact, pulses distal to a full-blown compartment syndrome are often normal. The management of compartment syndrome is surgical release of the involved compartments and delayed primary closure or skin grafting after swelling has subsided. The sequelae of an untreated compartment syndrome are, acutely, muscle necrosis and myoglobinuria resulting in renal shutdown and, chronically, muscle scaring, contractures, and nerve compression.

INITIAL MANAGEMENT OF PATIENTS WITH MULTIPLE INJURIES

The **emergency management of the multiply injured patient** is divided into two phases: the initial assessment and management and the secondary survey and management. When the multiply injured patient presents, the focus is on identification and management of life-threatening injuries. The first priority is to ensure that there is an **adequate airway**. This is done while an assistant stabilizes the head to prevent flexion or extension of the neck because all multiply injured patients are considered to have a cervical spine injury until proven otherwise. The mouth is opened, inspected, and cleared of loose bodies. The chin is lifted, and a nasal airway is inserted. If the patient is unable to protect the airway, the patient is intubated. The indication for an immediate cricothyroidotomy is **inability to secure the upper airway**, which is most frequently due to uncontrollable hemorrhage in the upper airway, fracture of the larynx, or displaced fractures of the facial bones, in particular the mandible.

After the airway has been established, the next priority is to ensure that the patient is **breathing**. If not, respiration is assisted with a bag and mask. Arterial blood gasses are drawn. Dark blood indicates decreased oxygenation. Assuming that the blood is arterial, that the upper airway is secured, and that the patient is ventilating, the cause of decreased oxygenation is usually a pneumothorax, a hemothorax, or a flail chest. The chest is inspected for open wounds and paradoxical motion. An open sucking wound suggests the diagnosis of pneumothorax. Paradoxical motion indicates a flail chest. The neck is inspected to determine whether the trachea is deviated. Deviation of the trachea indicates a pneumothorax on the side toward which the trachea is deviated. The chest is auscultated, percussed and gently palpated. Absence of breath sounds and increased tympany indicate a pneumothorax. Dullness suggests a hemothorax. Crepitus on palpation indicates fractured ribs and a flail chest. Pneumothorax is managed by covering the chest wound to prevent the ingress of air and by inserting a large-bore needle into the midclavicular line at the second intercostal space. Flail chest is managed by positive pressure ventilation.

The next priority after the upper airway and breathing is the **circulation**. Capillary refill and peripheral pulses are approximate measures of adequate circulation. Inadequate circulation indicates shock, which is assumed to be due to blood loss. External blood loss is controlled with application of sterile dressings and direct pressure. Tourniquets are almost never indicated for control of hemorrhage. Fluids and blood products are administered via large-bore lines. Initially, 2 L of Ringer's lactate is administered while blood is being typed and crossed. In absolute emergencies, type 0 rh-negative blood is administered. Military antishock trouser (MAST) suits are used to increase peripheral resistance. MAST suits have the added advantage of immobilizing lower extremity fractures and decreasing intrapelvic volume if there is a displaced pelvic fracture.

After the airway has been secured, ventilation has become adequate, and fluid resuscitation has started, the **secondary survey and management** begins. The secondary survey is a more detailed physical and radiographic examination of the patient. At the same time, procedures are performed: insertion of chest tubes (in place of an intercostal needle), intubation (oral if there is no cervical spine injury; nasotracheal if there is a cervical spine injury), catheterization of the bladder, and insertion of arterial and central lines. In addition, a detailed history of the injury is obtained from the patient or from witnesses of the injury.

The physical examination is performed in an orderly fashion, starting at the head and including the neck, eyes, ears, face, nose, mouth, chest, abdomen, rectum, bony pelvis, external genitalia, extremities, and neurologic system. The basic elements of the examination are inspection, auscultation, and palpation. In addition, the response to stimuli is noted (e.g., reaction of the pupils to light), and open wounds are examined.

Open wounds are managed acutely by removing foreign bodies and gross contaminants, obtaining material for anaerobic and aerobic cultures, and administration of broad spectrum antibiotics. The wounds are irrigated and covered with sterile dressings. **Fractures and dislocations** are reduced or aligned and splinted or placed in traction to facilitate transport. MAST suits temporarily immobilize the fractured pelvis.

Fractures and dislocations in the multiply injured patients are not immediately life threatening. They should be managed as soon as life-threatening injuries have been managed. **Early stabilization** (within 24 h of injury) of long bone fractures decreases the incidence of adult respiratory distress syndrome and fat embolus. The management of isolated fractures is straightforward. Multiple fractures are stabilized according to the following parameters: **debridement of open wounds** is a primary goal; **early mobilization** of the patient is a primary goal; therefore, stabilization of a tibial fracture is useless unless an associated fracture of the femur is also stabilized; and the **surgeon's facility with available techniques** is the major determinant of the duration and adequacy of the procedure (e.g., whether external fixation, intramedullary nailing, or plating of a grade 3 open tibia is the best procedure is dependent on the surgeon's facility with these techniques).

2 | Methods of Fixation

Clayton R. Perry

There are four basic methods used operatively to stabilize fractures: rigidly, with screws and plates; dynamically, with wires or lag screws; with intramedullary nails; and with external fixators. The distinction between these methods is not always clear (e.g., intramedullary nails and external fixators allow controlled motion through the fracture and thus could be considered a type of dynamic fixation). In this chapter, each of these basic methods of fracture fixation is described.

RIGID FIXATION

The Association for the Study of Internal Fixation (ASIF) group revolutionized fracture surgery by introducing techniques and implants that rigidly stabilized anatomically reduced fractures. Fixation is so stable that postoperative immobilization is not required, thus speeding rehabilitation and eliminating cast disease. This aspect of the ASIF method cannot be overemphasized: immobilizing an extremity in which a fracture has been reduced and stabilized is counterproductive. The primary disadvantages of rigid fixation are that an extended surgical exposure is necessary and consolidation of the fracture is by primary bone healing and is therefore prolonged. Stable fixation is achieved by using interfragmentary screws and plates.

Interfragmentary fixation with screws is performed so that a compression force is exerted across the fracture site. This is done by "lagging" the fragments together. In this technique, the reduced fracture is traversed by a screw. One fragment is fixed with the screw threads, and the second fragment lies under the head of the screw. Screw threads are functionally absent in the second fragment because the diameter of the hole equals the diameter of the screw threads or the portion of the screw in this fragment is smooth. As the screw is rotated, it advances, and the head of the screw moves the second fragment toward the first while applying compression across the fracture (Fig. 2-1).

Plates function in one of four ways: to neutralize forces across the fracture, to apply compression across the fracture, as a buttress, and as a tension band.

A **neutralization** plate isolates the fracture from extrinsic forces. It is applied after the fracture fragments have been lagged together. The plate is fastened to the bone without applying compression across the fracture site. An example of a neutralization plate is a one-third tubular plate used to stabilize a lateral malleolar fracture that has been lagged together with an interfragmental screw.

A **compression** plate applies a compressive force across the fracture. It can only be used to stabilize simple fractures because attempting to

FIG. 2-1   Lag-screw technique.

apply compression across a comminuted fracture results in shortening of the bone. The most frequently used method of applying compression is to fasten the plate to one fracture fragment and then insert screws into the second fragment. The screws in the second fragment are eccentrically located in the holes of the plate. Tightening the screws moves the plate, thereby compressing the fracture. Plates that are fabricated to perform this function are distinguished by oblong screw holes and are called *dynamic compression plates*. There are other methods of applying compression across a fracture (e.g., use of a compression device or a special clamp), but dynamic compression plates are by far the most commonly used method. An example of a compression plate is a dynamic compression plate used to stabilize a short oblique fracture of the tibia (Fig. 2-2).

A **buttress** plate functions as a buttress. That is, it prevents a fragment of bone from moving centrifugally, and it prevents shortening. The plate does not necessarily have to be fixed to the fragment to function as a buttress. An example of a buttress plate is a T-plate that stabilizes a split-depressed fracture of the lateral tibial plateau (Fig. 2-3). A type of buttress plate is the *antiglide plate* (Fig. 2-4). The antiglide plate is applied to an oblique fracture to prevent shortening. This technique is most commonly used to stabilize the fibula following an indirect fracture of the ankle.

A **tension band** plate is always applied to the tension side of the bone. It cannot be used on comminuted fractures. As the bone is axially loaded, the tension band plate prevents angulation at the fracture site. Directly under the plate, there are distraction forces across the fracture, and the plate is loaded in tension. The side of the fracture opposite the

FIG. 2-2   A compression plate used to stabilize a diaphyseal tibial fracture.

FIG. 2-3   A buttress plate used to stabilize a fracture of the lateral tibial plateau.

FIG. 2-4   An antiglide plate applied to the posterior aspect of the fibula will prevent shortening.

plate is loaded in compression. An example of a tension band plate is a dynamic compression plate applied to the lateral cortex of the femur, thereby stabilizing a transverse diaphyseal fracture.

DYNAMIC FIXATION

Dynamic fixation allows controlled motion between fragments after they have been stabilized. The disadvantage of dynamic fixation is that we occasionally underestimate or overestimate the amount of controlled motion that will occur. Underestimation leads to a fracture that is stabilized with its fragments distracted. Overestimation leads to uncontrolled collapse of a fracture and loss of reduction. The three techniques by which dynamic fixation is achieved are the tension band wire, sliding compression screw, and cerclage wires.

Tension band wires function similarly to tension band plates. They are always applied to the tension side of the bone. As the bone is loaded, distraction forces occur across the fracture directly under the wire and compression forces occur across the fracture through the opposite cortex. This method of stabilization can only be used for simple transverse fractures. If interfragmentary fixation is used to align the fracture prior to insertion of the tension band wire, it must allow for axial motion. Thus, if screws are used, the threads should not cross the fracture site; if Kirschner wires are used, they should be parallel with each other and with the axis along which compression is to occur. Tension band wires are used most frequently to stabilize fractures of the olecranon and patella.

Sliding compression screws are used to stabilize fractures around the hip. They allow controlled shortening of the fracture to a more stable position. Sliding compression screws are inserted parallel to the long axis of the femoral neck. They are either inserted directly through the lateral cortex (e.g., for a femoral neck fracture) or attached to a side plate on the lateral cortex of the femur (e.g., for an intertrochanteric fracture). Postoperatively, when the patient bears weight, the screws slide through the lateral cortex of the femur or through the side plate, and the fracture impacts until bone-to-bone contact across the fracture site prevents additional shortening. For these devices to function effectively, multiple screws, when used, must be parallel with each other; when adjunctive fixation is used, it must allow shortening (e.g., cerclage wires). The potential length that the fracture can shorten must not exceed the length that the device can shorten.

Cerclage wires are always used with other methods of fixation because they will not adequately stabilize a fracture when used alone. It is key that, as the fracture shortens or displaces, the cerclage wire tightens. Thus, these wires are an effective method of adjunctive fixation for intertrochanteric, subtrochanteric, and diaphyseal fractures of the femur but not for supracondylar fractures of the distal femur in which the fragments "telescope" together (Figs. 2-5 and 2-6).

FIG. 2-5 Tightened cerclage wires prevent shortening of a subtrochanteric fracture.

FIG. 2-6 Supracondylar fracture fragments "telescope"; therefore, cerclage wires do not prevent shortening.

INTRAMEDULLARY NAILS

The advent of intramedullary nails revolutionized the management of diaphyseal fractures of the femur and tibia. Today there are intramedullary nails designed to stabilize fractures of all long bones. They are usually inserted closed (i.e.,without opening the fracture site and using fluoroscopic guidance). The advantages of intramedullary nailing are a low incidence of implant failure due to the fact that they are load sharing versus load bearing, minimal soft tissue irritation due to their intramedullary location, a low incidence of infection because they are inserted without opening the fracture, and rapid healing by external callus. The disadvantages of intramedullary nailing are the difficulty of the technique, the frequency of insertion site symptoms, and that the use of intramedullary nailing is limited to diaphyseal fractures.

There are three parameters used to describe intramedullary nails: rigid or flexible, reamed or nonreamed, and dynamic or static.

The majority of intramedullary nails are **rigid**. One rigid nail is used to stabilize a fracture. On cross section, most rigid nails are hollow. Some are slotted along the length, whereas others are "closed section." Rigid nails are designed to approximate the shape of the bone that they are used to stabilize (e.g., femoral nails have an anterolateral bow that approximates that of the intact femur). They are inserted through a single insertion portal. For the femur there are two commonly used portals. The first is in the piriformis fossa, between the base of the femoral neck and the greater trochanter. The second is in the intercondylar notch of the distal femur. For the tibia, the portal is posterior to the patellar tendon. An example of a rigid nail is the Grosse–Kempf femoral nail.

Flexible intramedullary nails were distinct from rigid intramedullary nails in that more than one nail is used to stabilize a fracture; usually more than one insertion portal is used; they are smaller in cross section; and all flexible nails are solid. Flexible intramedullary nails control rotation through the fracture when more than one insertion portal is used and the tips are flared in the metaphysis. The major disadvantage of flexible intramedullary nails is that they cannot be statically locked; thus, they are indicated only for axially stable fractures. Examples of flexible intramedullary nails are Rush rods and Ender nails.

Reaming denotes sequential enlargement of the medullary canal with flexible drills. Enlarging the medullary canal has several advantages. It allows a larger intramedullary nail to be used, which is important in minimizing implant failure because the strength of the nail increases in proportion with the cube of its radius. In the management of nonunions, reaming reinjures the bone, theoretically stimulating the healing process to begin again. The primary disadvantage of reaming is that it is a tedious process. Reaming destroys the endosteal circulation, and this may be important in open fractures in which there has been periosteal stripping and in fractures that have been previously managed with plates and screws. In both instances, reaming may destroy the only remaining blood supply to the bone and result in segmental devascularization. Most rigid nails are reamed.

Dynamic nails are not fastened to the bone; however, they are fastened to either the proximal or distal fracture fragment. Dynamic nails act as intramedullary splints by aligning the fracture. A **static nail** is "locked" or fastened to the bone proximal and distal to the fracture, usually with screws that perforate the cortex and then go through the nail (Fig. 2-7). Placement of locking screws can be difficult and is done either freehand with fluoroscopic guidance or with the aid of guides that are fastened to the driving end of the nail.

FIG. 2-7   Radiograph of a healed femoral fracture stabilized with a statically locked nail. A figure of eight cables has been used to repair the extensor mechanism.

Nails that are fastened to the bone are called **locked**. Locked nails are either statically locked or dynamically locked. Static locking prevents shortening and rotation through the fracture site. However, it also prevents impaction at the fracture site and converts the nail into a load-bearing device; therefore, there is a high incidence of implant failure. Static locking extends the indications for intramedullary nails to fractures that are rotationally or axially unstable.

Dynamically locked nails are attached to the bone on only one side of the fracture. This method increases the stability of fixation of the locked fragment. In addition, the disadvantages of preventing impaction and of converting the nail into a load-bearing device are avoided.

The **reconstruction nail** is a specific type of locked nail used for proximal femur fractures. It is characterized by the proximal locking screw or screws being inserted up the femoral neck into the femoral head. Reconstruction nails can be locked distally, making them statically locked.

EXTERNAL FIXATION

External fixation is accomplished by driving pins through the bone proximal and distal to the fracture site. The pins are then fastened rigidly together with clamps and rods. These clamps and rods are known as the *external frame*. The ideal external frame is simple, stable, and allows access to open wounds.

The theoretical advantages of fracture management with external fixation are that the construct is relatively stable so that loss of reduction will not occur and that the risk of infection is minimized because surgical exposure of the fracture is minimized and an implant is not left in the wound. The practical advantage of external fixation is that it can be applied quickly, which is particularly important in the management of patients who have sustained multiple injuries that are unstable. An example of an external fixator used in this setting is application of a pelvic frame to a hemodynamically unstable patient with Melgaigne or "open book" pelvic fracture. The practical disadvantages of external fixation are infections of the pin sites and the high incidence of nonunion following its use for certain types of fractures (e.g., fractures of the tibial diaphysis).

There are two parameters by which external fixators are described: (1) whether they use large-diameter pins or small flexible wires to attach the external frame to the bone and (2) whether the fixator is static or dynamic. **Large-diameter pins** are 4 to 6 mm in diameter. They are threaded and are screwed into the bone through a predrilled hole. Large pins are attached to the external frame, which is either uniplanar or multiplanar. Uniplanar frames are simple frames used to manage diaphyseal fractures. They are applied quickly and do not obstruct access to the underlying extremity. Multiplanar frames are more rigid, more difficult to apply, and obstruct access to the extremity. They can be used for a greater variety of fractures than the simple unilateral frame (e.g., metaphyseal fractures).

Small wires are between 1.5 and 2.5 mm in diameter. They are drilled through the bone. Tension is applied across the wire to increase its rigidity, and the wire is attached to a ring that is placed around the extremity. The frames are called *small-wire circular fixators* and are always multiplanar (Fig. 2-8). The advantage of small-wire circular fixators is that they can be used to stabilize periarticular and intraarticular fractures. The disadvantages are that they are less stable than conventional fixators, they obstruct access to the extremity, and they are technically difficult to apply. In addition, unlike large pins, which are driven in only to the opposite cortex, small wires are driven through the extremity. Therefore, a thorough understanding of cross-sectional anatomy is necessary to minimize the risk to surrounding neurovascular structures.

FIG. 2-8   Clinical appearance of a small-wire circular external fixator.

Static frames are designed to immobilize a fracture or a joint and are used primarily in the management of trauma. They are not used to manipulate bone segments. In contrast, **dynamic frames** are used to manipulate bone segments and are used primarily in the management of nonunions, malunions, and to arthrodese joints. The external frame is made in such a way that it can be manipulated to lengthen or shorten the bone gradually through the nonunion and to correct angular deformity. In the most specialized example of this technique, an "internal lengthening" can be performed to fill in segmental defects of long bones.

SELECTED READINGS

Browner BD, Edwards CC: *The science and practice of intramedullary nailing.* Philadelphia, Lee and Febiger, 1987.
Maiocchi AB, Aronson J: *Operative principles of Ilizarov.* Baltimore, Williams and Wilkins, 1991.Muller ME: *AO manual of internal fixation*, 3rd ed. New York, Spring-Verlag, 1991.
Muller ME: *AO manual of internal fixation*, 3rd ed. New York, Spring-Verlag, 1991.

John A. Elstrom

The nonoperative techniques covered in this chapter are splints and casts, traction, and arthrocentesis.

SPLINTS AND CASTS

Splints and casts immobilize and support the injured extremity and thereby reduce pain, prevent injury of structures in the proximity of a fracture, and maintain alignment after reduction. Splinting and casting are also used postoperatively to provide additional stabilization when fixation is tenuous, reduce swelling, and maintain surrounding joints in a position of function (e.g., after open reduction of an ankle fracture to prevent equinus deformity). Splinting and casting are accomplished with plaster or synthetic materials such as fiberglass. Splints differ from casts in that splints are not circumferential and thus allow swelling of the extremity without a significant increase in pressure within the splint. Casts are circumferential, and swelling within the cast increases pressure, potentially resulting in a compartment syndrome or *pressure sores*. Casts tend to immobilize an extremity more completely than a splint.

Many of the **fundamental rules of splinting and casting** are identical. Ideally, at least one joint proximal and one joint distal to the injury are immobilized. Prior to immobilization, fractures are reduced, and, if possible, the extremity is placed in a position of function (e.g., the hand is immobilized in the clam-digger position, with the metacarpophalangeal joints in flexion and the interphalangeal joints in extension). The extremity is padded to prevent pressure sores and neurovascular compression. Incisions or wounds are covered with a sterile dressing. A layer of stockinette is applied, followed by cast padding appropriate to the type of material being used. Bony prominences (e.g., the posterior aspect of the heel and malleoli) and areas where nerves pass over bone (e.g., the medial elbow and the fibular neck) are protected with extra padding, foam, or felt. The splint or cast material is moistened with cold or room-temperature water to provide a prolonged setting time and decrease the heat of reaction, which could burn the skin as the material sets. This is especially important if the patient is anesthetized and cannot complain of pain. Fingertip indentation is avoided because it can result in pressure necrosis of the skin. Splints and casts covering damaged skin or surgical wounds should not be allowed to get wet.

The following **techniques of cast application** are used with plaster or synthetic materials. Plaster and fiberglass have different physical properties. It has been demonstrated that the intrinsic recoil of fiberglass results in potentially greater pressures on the skin. Plaster casts are undoubtedly safer in situations in which swelling is apt to be significant and the patient's skin is vulnerable (diabetes, stasis dermatitis, or peripheral vascular disease). It has been suggested that fiberglass casts be applied with a stretch–relax technique to address this pitfall. The polyurethane resin can be tacky, making it difficult to unwind the roll, and when the mesh is applied with the standard technique the material may be applied around the limb under substantial tension and lead to increased pressure. The stretch–relax technique involves pulling the fiberglass roll away from the limb to unwind the mesh. After the segment is unwound, the tension is relaxed and the mesh is laid on and around the limb. Only slight restretching is needed for contouring. To reduce pressure further, an anterior longitudinal cut can be made and the cast spread.

Fatigue prevents the patient from holding the **upper extremity** in the desired position during cast application. If an assistant is not available, a short or long arm cast is applied by using fingertip traction to the index and long fingers, with countertraction over the flexed elbow. The material is rolled on and carefully molded to prevent the cast from slipping or the fracture from displacing. **Short arm casts** are applied far enough proximally and with appropriate three-point molding to create an oval cross section to prevent the casts from sliding down the forearm like a glove. To prevent forearm rotation, the cast is extended above the elbow. To prevent elbow flexion and extension, the cast is extended to the proximal arm.

Casts are applied to the **lower extremity** with the patient sitting and the foot supported by a bolster or an assistant. The ankle is positioned in neutral to prevent equinus contracture. Because the limb changes in diameter, the padding is torn on the side of the larger diameter (i.e., proximal part of the padding) to conform the padding material to the limb. The padding is overlapped 50%. The cast material is then applied from the metatarsal heads to the upper limit of the cast. Short leg casts extend to the tibial tubercle. Patellar tendon–bearing casts are molded over the patellar tendon and patella but allow knee flexion. Long leg casts extend to the groin. Tucks in the cast material are taken on the side of the limb with the smaller diameter to conform the material to the limb. Longitudinal splints (i.e., a posterior splint at the ankle and medial and lateral splints at the knee) provide additional strength. Molding of the cast material along the medial aspect of the tibia and over the lateral malleolus increases stability. The cast is trimmed by removing excess material with scissors or a cast saw, pulling the stockinette over the edge of the cast, and wrapping it with additional cast material. Trimming of the cast should allow toe flexion and avoid pressure against the fifth toe. To prevent the cast from slipping on wood and linoleum floors, a cast shoe or rubber walking heel is applied. The rubber walking heel is advantageous when a limited axis of loading the lower extremity is desired (e.g., to avoid force transmission through fractured metatarsals). The rubber heel is placed proximal to the fracture.

A Gortex cast liner is currently available to allow bathing, pool swimming, and hydrotherapy while in a fiberglass cast. Because the exposure to water does not wet the liner but only the skin, rapid drying by evaporation prevents skin maceration. Casts covering damaged skin or surgical wounds would not be an appropriate use of this material.

The **technique of splinting** usually involves the use of a casting material that hardens after it is applied. However, there are other types of splints that are preformed. These preformed splints are used at the accident site (e.g., aluminum universal arm and leg splints, ladder splints, and inflatable splints) and seldom are left in place after the initial evaluation is completed. Preformed splints used for definitive management are the cervical collar, figure-of-eight clavicle splint, knee immobilizer, and ankle stirrup.

The **upper extremity** is splinted while the arm is in fingertrap traction or held by an assistant. Plaster or synthetic material 4–5 in. wide and 5–10 layers (sheets) thick are used. When plaster is used, the splint is conformed to the extremity with a gauze wrap and an Ace bandage. The material is applied from the metacarpal heads to the proximal extent of the splint. A short arm splint is applied to the volar surface of the forearm and extends to the olecranon. The sugar tongs splint starts on the volar surface of the hand and forearm and wraps around the elbow, ending on the dorsal surface of the hand. The thumb spica splint extends from the tip of the thumb along the radial aspect of the forearm to just below the flexion crease of the elbow. The radial styloid is padded to prevent injury to the superficial branch of the radial nerve.

The **lower extremity** is splinted with the patient sitting and the ankle in neutral. The ankle is splinted with a sugar tongs splint. The splint extends down the medial aspect of the leg under the foot and then back up the lateral aspect of the leg. When a posterior splint is applied, it must be thicker than the sugar tongs splint, and additional splints are used medially or laterally to provide additional strength. To prevent thermal injury, cold water is used, and excessively thick splints and heavy wrapping are avoided.

Complications of splinting and casting include pressure sores, burns, and skin irritation. **Pressure sores** occur when sensation is reduced (e.g., diabetic peripheral neuropathy); decreased sensation is a major concern when splinting and casting. To minimize the incidence of skin breakdown, bony prominences are padded, and the splint or cast is changed frequently. Pain underneath a splint or cast is a complaint that is taken seriously and is managed by windowing of the cast over the involved area or by cast removal and inspection of the skin.

Burns after the application of a splint or cast occur most commonly when plaster is used with warm water and the material is excessively thick. To minimize the incidence of burns, cold water and adequate padding are essential.

Skin irritation beneath the splint or cast can often be controlled with the use of mild analgesics such as aspirin and the use of a hair dryer set on room temperature to blow cool air underneath the cast. Powders and ointments should not be applied to the skin under the cast in hopes of drying or lubricating the skin.

TRACTION

Traction is used temporarily to splint or definitely manage fractures. Traction is applied through the skin (skin traction) or a pin inserted into a long bone (skeletal traction).

The disadvantage of **skin traction** is that it can result in skin break-down. The danger of skin breakdown limits the length of time it can be used and the amount of weight applied (10 lbs.). The advantage of skin traction is that it does not require insertion of a pin. Skin traction is applied through adhesive strips applied to the skin or, more frequently, a "Buck's" boot. Buck's traction is used to splint hip fractures temporarily before surgery. It employs a prefabricated soft synthetic boot held in place with Velcro straps through which 5–7 lbs. of weight is applied. A pillow is placed beneath the knee, slightly flexing it. The most common error is that the patient slides down in bed, and the weights rest on the ground or the boot lies against the end of the bed. A push box between the end of the bed and the opposite foot prevents the patient from sliding down in bed.

Skeletal traction is used most frequently to temporarily manage acetabular and femoral fractures and occasionally fractures of the distal humerus and distal tibia. More weight can be applied for a longer period of time through skeletal traction than through skin traction.

Basic **rules of skeletal traction** are as follows: the pin should be inserted at 90° to the long axis of the bone, skeletal traction is contraindicated when there is damage to the ligaments of the joint proximal to the pin site; radiographs in traction are obtained immediately after application as required for adjustments, and then weekly; and the neurologic and vascular status of the extremity is examined daily.

The **technique of pin insertion** is performed as follows: the area is shaved and scrubbed before pin insertion; local infiltration anesthesia (taking care to infiltrate the periosteum and skin on both sides) and parenteral sedation are used; pins are inserted from the side most vulnerable to neurovascular damage so that the point is accurately applied to the bone (e.g., lateral to medial in the distal femur and ulnar to radial in the proximal ulna); the skin is incised with a no. 11 blade; the pin is drilled by hand through the bone; the skin on the opposite side is incised as it is tented by the point of the pin; and stability of the pin is evaluated by pushing proximally and distally on one end of the pin to see if the bone moves with the pin—the "toggle test." Oblique placement of femoral traction pins for femoral fractures has been associated with an increased incidence of varus or valgus malalignment.

Pin selection is based on the following considerations: threads prevent the pin from loosening and sliding in the bone; threaded pins must have a larger caliber than smooth pins because the threads weaken the pin; smooth pins that are threaded in their midportions are especially useful; and threaded pins are not used when the pin will pass near a neurovascular bundle (e.g., through-and-through olecranon pin), for fear of the soft tissues being wrapped around the pin and causing a neurovascular injury. **Traction maintenance** consists of supporting the part distal to the pin, twice-daily cleaning of the pin sites with sterile saline or peroxide, sterile dressings, and release of skin under tension to prevent necrosis.

For **acetabular and femoral fractures,** the pins are inserted through the distal femur at the flare of the condyles or through the proximal tibia 2 cm posterior and 1 cm inferior to the tibial tubercle. As longitudinal traction is applied through the pin, the leg is supported with slings or in a frame. The frame used most frequently is the Thomas ring with a Pierson attachment. The Pierson attachment is an outrigger that slides up and down the Thomas frame to compensate for the length of the femur and allows knee flexion (Fig. 3-1). Depending on the size of the patient, 15–30 lbs. of longitudinal traction is appropriate initially.

The safest type of **olecranon** pin is a screw with an eyelet, inserted at 90° to the long axis of the ulna. A through-and-through pin can be used, but the ulnar nerve must be protected. Olecranon traction is supplemented with skin traction to support the hand and forearm. Five to ten pounds of longitudinal traction is applied initially (Fig. 3-2). The **calcaneal** pin is inserted 2 cm distal and 2 cm posterior to the medial malleolus. The leg is supported on a frame, and 5–10 lbs. of weight is applied initially.

FIG. 3-1   Skeletal traction using a Thomas splint and Pierson attachment.

FIG. 3-2 Overhead olecranon traction with a forearm support.

ARTHROCENTESIS

Arthrocentesis, or aspiration, of a swollen painful joint is both thera-peutic and diagnostic. Strict adherence to aseptic techniques is essential: the area through which the joint is aspirated is shaved and scrubbed, and sterile gloves are used. Local infiltration anesthesia is optional. Large joints are aspirated with a 19-gauge needle. Smaller joints of the fingers and toes are aspirated with a 22-gauge needle, but the smaller diameter makes obtaining fluid difficult. The larger the syringe, the more nega-tive pressure is generated, which tends to draw obstructive particles into the needle opening.

The **contraindications** to arthrocentesis are periarticular sepsis and uncorrected coagulopathy. Tubes for synovial fluid cell count, micro-scopic examination, and culture should be available in the event that an effusion suggestive of an acute inflammatory arthritis is found.

The **knee** is aspirated with the patient supine and the joint extended. The needle is directed posterior to the quadriceps tendon at the superior lateral pole of the patella. Alternatively, the knee can be aspirated with the patient sitting and the knee flexed. The needle is directed toward the center of the joint starting medial or lateral to the patellar tendon just above the articular surface of the tibia (Fig. 3-3).

FIG. 3-3   Aspiration of the knee. The needle is inserted medial or lateral to the patellar tendon at the level of the joint and directed posteriorly toward the center of the knee. (*Courtesy of Dr. Clayton R. Perry.*)

The **ankle** is aspirated through the interval between the extensor hallucis longus tendon and the medial malleolus or just proximal and medial to the tip of the lateral malleolus and below the level of the joint line.

Aspiration of the **hip** is done with the aid of fluoroscopy. The patient is supine and the hip is extended. A spinal needle is inserted lateral to the femoral artery and 2 cm distal to the inguinal ligament. It is directed toward the inferior aspect of the femoral head and neck. The resistance of the hip capsule is apparent as the needle enters the joint.

Shoulder aspiration is performed with the patient sitting and the humerus in neutral or slight external rotation. Unless the patient is unusually large, a 1.5-in. needle is used. The needle is inserted lateral to the coracoid process and below the acromioclavicular joint. It is directed posteriorly into the interval just medial to the biceps tendon and near the junction of the supraspinatous and subscapularis tendon (Fig. 3-4).

The **elbow** is aspirated with the patient sitting and the elbow in 80° of flexion. A tense hemarthrosis can often be palpated in the interval between the lateral epicondyle, radial head, and olecranon. The needle is passed medially through the center of this triangular area (Fig. 3-5).

FIG. 3-4 Aspiration of the shoulder. The needle is inserted lateral to the coracoid and directed posteriorly. (*Courtesy of Dr. Clayton R. Perry.*)

FIG. 3-5 Aspiration of the elbow. The epicondyle, tip of the olecranon, and radial head form a triangle. The needle is inserted into the center of this triangle. (*Courtesy of Dr. Clayton R. Perry.*)

SELECTED READINGS

Davids JR, Frick SL, Skewes E, et al: Skin surface pressure beneath an above-the-knee cast: plaster casts compared with fiberglass casts. *J Bone Joint Surg* 79A:565–569, 1997.
Marson BM, Keenan MAE: Skin surface pressures under short leg casts. *J Orthop Trauma* 7:275–278, 1993.

4

Anesthetic Techniques

Carl H. Nielsen

Physicians without specialty training in anesthesiology may safely employ the following techniques of sedation and regional anesthesia for short surgical procedures, provided a few basic rules are followed. Drugs must never be administered to a patient without a plan for establishment of an airway, administration of oxygen, and immediate management of an overdose or side effect of the administered drug. The following recommendations apply only to healthy, nonpregnant patients without allergy to the drugs.

SEDATION

Midazolam (Versed®) has a wide margin of safety, but it may cause respiratory depression with rapid injection and/or overdose. Dosage must be reduced for geriatric patients. Midazolam is administered intravenously (IV), and 0.03 mg/kg is used as a single dose. The dose may be repeated after 5 min if the patient needs additional sedation. Midazolam has no analgesic properties. Mental function may be impaired for hours after midazolam administration.

ANALGESIA

Opioids rarely provide complete analgesia for even minor procedures, but used as adjuncts to sedation and/or regional anesthesia they add to patient comfort. All opioids are potent dose-dependent respiratory depressants. Avoid intramuscular injection because duration of onset is slow and variable. Intravenous bolus of 2.5 mg morphine, 25 mg meperidine, or 50 µg fentanyl is used. The bolus dose may be repeated to a total of 10 mg morphine, 100 mg meperidine, or 100 µg fentanyl.

REGIONAL ANESTHESIA

Infiltration techniques inhibit excitation of sensory nerve endings and provide sensory anesthesia. Intravenous regional anesthesia is usually classified as an infiltration block, although the exact mechanism of action is unclear. Peripheral nerve block involves reversible block of nerve action potentials along all types of nerve fiber and is called *conduction anesthesia*.

Bier Block

Bier block, or intravenous regional anesthesia (IVR), is a suitable technique for operative procedures on the hand and forearm, with duration of less than 1 h. This technique may also be used for foot and lower leg anesthesia, but the quality of anesthesia is not as good for the lower extremity as for the upper extremity. The following diseases of the limb are contraindications for the use of IVR: infection; malignant tumor; and vascular insufficiency.

A 20- or 22-gauge canula is placed and secured in a distal vein on the limb to be anesthetized. A tourniquet is placed as proximally on the limb as possible; for longer lasting procedures, two tourniquets or a double tourniquet must be used. The limb below the tourniquet is exsanguinated by compression. The tourniquet is inflated to a pressure 100 mmHg above the systolic blood pressure. The source of the pressure must be calibrated and must continuously maintain the desired preset pressure. A regular cuff, sphygmomanometer, and bulb with release valve are inadequate as a tourniquet for IVR. Immediately after exsanguination, a single dose of 50 mL 0.5% (250 mg) lidocaine (Xylocaine®) is injected into the indwelling canula. Complete IVR of the leg requires about 75 mL of local anesthetic. Use lidocaine only from a sealed single-dose vial without epinephrine. The canula may be removed after the injection, and satisfactory anesthesia is obtained within 10 min. When two tourniquets are used, the distal one is deflated at this point. Should the patient complain about tourniquet pain before the completion of the operation, the distal cuff is inflated and about 20 s later the proximal cuff is deflated (Fig. 4-1). At completion of the operation, the tourniquet is deflated. This is not done until at least 15 min has elapsed after injection. Early release of the tourniquet may bring about a systemic reaction to the lidocaine.

Nerve Block

The following nerve blocks are all performed with 1 to 1.5% lidocaine, 1 to 1.5% mepivacaine (Carbocaine®), or 0.5% bupivacaine (Marcaine®). Distal blocks (i.e., of fingers and toes, wrist and ankle) must never be performed with local anesthetics containing epinephrine because of the risk of prolonged vasospasms. When epinephrine is used for prolongation of peripheral nerve blocks, the optimal concentration is 1:200,000, which is equivalent to 5 µg epinephrine per milliliter of local anesthetic. When small amounts of local anesthetics are injected, multiple-dose vials are appropriate. When larger amounts of local anesthetics are injected, the single-dose vial is used. The difference is that single-dose vials contain no preservatives, whereas multiple-dose vials do.

Digital Nerve Block

Four nerves innervate each finger and toe: two are palmar/plantar and two are dorsal. Block of these four nerves provides adequate anesthesia for minor operations. The injection may be performed at the base of the digit, but an injection about 1 cm farther proximal is less painful. Despite anesthesia of half of the two digits next to the anesthetized digit, it is the preferred method (Fig. 4-2).

FIG. 4-1 Bier block. (*A*). The distal tourniquet is deflated and anesthetic injected. If there is tourniquet pain, the distal tourniquet is inflated (*B*) and the proximal tourniquet is deflated (*C*).

A 23-gauge 1-inch-long needle is advanced from the dorsal side to the palmar/plantar fascia so the needle tip can be palpated. It is retracted 2 mm, and 3 mL of local anesthetic is injected. The needle is retracted so that the tip is just below the subcutaneous tissue, and another 2 mL is injected. The procedure is repeated on the other side of the digit.

Wrist Block

Blocks of one, two, or all three nerves at the wrist will provide adequate anesthesia of the part of the hand innervated by the blocked nerve(s).

The **median nerve** runs in the wrist between the palmaris longus and flexor carpiradialis tendons. It is blocked approximately 2 cm proximal to the proximal wrist crease. With the hand slightly dorsiflexed, a 23-gauge 1-inch needle is advanced perpendicular to the skin between

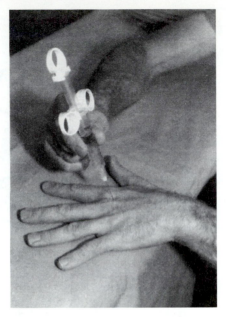

FIG. 4-2   Digital nerve block.

these two tendons, and the area is infiltrated with 5 to 8 mL of local anesthetic (Fig. 4-3). If there is paresthesia, the needle is stopped and the entire volume is injected. If there is no paresthesia, the local anesthetic is deposited with a fanwise injection. This block is not used in patients with carpal tunnel syndrome and is not performed distally at the level of the carpal tunnel.

The **ulnar nerve** is blocked approximately 6 cm proximal to the proximal wrist crease, just to the radial side of the tendon of the flexor carpiulnaris. The nerve is on the ulnar side of the ulnar artery. A 23-gauge 1-inch needle is inserted perpendicular to the skin, and 8 to 10 mL of local anesthetic is injected. If the block is performed less than 6 cm proximal to the wrist, it will not include the dorsal branch of the ulnar nerve; a block of this branch must be performed with a subcutaneous ring of anesthesia around the ulnar aspect of the wrist, starting from the flexor carpiulnaris tendon. Five milliliters of local anesthetic is used for this block.

The **radial nerve** is blocked with infiltration under the brachioradialis tendon 8 cm proximal to the proximal wrist crease. Alternatively,

FIG. 4-3   Median nerve block at the wrist.

the radial nerve is blocked with a subcutaneous ring of anesthesia. The ring starts at the radial aspect of the wrist at the flexor carpiradialis and continues around the wrist dorsally to the styloid process of the ulna. Both methods require approximately 5 to 8 mL of local anesthetic.

Elbow Block

The **ulnar nerve** is blocked 3 cm proximal to its course in the groove behind the medial epicondyle. A 23-gauge 1-inch needle, pointed either distally or proximally, is advanced at a 45° angle to the course of the nerve; 5 to 8 mL of local anesthetic is injected around the nerve.

The **median nerve** lies on a line drawn on the anterior elbow between the two epicondyles on the medial side of the brachial artery and is easily palpated in thin individuals. The block is performed at this level with a 23-gauge 1-inch needle. When paresthesia is encountered, 5 to 8 mL local anesthetic is injected (Fig. 4-4). A subcutaneous infiltration is required to block the cutaneous branches to the forearm.

To find the **radial nerve**, a line is drawn from the most prominent point of the humeral head to the lateral epicondyle. The nerve crosses the humerus one-third up from the lateral epicondyle. It can be palpated on the bone, and the block is performed with a 23-gauge 1-inch needle and 5 to 8 mL of local anesthetic. Alternatively, the radial nerve is blocked with the lateral cutaneous nerve of the forearm, as described next.

The **lateral cutaneous nerve** of the forearm is a continuation of the musculocutaneous nerve and perforates the deep fascia on the lateral side of the biceps muscle just proximal to the elbow. The lateral cuta-

FIG. 4-4 Median nerve block at the elbow.

neous nerve and the radial nerve can both be blocked with a 23-gauge 1.5-inch needle inserted between the brachioradialis muscle and the biceps tendon (Fig. 4-5). The needle is directed proximally toward the anterior lateral surface of the lateral epicondyle, and 3 mL of local anesthetic is injected just above the periosteum. Bone contact is made two more times, and 3 mL is injected each time above the periosteum. An additional 5 mL of local anesthetic is injected as the needle is withdrawn. If paresthesia is elicited, 5 to 8 mL of local anesthetic is injected, and no further bone contact is necessary. A subcutaneous ring of 5 mL of local anesthetic from the biceps tendon to the brachioradialis muscle will provide anesthesia of the superficial branches of the musculocutaneous nerve.

Ankle Block

Foot operations lasting less than 2 h can be done with an ankle block. The block provides anesthesia for a tourniquet at the level of the malleoli. A common mistake is to block the ankle too distally. Injections 1 to 2 cm above the malleoli provide a more complete block. The block is a conduction block of the five nerves that innervate the foot: three on the dorsal side and two on the plantar side. The block is performed with a 23-gauge 1-inch needle, and 5 to 10 mL local anesthetic is infiltrated around each of the nerves, as described in the following section.

The **saphenous nerve** is blocked at the greater saphenous vein 1 to 2 cm above the medial malleolus (Fig. 4-6).

The **deep peroneal nerve** is blocked around and deep to the dorsalis pedis artery. Alternatively, the infiltration is performed between the tib-

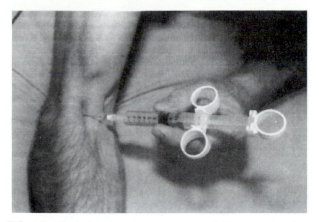

FIG. 4-5   Block of the lateral cutaneous and radial nerves at the elbow.

FIG. 4-6   Saphenous nerve block.

ialis anterior and the extensor hallus longus tendons; flexion of the first and second toes improves visualization of the two tendons (Fig. 4-7).

The **superficial peroneal nerve** is blocked with subcutaneous ring infiltration from the anterior edge of the tibia to the anterior edge of the fibula (Fig. 4-8).

FIG. 4-7   Deep peroneal nerve block.

FIG. 4-8   Superficial peroneal nerve block.

The **sural nerve** is blocked with subcutaneous fan-wise infiltration between the Achilles tendon and fibula (Fig. 4-9).

The **tibial nerve** is blocked with a needle advanced just lateral to the posterior tibial artery toward the posterior surface of the tibia. The needle is retracted 1 cm after contact with the tibia, and the anesthetic is injected (Fig. 4-10).

FIG. 4-9 Sural nerve block.

FIG. 4-10 Tibial nerve block.

Hematoma Block

Spread of local anesthetic to the nerve fibers supplying soft tissue and periosteum around a fracture is obtained with a hematoma block. This technique is contraindicated if there is any risk of contamination of the fracture site from the skin puncture.

A large-bore needle, (e.g., 19 gauge, 1.5 inches) is used for this block because it is important to withdraw blood from the fracture hematoma and replace it with local anesthetic. This method provides better anesthesia and reduces the risk of a high compartment pressure. After aspiration of the hematoma, 10 to 15 mL 1% lidocaine is injected. When there is an associated distal radioulnar joint injury, 5 to 8 mL 1% lidocaine is injected into the radioulnar joint in addition to the hematoma block.

5

Radiologic Evaluation

John A. Elstrom

This chapter deals with the terminology used to describe the radiologic appearance of a long bone fracture. As can be seen from the illustration shown in Fig. 9-2, fractures are described as involving the proximal or distal metaphysis (these fractures are often intraarticular) and fractures that involve the diaphysis (these are usually divided into fractures of the proximal, middle, and distal thirds). The fracture line itself may be transverse, oblique (a spiral fracture is a long oblique fracture), segmental, and comminuted. The fracture is determined to be closed or open depending on whether the fracture site communicates with the external environment through a wound that can be due to either the bone puncturing the skin or an external force penetrating the skin (such as a bullet in a gunshot wound).

To describe the radiologic appearance of a fracture adequately, one must have two views at right angles to each other: an anteroposterior (AP) radiograph and true lateral radiograph. (Oblique radiographs are necessary when the fracture involves the metaphysis or articular components.) The second requirement is the knowledge of the anatomic structures involved (an anatomy text or a text dealing with fractures is frequently useful in this case).

The description of fracture displacement presents several problems. Inadequate x-rays often result in fracture lines being missed and the displacement of a fracture being underestimated. The two major sources of confusion in describing fractures arise from the description of the direction of displacement or angulation and what is actually meant by **displacement**. A fracture of the distal radius in which the distal fragment is angulated dorsally is, in fact, angulated volarly (palmarward) at the fracture site (Fig. 5-1). The reverse fracture in which the distal fragment is angulated volarward is angulated dorsally at the fracture site. The term *displacement* creates another problem. Any fracture that is angulated, even though there is continuity between the bone ends, is a displaced fracture. Displaced fractures usually require reduction. A fracture should be described as having the bone ends in continuity as in a greenstick fracture, having complete loss of continuity as in a fracture of both bones of the forearm with bayonnette apposition, or retaining partial continuity as in the case in which the bone ends are still in contact but the cortical alignment is offset. An adequate description is important to the treating surgeon because fractures that retain some continuity can frequently be reduced in the emergency room, whereas fractures that have lost end-to-end continuity require reduction with a general or regional anesthetic and often require open reduction and in-

FIG. 5-1   A dorsally displaced, dorsally angulated fracture of the distal radius that has complete loss of continuity between the bone ends and is in bayonette apposition with shortening. There is volar angulation at the fracture site.

ternal fixation. Thus fractures can be angulated and in continuity; aligned with bayonnette apposition, or shortening and not in continuity.

With regard to the hip joint, displaced fractures of the femoral neck in which the femoral neck has moved superiorly in relation to the femoral head often require prosthetic replacement in the elderly, osteoporotic patient and immediate reduction and internal fixation in the younger patient in whom an attempt should be made to preserve the femoral head. An impacted fracture of the femoral neck only occurs when the femoral neck has moved under the femoral head (Fig. 5-2). This term is **valgus displacement of the femoral head** and usually signifies a stable position in which the femoral head can be fixed internally. The opposite position, described as a **varus displacement of the femoral head**, is unstable and should not be described as being impacted (Fig. 5-3). Fractures of the base of the femoral neck adjacent to the intertrochanteric line are fixed internally just like an intertrochanteric fracture and must be differentiated from subcapital and transcervical fractures.

Involvement of the joint surface in the fracture is important, especially when there is displacement; frequently, additional studies such as a magnetic resonance imaging (MRI) or computed tomography (CT) are required. Displaced intraarticular fractures frequently require open reduction and internal fixation.

Additional terms used to describe the x-ray appearance of a fracture include **avulsion** fracture, where the patella or olecranon is pulled apart by muscle, tendon, or ligament (Fig. 5-4). Impaction of a fracture de-

FIG. 5-2   An impacted fracture of the femoral neck that was pinned in situ. The femoral neck has moved under the femoral head in a valgus configuration.

FIG. 5-3   A fracture of the femoral neck in which the femoral neck is moved superiorly in relation to the femoral head. This varus displacement is unstable and frequently is treated with prosthetic replacement.

scribes a situation in which muscle forces draws the distal fragment onto the proximal fragment, usually in a situation about the metaphysis in which the bone is rather osteopenic such as the distal radius (Fig. 5-5). **Depression** of a fracture describes a situation in which the joint surface is impressed into the metaphyseal area, such as commonly occurs in a fracture of the tibial plateau or the articular surface of the dis-

FIG. 5-4   An avulsion fracture of the olecranon with subluxation anteriorly (volarward) of the radius and ulna.

FIG. 5-5   An impacted fracture of the distal radial metaphysis without significant angulation and without loss of continuity between the bone ends.

tal tibia after a fall from a height. Fractures may be described as **pathologic** if there is a process affecting the strength of the bone such as metastatic carcinoma. There are those fractures that frequently do not appear on the initial x-rays. **Stress** fractures are associated with pain and localizing tenderness due to repetitive stresses such as running or a new exercise activity. Stress fractures frequently occur in the pubic rami, the femoral neck, the tibial shaft, and the metatarsals. **Occult** fracture of the navicular is diagnosed by tenderness in the snuff box and the appearance of the fracture either on an AP radiograph with the wrist in ulnar deviation or by special imaging studies such as a bone scan or MRI. Fracture of the **hook of the hamate** is diagnosed by tenderness over the hook of the hamate and the appearance of a fracture on a carpal tunnel view or on a MRI.

With regard to **joint dislocations**, the joint is dislocated when there is complete loss of contact between the two articular surfaces involved. **Joint subluxation** is a situation in which the two articular surfaces no longer have their normal congruous alignment, but the articular surfaces are still in partial contact. **Diastasis** is a form of joint subluxation in which there is widening of an articulation, such as can occur after ankle injury, when the deltoid ligament and the distal tibiofibular ligaments rupture, and often is associated with an easily overlooked fracture proximally in the fibula. Diastasis also occurs with injury to the symphysis pubis—widening it. The direction of a dislocation or subluxation is usually determined by the displacement of the distal part. The humeral head is displaced anterior to the glenoid and posterior to the glenoid in shoulder dislocations. Dislocation is not infrequently associated with a fracture. Significant fracture dislocations occur most frequently about the shoulder, wrist, proximal interphalangeal joint, hip, ankle, and foot. These injuries are important to identify because the treatment is more complicated and frequently needs to be performed on an emergency basis.

SELECTED READING

Schultz RJ: *The Language of Fractures*, 2d ed. Baltimore, Williams & Wilkins, 1990.

6 Fracture Healing and Bone Grafting

Michael E. Joyce   Clayton R. Perry

In this chapter we describe fracture healing at the clinical, radiographic, biomechanical, cellular, regulatory (i.e., growth factors), and biochemical levels. In addition, bone grafting, a surgical procedure that stimulates fracture healing, is described.

FRACTURE HEALING

The **clinical** course of fracture healing is predictable. Failure to progress clinically is an indication of delayed union or impending nonunion. Initially, all fractures are characterized by pain because of disruption of nerve endings in the periosteum and surrounding soft tissue. Other findings at the time of injury include abnormal motion, soft tissue swelling, warmth, and redness. Characteristically, motion through the fracture exacerbates pain. Conversely, immobilization of the fracture with splinting or internal fixation decreases pain. Fractures managed with splinting gradually become less painful as they heal, and usually at 2 weeks there is minimal pain. Initially, the patient may have the sensation of a "click" or "pop" as the fractured bone ends move over each other, but this sensation gradually disappears during the subsequent 2–4 weeks. Concurrently, a fusiform mass becomes evident around the fracture, representing external callus. When the fracture site is stressed, a feeling of discomfort is elicited, and a "spring" is present (i.e., there is slight motion of the fracture fragments, but they return to their initial position). Gradually, the discomfort and spring decrease and eventually disappear 6–12 weeks after injury. At this point, the fracture is clinically healed. Remodeling is a prolonged process, resulting in a variable decrease in the size of the external callus mass.

This is the normal healing sequence that is followed when the fracture has been managed with an intramedullary rod or a splint. However, when the fracture has been stabilized rigidly (i.e., with a plate and screws), the presence of callus, motion, and pain are signs of failure of fixation.

The rate at which fracture healing proceeds is decreased in elderly patients and increased in children. Medical conditions (diabetes mellitus) or medications (Prednisone) prolong fracture healing. Different bones in the body heal at different rates (e.g., tibia vs. radius). Similarly, different regions of the same bone heal at different rates (e.g., metaphysis vs. diaphysis). The type of injury has a profound effect on the rate of fracture healing. Soft-tissue injury and bone loss are associated with a decreased rate of healing.

The initial **radiographic** sign of healing is the appearance of callus. This occurs 2–4 weeks after fracture. Initially, ossification is seen at the periphery of the callus, which gradually moves centripetally. As the callus matures, it develops trabeculae and a cortex. Necrotic bone becomes relatively radiodense, appearing whiter than the surrounding bone because of the hyperemia and resulting osteopenia of living bone. The appearance of callus around fractures that have been rigidly stabilized indicates failure of fixation. Trabeculae crossing the fracture site is the radiographic indication of a healed fracture that has been rigidly stabilized.

The restoration of strength, or the **biomechanical** healing of fractures, is divided into four stages. The first stage is at the time of injury, when the only mechanical strength is due to the stability attributable to the interdigitation of the fracture fragments. The second stage starts with the formation of a soft callus. The soft callus is cartilage and provides only a fraction of the normal strength of the bone. In the third stage, soft callus ossifies and is replaced by a hard callus comprised of woven bone. The hard callus is detectable radiographically and results in full restoration of strength. The fourth stage is remodeling of the hard callus into compact and cortical bone that results in restoration of the architecture.

On the **cellular level**, there are five stages of fracture healing. Stage 1, healing response to injury, occurs immediately after fracture, when a hematoma forms at the fracture site. Soft tissue surrounding the fracture is invaded by monocytes and inflammatory cells. Within the first 24 h, cells in the deep layer of the periosteum begin to proliferate.

Stage 2, intramembranous ossification, occurs within 3 days after fracture. New bone matrix is synthesized by osteoblasts located adjacent to the fracture site and below the proliferating periosteal cells. The bone that forms in this area does so without a cartilaginous intermediate, a process termed *intramembranous ossification*. The area of subperiosteal bone formation determines the area of hard callus formation.

Stage 3, chondrogenesis, occurs within 10 days after fracture. Chondrocytes appear within the granulation tissue in the immediate vicinity of the fracture gap. Mesenchymal cells, presumably chondrocyte precursors, are found within granulation tissue bordering the advancing chondrogenic front. Chondrogenesis occurs as the newly differentiated chondrocytes mature within the enlarging cartilaginous matrix. This process continues until the fibrous tissue within this soft callus is replaced by cartilage, thereby bridging the fracture gap.

Stage 4, endochondral ossification, takes place within 14 days after fracture. Chondrocytes begin to hypertrophy within the soft callus adjacent to subperiosteal bone. The surrounding extracellular matrix calcifies before vascular invasion and repopulation with osteoblasts. This process (identical to that which occurs at the growth plate) continues until the fracture gap has been bridged. Remodeling eventually restores the normal bone architecture.

Stage 5, remodeling, involves the simultaneous removal and replacement of bone. Removal is accomplished by osteoclasts, and replacement is accomplished by osteoblasts. Osteoblasts accompanying the blood vessels lay down lamellar bone, forming a new osteon. In trabecular bone, the osteoclasts and osteoblasts line the surface of the trabeculae. Remodeling results in "primary bone healing" (i.e., the bridging of a fracture by osteons) when cortical bone ends are rigidly and anatomically reduced and in "creeping substitution" (i.e., the ingrowth of blood vessels and bony trabeculae) when cancellous bone ends are reduced rigidly.

The **regulation** of cellular proliferation, differentiation, chemotaxis, and the synthesis of extracellular matrix is not fully understood; but it is clear that a class of peptides, termed **growth factors**, plays a central role. Their role in the regulation of fracture healing has been deduced by their localization within fracture callus by immunohistochemistry.

Growth factors arrive at the fracture callus by two pathways. First, they can be delivered by the blood stream (e.g., released by platelets into the fracture hematoma). Second, they can arrive through synthesis by cells within the fracture callus.

Platelet-derived growth factor (PDGF) is released from platelets and macrophages in the earliest stage of wound healing, suggesting an important role for PDGF in the initiation of fracture repair. At the initiation of fracture healing, PDGF acts as a stimulator of mesenchymal cell proliferation and as an initiator of new matrix formation during fracture repair. PDGF stimulates type I collagen synthesis and intramembranous bone formation. Other mitogenic factors (e.g., transforming growth factor β [TGFβ] and insulinlike growth factor II) further stimulate the primitive mesenchymal cells to proliferate.

Maturation factors such as bone morphogenic protein (BMP), TGFβ, acidic fibroblast growth factor (AFGF), and basic fibroblast growth factor (BFGF) stimulate differentiation of primitive mesenchymal cells to different specialized cell lines. BMP induces differentiation of osteoblasts. TGFβ has a more complex and central role as a modulator of fracture healing. Differing concentrations at different stages of healing stimulate fibrocytes, chondrocytes, or osteocytes. The exclusive intracellular immunostaining of AFGF suggests that its synthesis and action are through autocrine regulatory pathways within the fracture callus. BFGF induces the differentiation of chondrocytes and osteoblasts and neovascularization by promoting endothelial cell proliferation and capillary cell differentiation.

The **biochemical** composition of the healing fractures evolves as it matures. Collagen synthesized by fibroblasts (types III and V) is replaced by collagen synthesized by chondrocytes (types II and IX) and in turn is replaced by collagen synthesized by osteoblasts (type I). Initially, the proteoglycan composition of the extracellular matrix is primarily dermatan sulfate. By the second week, chondroitin sulfate predominates. As healing progresses, the concentration of proteoglycan in the fracture callus decreases and the proportion of monomeric proteoglycan increases. Activity and concentrations of various enzymes also change throughout the healing process. Enzymes are key in the process of deposition of hydroxyapatite (alkaline phosphatase) and degradation of macromolecules, such as early types of collagen and proteoglycans (collagenase and proteoglycanase). In addition to collagen, proteoglycan, and enzymes, there are numerous types of molecules that play roles in modulating responses (e.g., enzyme inhibitors or activators), form basic building blocks, perform specialized functions such as acting as a nidus of calcification, or are simply debris.

BONE GRAFT

Bone graft is an avascular source of the osteoconductive and osteoinductive matrices. **Osteoconductive** matrix is defined as a material that provides a "scaffold" for bone ingrowth. Allogenic bone grafts are harvested postmortem and preserved by desiccation or freezing. They are used to manage large bone defects, but they are only osteoconductive. **Osteoinductive** matrix is defined as a material that induces mesenchymal cells to differentiate into osteoblasts and chondroblasts. Autologous bone graft is osteoinductive. Bone morphogenic protein is one of the factors present that stimulates bone formation de novo in a variety of mesenchymal-rich tissues including muscle. Autografts also supply mesenchymal cells, which have osteogenic potential. These cells reside in the marrow and surrounding trabecular network of cancellous bone; although the majority die during the grafting procedure, some remain viable.

7

Injuries of the Glenohumeral Joint

John A. Elstrom   *Clayton R. Perry*

This chapter reviews dislocations of the humeral head from the glenoid fossa and fractures of the proximal humerus.

ANATOMY

The **proximal humerus** consists of the head, greater and lesser tuberosities, and anatomic and surgical necks. The head is approximately half a sphere and is covered with hyaline cartilage. When the axis of the distal humerus is at 0° in the coronal plane, the humeral head is directed posteriorly 15°. The **greater tuberosity** is the insertion of the supraspinatus superiorly and the infraspinatus and teres minor posteriorly. It is the most lateral bony projection of the shoulder. The **lesser tuberosity** is anterior and is the insertion site of the subscapularis. The long head of the biceps lies in the intertubercular groove between the two tuberosities. The anatomic and the surgical neck refer to the constrictions around the base of the humeral head and the metaphysis just distal to the tuberosities, respectively. The anterior and posterior circumflex humeral arteries and the axillary nerve circle the proximal humerus at the level of the surgical neck. The vascular supply of the humeral head is through the anterior lateral ascending artery, which originates from the anterior humeral circumflex artery. The anterior lateral ascending artery runs proximally along the lateral aspect of the intertubercular groove and enters the humeral head through foramina along its course.

The function of the **glenoid** is to serve as a fulcrum against which the muscles of the shoulder work to move the humerus. The glenoid forms a shallow cavity with an articular surface covered with hyaline cartilage. The articular surface of the glenoid is one-third the area of the articular surface of the humeral head.

The **glenohumeral articulation** is a multiaxial ball-and-socket joint with a remarkable range of motion. Stability is dependent on passive and active mechanisms. Passive mechanisms of stability include the glenoid labrum, the coracoacromial ligament, the capsule, and the glenohumeral ligaments. The **glenoid labrum** deepens the glenoid fossa and consists of dense fibrocartilage. It is frequently detached from the rim of the glenoid during an anterior dislocation of the shoulder. The supraspinatus tendon, **coracoacromial ligament**, and acromion form the roof of the glenohumeral articulation and with other components of the rotator cuff prevent proximal migration of the humeral head. The capsule of the glenohumeral articulation is large and redundant. This allows the range of motion of the shoulder but imparts minimal stability. The three glenohumeral ligaments are intracapsular (i.e., thickenings of the capsule) and are major passive stabilizers of the joint. These ligaments are called the **superior, middle, and inferior glenohumeral ligaments**. They differ in size and shape but serve as primary restraints to anterior translation of the humeral head on the glenoid. The anterior superior aspect of the shoulder capsule and subscapularis tendon limit posterior glenohumeral translation, even when the entire posterior capsule has been divided. An intact rotator interval is felt to be a major stabilizer opposing posterior and inferior humeral displacement on the glenoid. The **coracohumeral ligament** appears to be a fold in the anterior superior glenohumeral capsule that becomes prominent with inferior translation of the humeral head.

Active glenohumeral stability is due to the muscles of the rotator cuff and the long head of the biceps. The muscles of the **rotator cuff** (i.e., the subscapularis, supraspinatus, infraspinatus, and teres minor) function to maintain the humeral head in the glenoid, preventing dislocation, and the deltoid, pectoralis major and minor, teres major, and latissimus dorsi abduct, extend, flex, and rotate the humerus.

DISLOCATIONS OF THE GLENOHUMERAL ARTICULATION

Dislocations of the glenohumeral articulation are classified according to the position of the humeral head in relation to the glenoid, the duration or number of times the glenohumeral joint has been dislocated, and the etiology of the dislocation.

The humeral head is dislocated anteriorly, posteriorly, inferiorly, or superiorly. The majority of glenohumeral dislocations are **anterior**. The humeral head is most commonly subcoracoid, although it may also be subclavicular, subglenoid, or intrathoracic (Fig. 7-1). Posterior dislocations are rare, with the humeral head usually subacromial or occasionally subglenoid (Fig. 7-2). **Posterior dislocations** are difficult to diagnose and may be overlooked without a careful physical examina-

FIG. 7-1   Anterior glenohumeral dislocation.

FIG. 7-2   Posterior glenohumeral dislocation.

tion and an axillary radiograph or computed tomographic (CT) scan of the involved shoulder. **Inferior dislocations** are known as traumatic **luxatio erecta** (Fig. 7-3). Superior dislocations are rare and result from a superiorly directed axial load applied to the arm. The humeral head is driven superiorly, disrupting the rotator cuff and often fracturing the acromion.

Glenohumeral dislocations are further classified as acute, chronic, or recurrent. We arbitrarily define **acute dislocations** as being dislocated 2 days or less and **chronic dislocations** as being dislocated more than 2 days. Most dislocations are acute because the patient immediately seeks attention due to pain. However, glenohumeral dislocations are occasionally neglected, especially by the elderly. A dislocation is defined as **recurrent** when it has occurred previously.

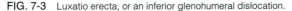

FIG. 7-3   Luxatio erecta, or an inferior glenohumeral dislocation.

Glenohumeral dislocations are classified according to their etiology as being atraumatic, acquired, or traumatic. The **atraumatic** dislocation is associated with ligamentous laxity and is an ill-defined event in which self-reduction occurs. Management of the initial atraumatic dislocation does not affect the outcome. The **acquired** dislocation results from repeated minor injuries that typically take place in sports such as weight lifting, and it occurs during a minor injury that would not dislocate a normal shoulder. Manipulative reduction is required, but initial management with immobilization is not effective in preventing recurrences. This group includes a significant portion of patients with shoulder instability. The **traumatic** dislocation results from a violent injury and requires manipulative reduction. Management of the initial traumatic dislocation by reduction and prolonged immobilization is effective in preventing recurrent injury. We are concerned primarily with traumatic dislocations.

Associated Injuries

Injuries associated with traumatic dislocations include fracture of the glenoid or proximal humerus, injuries of the rotator cuff, arterial disruption, and nerve injuries. Fractures associated with glenohumeral dislocations include fracture of the humeral neck, fracture of the glenoid rim, impaction fracture of the humeral head, and fractures of the greater and lesser tuberosities.

Careful review of the radiographs determines the presence of these fractures. The most clinically significant is an undisplaced fracture of the humeral neck, which may displace during attempted reduction of the dislocation. In this situation, to minimize the probability of displacement, reduction is performed under general anesthesia with muscle relaxation and is monitored fluoroscopically. Displaced fractures of the humeral neck associated with glenohumeral dislocation usually require open reduction and internal fixation; these are covered in "Fractures of the Proximal Humerus." Fracture of more than 25% of the glenoid may result in chronic instability. Impaction fractures of the humeral head are equivalent to fractures of the glenoid rim. These fractures are known as the Hill–Sachs lesion and contribute to glenohumeral instability. The **Hill–Sachs lesion** is seen on the anteroposterior radiograph when the arm is maximally internally rotated. Fractures of the greater and lesser tuberosities are avulsions of the insertions of the supraspinatus, infraspinatus, teres minor, and subscapularis muscles. Frequently, these fractures reduce when the glenohumeral joint is reduced. If not, open reduction and internal fixation is indicated.

The presence of a **rotator cuff tear** is determined by physical examination (e.g., inability to initiate abduction of the glenohumeral joint). In questionable cases, arthrography, magnetic resonance imaging, and electromyography are helpful in determining the etiology of persistent weakness of the rotator cuff following reduction.

Rupture of the axillary artery is more likely to occur following a high-energy injury, in older patients, and in association with a brachial plexus injury. Physical signs include an expanding hematoma in the axilla and absent pulses at the elbow and wrist. Rupture of the axillary artery is an absolute surgical emergency.

The neurologic injury most frequently associated with glenohumeral dislocation is stretching of the **axillary nerve**, resulting in a transient palsy. Injury is ruled out when voluntary contractions of the anterior and middle portions of the deltoid muscle are elicited. This is not possible until the patient's pain is controlled by reduction of the dislocation. Sensory testing of the axillary nerve is unreliable. The radial, median, ulnar, and musculocutaneous nerves are examined to determine whether a brachial plexus injury is present.

Diagnosis and Initial Management

History and Physical Examination

Determine when the injury occurred and whether it is recurrent. The traumatic anterior dislocation results from a direct blow or from abduction and external rotation of the arm. The traumatic posterior dislocation results from a convulsion or a fall forward onto a flexed arm. There is no clearly defined injury causing atraumatic dislocation. Acquired dislocations are characterized by a history of repeated minor injuries.

Traumatic dislocations are painful. Anterior dislocations are characterized by external rotation of the arm. The area beneath the acromion is hollow due to displacement of the humeral head. The diagnosis of posterior dislocation is frequently missed because of the rarity of this injury and its subtle radiographic findings. This dislocation may be mistaken for adhesive capsulitis. The physical findings are key to the diagnosis. Posterior dislocations are characterized by internal rotation and adduction of the arm. The internal rotation is most obvious when the patient flexes both elbows to 90°. The normal anterior contour of the shoulder is absent, and there is a posterior fullness on the side of the dislocation, best seen by standing behind the seated patient. The physical examination of the patient with luxatio erecta is dramatic, with the humerus locked in greater than 90° of abduction.

Radiographic Examination

Radiographic examination of the injured shoulder confirms the direction of the dislocation and determines the existence of associated fractures. Three radiographic projections are essential. The scapular, or true, anteroposterior view is taken with the cassette parallel to the plane of the scapula, and the beam is directed perpendicular to the scapula (Fig. 7-4). Normally, this view indicates the parallel articular surface of the humeral head and the glenoid fossa. Following an anterior or posterior dislocation, the parallelism between the articular surfaces is lost,

FIG. 7-4   Scapular anteroposterior radiograph and shoulder anteroposterior projections.

and the images are superimposed (Fig. 7-5). The scapular lateral is taken with the cassette placed against the lateral surface of the shoulder at a right angle to the plane of the scapula (Fig. 7-6). The beam is directed from medial to lateral and parallel to the surface of the scapula. As seen on the scapular lateral projection, the glenoid is found at the intersection of the body, spine, and acromion. The axillary view is taken by placing a rolled cassette in the axilla and directing the beam distally (Fig. 7-7). Alternatively, the cassette is placed proximal to the shoulder with the patient supine, the arm is abducted, and the beam is directed through the axilla from distal to proximal. The patient requires analgesia to obtain a satisfactory axillary radiograph.

Other radiographic studies of use are an anteroposterior view of the shoulder and a CT scan. CT scans are particularly useful in cases in which an adequate axillary view cannot be obtained (Fig. 7-8).

Initial Management

Chronic dislocations do not require acute reduction and should be reduced only after the patient has been anesthetized. Acute dislocations are reduced immediately. Failure to reduce an acute dislocation is a surgical emergency. Prior to reduction, venous access is established, the patient is sedated, and intravenous analgesics are administered, as described in Chapter 4. Alternatively, intraarticular lidocaine can be used. In this technique, 20 mL 1% lidocaine is injected with a 1.5-inch 20-gauge needle 2 cm inferior and lateral to the acromion in the sulcus formed by the absent humeral head; the needle is directed slightly caudad. Care must be taken to avoid the axillary nerve. The reduction maneuver used is determined by the type of dislocation. Anterior dislocations are reduced with straight traction in line with the humerus. Gentle internal and external rotation of the arm will relocate the

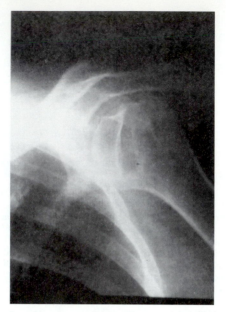

FIG. 7-5   Superimposition of humeral head on glenoid indicates posterior dislocation.

humeral head. Countertraction is applied by an assistant by a sheet wrapped around the chest. The traction is firm and consistent. It is important not to attempt to force the humeral head back into place because this will result in muscle spasm, making reduction more difficult and traumatic. Other methods of reduction of anterior dislocations that bear

FIG. 7-6   Scapular lateral view.

FIG. 7-7   Method of obtaining an axillary radiograph.

mention include Stimson's method, the Hippocratic method, and Kocher's method. **Stimson's method** involves hanging 5 to 10 lbs of weight from the arm of the prone patient. After 10 to 20 min, gentle internal and external rotation of the arm will relocate the humeral head. Stimson's method is useful as a last resort for dislocations that are difficult to reduce by other methods. The **Hippocratic method** involves applying lateral traction through the arm and countertraction by placing the foot in the axilla. The Hippocratic method is useful if no one is avail-

FIG. 7-8   Computed tomography indicates bilateral posterior fracture dislocations of the shoulder.

able to assist in the reduction. **Kocher's method** involves applying traction to the arm and then adducting and internally rotating the arm, levering the humeral head over the glenoid. This method is no longer used because of the risk of fracturing the proximal humerus. Posterior dislocations are reduced with gentle traction through the arm and applications of anteriorly directed pressure to the humeral head. Stimson's method will usually reduce posterior dislocations. **Luxatio erecta** is reduced with traction along the line of the arm. Countertraction is applied by an assistant.

Following reduction of the shoulder, a focused neurovascular examination is performed, with emphasis on assessment of the axillary nerve and rotator cuff. The shoulder is then immobilized in a stable position. Immobilization is usually performed with the arm held against the body in a sling and swathe. In this position, the arm is internally rotated and adducted. Uncomplicated anterior dislocations are always stable in this position, but a posterior dislocation may not be stable. When the humeral head is unstable posteriorly immobilization should be carried out in a position that holds the arm in a position of slight external rotation. Axillary and scapular anteroposterior and lateral radiographs are obtained to ensure the adequacy of reduction. Instability or an incongruous reduction may indicate a displaced glenoid rim fracture or a loose body that requires reduction and fixation or removal. A CT scan is useful in determining the cause of instability or an incongruous reduction.

Definitive Management

The definitive management of traumatic dislocation of the glenohumeral joint is based on whether the dislocation is acute, chronic, or recurrent. Management of all acute traumatic dislocations, regardless of the direction of dislocation, has two components: immobilization followed by rehabilitation. There is no benefit achieved from prolonged immobilization of the shoulder following a recurrent dislocation. Patients with recurrent dislocations require a reconstructive procedure to prevent future dislocation.

Acute traumatic dislocation (anterior, posterior, and inferior) is reduced and immobilized as described in the "Initial Management" section. Prolonged immobilization (4 to 6 weeks) reduces the incidence of recurrence. The sling and swathe is loosened for range-of-motion exercises of the elbow. Isometric exercises in the sling and swathe are begun at 2 to 3 weeks. At 4 to 6 weeks, all immobilization is discontinued, and strengthening exercises are initiated.

An unstable reduction, or irreducible dislocation, is an indication for immediate surgery. Unstable reduction is usually due to a glenoid rim fracture, or more commonly, a humeral head defect. A large rotator cuff tear can also be a factor in instability. Irreducible dislocation is due to soft tissue or bony interposition. The displaced glenoid rim fracture is reduced from an anterior approach for an anterior defect or a posterior approach for a posterior defect and is stabilized with screws. If comminution prevents adequate stabilization, the *coracoid process* or a block of autogenous iliac crest is used to reconstruct the glenoid rim. Humeral head defects are managed by transferring the subscapularis into the anteromedial defect (posterior dislocation) or infraspinatus into the posteromedial defect (anterior dislocation).

Management of **chronic traumatic posterior dislocation** depends on the activity and health of the patient, length of time that the glenohumeral joint has been dislocated, and size of associated humeral head defect.

Reduction is not attempted if the patient is inactive or a poor surgical candidate.

When the dislocation is less than 4 weeks old and the defect involves less than 20% of the articular surface of the humeral head, closed reduction is attempted. If successful, the shoulder is immobilized for 6 weeks as described for acute posterior dislocation. In cases in which closed reduction is not successful, open reduction by an anterior approach and transfer of the subscapularis or lesser tuberosity into the humeral defect is performed.

When the dislocation is more than 4 weeks old or the defect involves more than 20% of the articular surface of the humeral head, open reduction is performed from an anterior approach, and the lesser tuberosity is transferred into the defect. Postoperatively, the shoulder is immobilized for 6 weeks. Very old posterior dislocations or dislocations associated with large (greater than 50%) defects of the humeral head and glenoid are managed with arthroplasty or rarely arthrodesis and bone grafting. Associated axillary nerve palsy or massive rotator cuff tear with a chronic dislocation would be an indication for arthrodesis.

Chronic traumatic anterior dislocation of the shoulder is rare and occurs in the confused elderly or in patients with an impaired level of consciousness. The criteria for attempting a closed reduction include a history of dislocation of less than 4 weeks, the patient's level of activity, and the patient being healthy enough to undergo general anesthesia. Severe osteoporosis, arteriosclerosis, and other fractures around the shoulder joint are relative contraindications for reduction. If closed reduction is not possible, open reduction is indicated in the appropriate patient with significant disability. Arthrodesis or arthroplasty with bone grafting of a deficient glenoid may be necessary.

Complications

The complications unique to glenohumeral dislocation are recurrent dislocation and adhesive capsulitis. **Recurrent dislocation** is more common in patients who sustained their first dislocation when they were younger than age 30 years, and if there were no associated fractures of the greater and lesser tuberosities of the humerus. Management of recurrent dislocation starts with determining which lesions are contributing to instability. These lesions are then corrected surgically. Procedures have been designed to change the version of the humeral head or glenoid, fill defects of the glenoid rim or humeral head, limit external and internal rotation, and repair and reinforce the anterior capsule. Procedures that repair and reinforce the capsule are felt to be superior. The treatment of recurrent anterior instability in the elderly may necessitate a rotator cuff repair.

Adhesive capsulitis of the shoulder (also know as *frozen shoulder*) can follow any upper extremity injury. It occurs more frequently in older patients and is marked by painful limitation of motion of the glenohumeral joint. Before the diagnosis of adhesive capsulitis is accepted, following a shoulder injury radiographs must be obtained that show that this is not an unrecognized posterior dislocation. Management of true adhesive capsulitis is aggressive and employs physical therapy, joint injection with local anesthetic and steroids, and as a last resort arthroscopic expansion of the joint with Ringer's lactate and a gentle closed manipulation.

FRACTURES OF THE PROXIMAL HUMERUS

The proximal humerus is proximal to the insertion of the pectoralis major.

Classification

Fractures of the proximal humerus are classified according to whether there is significant displacement, if there is displacement, the number of fragments, and whether there is an associated dislocation.

Undisplaced fractures are displaced less than 1 cm or angulated less than 45° regardless of the fracture pattern or the number of fragments.

Displaced fractures occur along predictable anatomic lines, producing similar patterns of fractures. These anatomic lines are the anatomic neck, the surgical neck, the greater tuberosity, and the lesser tuberosity. Displaced fractures are further classified into three groups according to the number of major fragments present (i.e., two-part, three-part, and four-part fractures).

Two-part fractures occur in four patterns: fracture through either the anatomic or surgical neck, and fracture of either the greater or lesser tuberosity (Figs. 7-9 to 7-12). The vascularity of the head is at risk following a fracture of the anatomic neck. **Three-part fractures** occur in two patterns: fracture of the surgical neck with a fracture of either the greater or lesser tuberosity (Figs. 7-13 and 7-14). Because either the greater or lesser tuberosity remains attached to the head fragment, there

FIG. 7-9   Fracture through the anatomic neck.

FIG. 7-10   Fracture through the surgical neck.

is marked rotation of the head due to unopposed muscle pull (i.e., if the greater tuberosity remains attached, the head is abducted and externally rotated; if the lesser tuberosity remains attached, the head is internally rotated). **Four-part fractures** occur in one pattern: fracture of the anatomic neck and fracture of the greater and lesser tuberosities

FIG. 7-11   Fracture of the greater tuberosity.

FIG. 7-12   Fracture of the lesser tuberosity.

(Fig. 7-15). The vascular supply of the head is disrupted following four-part fracture.

Fracture dislocations are characterized by a dislocation of the glenohumeral articulation and an associated fracture of the proximal humerus. The fracture may be an undisplaced or displaced fracture (Fig.

FIG. 7-13   Fracture of the surgical neck and greater tuberosity.

FIG. 7-14   Fracture of the surgical neck and lesser tuberosity.

7-16). The displaced fracture that is most frequently associated with a dislocation is a two-part fracture involving the greater tuberosity.

Associated Injuries

Injuries of the axillary nerve, brachial plexus, and axillar artery and vein are frequently associated with fractures of the proximal humerus. The diagnosis of these injuries is covered in "Dislocations of the Gleno-humeral Articulation."

FIG. 7-15   Four-part fracture.

FIG. 7-16   Posterior fracture (two-part) dislocation.

Diagnosis and Initial Management

History and Physical Examination

There is pain that limits motion localized to the shoulder. Acutely, the appearance of the shoulder is relatively normal. It has a normal contour, and because of the overlying muscles there is no discernible swelling or ecchymosis. Within several days, a large ecchymosis appears around the shoulder and distally.

Radiographic Examination

The three essential projections are the scapular anteroposterior, the scapular lateral, and the axillary.

Supplemental views (e.g., the anteroposterior projection with the humerus in differing degrees of rotation and the transthoracic lateral) are frequently of value and are obtained at the surgeon's discretion. CT scans are of value in the evaluation of complex fracture dislocations or to assess the glenoid rim.

Initial Management

Initial management of undisplaced fractures consists of immobilization in a sling and swathe. Displaced fractures of the surgical or anatomic neck, regardless of whether there is a fracture of the greater or lesser tuberosities that is to be managed nonoperatively, are placed in a collar and cuff. The collar and cuff is designed to exert constant traction (the weight of the arm) through the fracture. Displaced isolated fractures of the greater or lesser tuberosity managed nonoperatively are placed in a sling. Fractures that are to be managed operatively are placed in a sling, and ice is applied to minimize swelling. The initial management of fracture dislocations is dependent on the location of the fracture. If there is an isolated fracture of the greater or lesser tuberosity, closed reduction is attempted in the emergency room. Dislocations with isolated fractures of the greater or lesser tuberosities are infrequently associated with occult fractures of the anatomic or surgical neck. Adequate images must be obtained before reduction is attempted. If there is a fracture of the anatomic or surgical neck, reduction is performed with general anesthesia and image intensification. Open reduction and internal fixation may be required to prevent fracture displacement.

Definitive Management

The definitive management is dependent on the type of fracture. Undisplaced fractures are managed as described in the "Initial Management" section.

Displaced Fractures

Displaced two-part fractures of the surgical neck and lesser tuberosity should be managed operatively. Manipulative reduction of surgical neck fractures can be accomplished with general anesthesia, but the fracture frequently displaces due to muscle forces when the patient awakens. Open reduction is done from the deltopectoral approach, and stabilization is done with a plate and screws or modified Ender's rods.

In this technique, two rods with an additional hole drilled above the eyelet are introduced through longitudinal incisions in the supraspinatus tendon insertional area, and then a heavy suture or wire is brought through these holes and under the supraspinatus tendon and passed through a drill hole in the distal fragment in a figure-of-eight tension band construct to provide stability. This technique has been described by Cuomo et al. (1992; Fig. 7-17).

Anatomic neck fractures are reduced and stabilized in young patients with high demands. Hemiarthroplasty is performed in elderly patients with osteopenic bone and fewer demands. The fracture is approached through the deltopectoral interval. Screws or screws and plates are used to stabilize the fracture once it has been reduced. Fractures of the greater

FIG. 7-17 Modified Ender's intramedullary fixation of a fracture of the proximal humerus supplemented with a tension band suture.

tuberosity are approached through a deltoid splitting approach and then reduced and stabilized with screws and washers.

The majority of displaced two-part fractures of the surgical neck or of the lesser tuberosity is managed nonoperatively. Surgical neck fractures are managed in a collar and cuff. An axillary pad can be added to correct medial displacement of the distal fragment. If the distal fragment cannot be reduced and it remains medially displaced, open reduction through the deltopectoral interval and stabilization with a plate and screws are indicated.

Displaced fractures of the lesser tuberosity are avulsion injuries of the subscapularis and should be repaired. These fractures can be associated with an undisplaced fracture of the surgical neck and result in limitation of internal rotation and weakness of internal rotation with a positive lift off test if not repaired.

Three-part fractures are almost always managed operatively because of the associated rotary deformity. They are approached through the deltopectoral interval, reduced, and stabilized with plate and screws if the bone is adequate. Three- and four-part fractures frequently occur in osteopenic bone, and stable fixation can be difficult to achieve with plate and screws. Polymethylmethacrylate (PMMA) can be used to supplement fixation in osteopenic bone. When PMMA is used, the fracture is grafted with autogenous cancellous bone to stimulate healing. Alternatively, the modified Ender's nail technique, open reduction and limited internal fixation, external fixation using the Hoffmann device as described by Ko and Yamamoto (1996), or pin fixation with three crossed pins and suture repair of the displaced tuberosities can be attempted.

A technique for nonunions of the surgical neck of the humerus using an intramedullary bone peg, plate and screw fixation, and cancellous bone grafting as described by Walch et. al. (1996) may also be applicable. In this technique, a 6- to 10-cm corticocancellous bone graft from the iliac crest is impacted into the distal humeral fragment and plugged into the humeral head. An external T-plate completes the stabilization.

Techniques using solely wire or a heavy suture passed through the tendinous insertions of the rotator cuff on the tuberosities and fixed in a figure-of-eight fashion to the distal shaft fragment frequently prove inadequate and are not recommended.

The following technique was developed at Cook County Hospital by Dr. Robert F. Hall, Jr., and is described in detail. It mimics the fixation of an intertrochanteric hip fracture because it is done under x-ray control in patients with osteopenia and fracture comminution. The patient is positioned supine on an operating room table that has a radiolucent extension. The imaging machine must visualize the shoulder joint and proximal humerus. A deltopectoral approach is used, by opening the interval from the clavicle to the deltoid insertion. The deltoid insertion can be mobilized, if needed, for additional exposure. A preliminary reduction is done under direct vision and the C-arm, which is angled about 45° off the longitudinal axis of the patient, is brought into the operative field. The fracture reduction is checked for adequacy and adjusted, if necessary. If possible, the reduced fracture is held with a bone clamp. The arm is allowed to rest on the imaging camera, which has been draped sterilely, and the arm is stabilized by an assistant. An internal fixation device such as a T-plate or the Synthes 90° Cannulated LC-Angle Blade Plate is placed along side the humeral shaft and neck, and an image is made to check its position. If a T-plate is used and the position is satisfactory, a 3.2-mm drill hole is placed in the humeral shaft to fix the plate to the proximal humeral shaft with a 4.5-mm cortical screw. A 3.2-mm drill is then placed through the plate into the humeral head. This is done under image control to check the angle of the drill and the depth of penetration. After length assessment, a 6.5-mm cancellous screw is placed in the humeral head. Similarly, a second cancellous screw is placed more posteriorly in the humeral head. The two screws are angled slightly toward each other to keep them in the humeral head. The remaining shaft screws are then placed. Final images are obtained to check the fracture for reduction, screw length, and position. If satisfactory fixation is obtained, Codman exercises are started the day following surgery.

The 90° Cannulated LC-Angle Blade Plate uses a blade plate drill guide through which a 2.0-mm threaded guidewire is inserted until the tip engages subchondral bone. Image intensification confirms placement. The guidewire is designed to orient the blade at 90° to the shaft of the bone. The most proximal screw hole permits insertion of an oblique 4.5-mm lag screw into the far cortex of the proximal fragment for more stable fixation of the humeral head (Fig. 7-18).

The results of prosthetic replacement are mediocre at best, with adequate pain relief in only three of four patients and flexion limited to about 100°. These patients frequently have difficulty using the hand above shoulder level and carrying more than 10 to 15 lbs.

The management of four-part fractures is dependent on the demands of the patient and the degree of osteopenia present. These fractures frequently occur through osteopenic bone in sedentary patients with very limited demands. In these cases, four-part fractures are managed nonoperatively in a sling, with the clear understanding that the mobility and strength of the shoulder will be severely limited. In more active patients with osteopenic bone, a hemiarthroplasty is performed. The goal of hemiarthroplasty is a strong painless shoulder with a relatively limited range of motion. In patients younger than age 50 years with bone of normal density, open reduction and stabilization are attempted. There is a high incidence of avascular necrosis and nonunion following this procedure, but it provides the patient a chance for the best result.

A

FIG. 7-18   *A, B.* Anteroposterior and axillary views of comminuted three-part fracture of the proximal humerus.

B

FIG. 7-18   *Continued.*

C

FIG. 7-18 *C, D.* Radiographs following reduction and fixation with the 90° Cannulated LC-Angle Blade Plate.

D

FIG. 7-18   *Continued.*

Whether a hemiarthroplasty or reduction and internal fixation is performed, the surgical approach is through the deltopectoral groove. When a hemiarthroplasty is performed, essential steps include the restoration of proper humeral length and retrotorsion and reattachment of the tuberosities beneath the prosthetic head to the humeral shaft and each other with wires or heavy suture so that healing occurs between them and minimizes the chance of late displacement. The humeral head is used as a source of cancellous graft.

Fracture Dislocation

The most commonly encountered fracture dislocation is an anterior dislocation and a fracture of the greater tuberosity. As described in the "Initial Management" section, a gentle atraumatic reduction is performed in the emergency room. If the greater tuberosity remains displaced, it is reduced and stabilized operatively. Two-part fracture dislocations through the anatomic or surgical neck and all three- and four-part fracture dislocations are managed operatively. Closed reduction is not attempted because the brachial plexus and axillary artery may be injured. The fracture is approached through the deltopectoral interval. Two- and three-part fractures are reduced and stabilized with plates and screws (Fig. 7-18). Four-part fractures are managed with a hemiarthroplasty.

Rehabilitation of the shoulder following fracture is extremely important. Depending on the patient's comfort level and the stability of fixation, pendulum exercises are begun at 2 to 3 weeks. Gentle, passive-assisted abduction and external and internal rotation exercises are added at 3 to 4 weeks. Usually at 6 to 8 weeks, enough healing has occurred so that active range-of-motion and strengthening exercises can be initiated.

Complications

Malunion is the most common complication of displaced proximal humeral fractures and results from nonoperative treatment and inability to obtain or maintain an operative reduction. The treatment of malunion by osteotomy or prosthetic replacement is difficult and often unrewarding. Avascular necrosis of the humeral head, nonunion, intraarticular adhesions, and posttraumatic arthritis are complications of proximal humerus fractures. Avascular necrosis is not always symptomatic. In cases in which avascular necrosis is symptomatic, it is usually managed with hemiarthroplasty. Nonunion is managed with open reduction, stabilization, and autogenous cancellous bone grafting. The management of intraarticular adhesions is covered in the section "Dislocations of the Glenohumeral Articulation." Posttraumatic arthrosis is managed with arthroplasty if symptoms warrant. Arthrodesis is recommended only for a painful shoulder with paralysis of the deltoid or the rotator cuff.

SELECTED READINGS

Dislocations of the Humeral Head from the Glenoid Fossa
Gonzalez D, Lopez RA: Concurrent rotator cuff tear and brachial plexus palsy associated with anterior dislocation of the shoulder: A report of two cases. *J Bone Joint Surg* 73A:620–621, 1991.
Matthews D, Roberts T: Intraarticular lidocaine versus intravenous analgesic for reductions of acute anterior shoulder dislocations. *Am J Sports Med* 23:5458, 1995.
Rowe CR, Zarins B: Chronic unreduced dislocations of the shoulder. *J Bone Joint Surg* 64A:495–505, 1982.
Wirth MA, Groh GI, Rockwood CA: Capsulorrhaphy through an anterior approach for treatment of atraumatic posterior glenohumeral instability with multidirectional laxity of the shoulder. *J Bone Joint Surg* 80A:1570–1578, 1998.

Fractures of the Proximal Humerus
Beredjiklian PK, Iannotti JP, Norris TR, Williams GR: Operative treatment of malunion of a fracture of the proximal aspect of the humerus. *J Bone Joint Surg* 80A:1484–1497, 1998.
Cuomo F, Flatow EL, Mayday MG, Miller SR, McIlveen SJ, Bigliani LU: Open reduction and internal fixation of two- and three- part displaced surgical neck fractures of the proximal humerus, *J Shoulder Elbow Surg* 1:287–295, 1992.
Goldman RT, Loval KJ, Cuomo F, et al: Functional outcome after humeral head replacement for acute three- and four- part proximal humeral fractures. *J Shoulder Elbow Surg* 4:81–86, 1995.
Jupiter JB, Mullaji AB: Blade plate fixation of proximal humeral nonunions. *Injury* 25:301–303, 1994.

Ko J-Y, Yamamoto R: Surgical treatment of complex fracture of the proximal humerus. *Clin Orthop* 327:225–237, 1996.

Neer CS II: Displaced proximal humerus fractures. Part I: Classification and evaluation. *J Bone Joint Surg* 52A:1077–1089, 1970.

Walch G, Badet R, Nove-Josserand L, et al: Nonunions of the surgical neck of the humerus:surgical treatment with an intramedullary bone peg, internal fixation, and cancellous bone grafting, *J Shoulder Elbow Surg* 5:161–168, 1996.

8

Fractures and Dislocations of the Clavicle and Scapula

John A. Elstrom

This chapter reviews fractures of the clavicle, injuries of the sternoclavicular and acromioclavicular joints, and fractures of the scapula.

ANATOMY

The clavicle is the strut that connects the upper extremity to the chest. It stabilizes and serves as a fulcrum for the scapula. Without the clavicle, contraction of muscles that cross the glenohumeral joint (e.g., the pectoralis major) would pull the proximal humerus to the chest instead of lifting the arm.

The **clavicle** is S-shaped when viewed from above. The flat acromial end is covered by the deltoid origin anteriorly and the trapezius insertions posteriorly. The round sternal end gives rise to the origins of the pectoralis major anteriorly and the sternocleidomastoid posteriorly.

The **scapula** is a flat triangular bone located on the posterior aspect of the chest. It has three bony processes: the coracoid process; the spine; and the continuation of the spine, the acromion. It has two articulations: the acromioclavicular joint and the glenohumeral joint. The scapula is buried in muscles. The costal, or anterior, surface is covered by the subscapularis muscle. The posterior surface is covered by the supra- and infraspinatus muscles. The spine is the origin of the posterior deltoid and the insertion of the trapezius. The short head of the biceps, the coracobrachialis, and the pectoralis minor originate from, and insert on, the coracoid process. The trapezius and levator scapulae elevate the scapula. The serratus anterior moves the scapula anteriorly, holding it against the chest wall. Paralysis of the serratus anterior results in "winging" of the scapula.

The **acromioclavicular joint** is a diarthrodial plane joint. Its articular surfaces are covered by fibrocartilage and separated by a meniscus. The joint is stabilized by weak acromioclavicular ligaments, the deltoid and trapezius muscles, and the coracoclavicular ligaments (i.e., the trapezoid and conoid ligaments). The range of motion through the acromioclavicular joint is 20°, with most of it occurring in the initial 30° of shoulder abduction.

The **sternoclavicular joint** is a diarthrodial saddle joint. Its surfaces are covered with fibrocartilage, and the joint is completely divided by an articular disc. This disc attaches to the articular border of the clavicle, first rib, and joint capsule. The sternoclavicular joint is strengthened by anterior and posterior sternoclavicular ligaments, the interclavicular ligament running between the clavicles behind the sternum, and by the costoclavicular ligament running between the first rib and the clavicle. The clavicle abducts or elevates about 40° through the sternoclavicular joint. This motion occurs throughout shoulder abduction up to 90°. The medial physis of the clavicle fuses around the age of 25 years; therefore, epiphyseal separations rather than true sternoclavicular dislocations occur in patients younger than 25 years of age. This is important because physeal injuries will remodel, and joint dislocations will not.

Behind the sternoclavicular joint are the major blood vessels and the trachea and esophagus. The brachial plexus and subclavian artery continue laterally, posterior to the clavicle, passing over the first rib and anterior to the scapula just distal to the coracoid. The costoclavicular space may be decreased by a fracture of the first rib or medial portion of the clavicle, resulting in acute neurovascular injury or late compression. The axillary nerve passes below the neck of the glenoid and is frequently injured in shoulder dislocations. The suprascapular nerve passes through the scapular notch just medial to the base of the coracoid under the transverse scapular ligament.

FRACTURES OF THE CLAVICLE

Classification

Clavicle fractures are classified, according to location, as distal, middle, and proximal third fractures. The mechanism of injury is either a direct blow or an axial load resulting from a fall or blow on the lateral aspect of the shoulder.

Distal third fractures are further classified into three types (Fig. 8-1). Type I fractures are the most common and occur between intact coracoclavicular and acromioclavicular ligaments. The ligaments hold the fragments in alignment. Type II fractures are characterized by disruption of the coracoclavicular ligaments. The weight of the arm pulls the distal fragment inferiorly and the trapezius and sternocleidomastoid pull the proximal fragment superiorly. Type III fractures are intraarticular, usually undisplaced, and frequently become evident years later as posttraumatic arthritis.

Middle third fractures are the most common type of clavicle fracture. The proximal fragment is displaced superiorly by muscle pull; the distal fragment is displaced inferiorly by the weight of the arm.

Fractures of the proximal third of the clavicle, excluding injuries of the sternoclavicular joint, are uncommon and frequently pathologic.

Diagnosis and Initial Management

History and Physical Examination

The clavicle is subcutaneous; therefore, swelling and deformity are obvious, and tenderness on palpation reveals the site of the injury.

FIG. 8-1 The three types of distal clavicle fracture: (*A*) type I, (*B*) type II, and (*C*) type III.

Radiographic Examination

Radiographic confirmation and evaluation of fractures of the clavicle are done with anteroposterior and 45° cephalic tilt views with the patient upright. Radiographs of proximal third fractures may occasionally have to be augmented with computed tomography (CT). In fractures of the distal third of the clavicle anteroposterior, radiographs of both acromioclavicular joints with the use of 5- to 10-lb. weights are obtained to determine the presence of ligamentous disruption.

Initial Management

Initial management consists of a sling.

Associated Injuries

Associated injuries to the chest, brachial plexus, and major vessels are ruled out by history and physical examination. Visceral injury is associated with high-energy trauma, an open fracture, and fracture of the first rib or scapula. Scapulothoracic dissociation is a devastating injury associated with clavicle fracture or dislocation. The diagnosis is confirmed by lateral displacement of the scapula, with an associated injury of the clavicle, acromioclavicular joint, or sternoclavicular joint. There is frequently an associated injury of the brachial plexus or axillary artery.

Definitive Management

Open reduction and internal fixation of **fractures of the distal third of the clavicle** are indicated if there is superior displacement of the proximal fragment due to disruption of the coracoclavicular ligaments or if there is intraarticular displacement. Type I and undisplaced type III distal clavicle fractures are managed symptomatically with a sling. The figure-of-eight splint has no value for fractures of the distal third. Type II distal clavicle fractures and the rare displaced type III fractures are managed with open reduction and internal fixation. The distal clavicle is exposed through an incision over its anterior subcutaneous border. The fracture is stabilized with a "T", or one-third tubular, plate.

Fractures of the middle and proximal third of the clavicle are treated with manipulative reduction and immobilization with a figure-of-eight splint that holds the shoulders dorsally. The figure-of-eight splint is applied and tightened with the shoulders retracted. The splint will stretch and loosen; therefore, it must be tightened every morning for the first few days. A sling supports the arm the first week. After 4 or 5 weeks, fracture healing has usually progressed to the point where immobilization is no longer required.

Indications for primary open reduction of middle and proximal third clavicle fractures include the threat of skin penetration by fracture fragments, initial fracture shortening of 2 cm or more, irreducible displacement (e.g., button holing of the proximal fragment), neurovascular compromise, open fractures, and fractures associated with other injuries of the shoulder girdle (e.g., displaced extraarticular fractures of the glenoid neck and scapulothoracic dissociation). Exposure of the clavicle is through an incision just inferior to the clavicle. A 3.5-mm reconstruction or dynamic compression plate is contoured and placed on the flat superior surface of the clavicle. Autogenous cancellous grafting is required with extensive comminution, devitalized bone fragments, or loss of continuity. Postoperatively, the arm is supported in a sling until callus formation is evident at about 4 weeks.

Complications

Complications consist of nonunion, malunion, and neurovascular compromise.

Nonunion of fractures of the middle third of the clavicle occur more frequently following high-energy injuries. Atrophic nonunions are radiographically obvious. Tomography or fluoroscopic examination may be required to demonstrate the more common hypertrophic nonunion. Management of symptomatic nonunions includes open reduction, internal fixation, and bone grafting.

Malunion of middle third clavicular fractures is usually a cosmetic problem. Symptomatic shortening or angulation resulting in tenting of the skin is managed with osteotomy and bone grafting, with internal fixation to restore clavicular length or resection of protruding bone ends.

Neurovascular complications result from displacement of the fracture fragments at the time of injury, from associated injuries (e.g., first rib fracture), and from late sequelae associated with hypertrophic callus. Subclavian vein obstruction between the clavicle and first rib is characterized by engorgement of the veins in the ipsilateral upper extremity. Angiography, electromyography, and magnetic resonance imaging (MRI) are useful in determining the extent of neurovascular compromise. These complications are managed in conjunction with a thoracic surgeon.

FRACTURES OF THE SCAPULA

Fractures of the scapula are rare and often associated with other severe injuries. As a result, nearly 50% of injuries is overlooked initially. The most common associated injury is fracture of the ipsilateral ribs, with hemopneumothorax occurring in approximately one-third of high-energy injuries.

Classification

The most important factor in classifying a scapular fracture is whether it was caused by high-energy (e.g., an automobile accident) or low-energy (e.g., avulsion of a muscle insertion) trauma. Comminution and displacement, the "burst fracture," indicate high-energy trauma. Scapular fractures are further classified according to the location: fractures of the body and spine, the glenoid neck (extraarticular), the acromion, the coracoid process, and the glenoid (intraarticular). Intraarticular fractures of the glenoid are subdivided into undisplaced and displaced fractures. Displaced fractures are simple (i.e., part of the glenoid is intact) or complex (i.e., the entire articular surface of the glenoid is fractured; Fig. 8-2).

Diagnosis and Initial Management

History and Physical Examination

Pain is localized in the shoulder and back. The arm is adducted and protected against motion. Ecchymosis and swelling are minimal due to the location of the scapula beneath layers of muscle. Loss of active abduction and forward elevation of the arm, known as *pseudoparalysis of the rotator cuff*, is often associated with scapular fracture and is the result of intramuscular hemorrhage and pain.

Radiographic Examination

Radiographic evaluation of the scapula includes true anteroposterior and lateral views of the scapula and an axillary view. The anteroposterior view of the scapula will show fractures of the glenoid and glenoid

FIG. 8-2   The six types of scapular fractures: (*A*) fracture of the body, (*B*) extraarticular fracture of the neck of the glenoid, (*C*) fracture of the acromion, (*D*) fracture of the coracoid, (*E*) simple fracture of the glenoid, and (*F*) complex fracture of the glenoid.

FIG. 8-2 *Continued.*

FIG. 8-2 *Continued.*

FIG. 8-2 *Continued.*

neck. Lateral scapular views show fractures of the scapular body and acromion. The axillary view will show fractures of the coracoid and glenoid. MRI, CT, and anteroposterior and lateral chest radiographs provide additional information.

Initial Management

The initial management consists of a sling.

Associated Injuries

The most important factor in the initial management of scapular fractures is that high-energy fractures are associated with life-threatening visceral injuries. The most common associated visceral injuries include hemopneumothorax, pulmonary or cardiac contusion, aortic tear, brachial plexus injury, axillary artery injury, and closed head injuries. The most common associated osseous injuries are fractures of the ribs and clavicle. Fracture of the first rib is frequently associated with injury of the brachial plexus and subclavian vessels.

Definitive Management

Management of **fractures of the body and spine** is usually nonoperative. The muscles surrounding the scapula prevent further displacement. A sling and ice are used for the first few days to control pain. As the pain subsides, pendulum exercises in the sling are initiated. Healing is rapid, and usually after 4 weeks, active motion can be initiated. Burst fractures with proximal displacement of the lateral margin of the body may impinge on the glenohumeral joint capsule. When this occurs, the fracture is reduced and stabilized or the offending bony spike is osteotomized.

Extraarticular fractures of the glenoid neck are the second-most common type of scapular fracture and occur when the humeral head is driven into the glenoid fossa. A CT scan may be necessary to confirm that the fracture does not involve the joint. Reduction is not attempted. The arm is supported in a sling, and management is as described for fracture of the body and spine. The prognosis is good for near full return of function.

Fractures through the neck of the glenoid with an associated clavicular fracture are unstable because of loss of the suspensory function of the clavicle. The weight of the arm pulls the glenoid fragment distally, resulting in deformity and ultimate loss of function. Open reduction and internal fixation of the fractured clavicle is recommended. Open reduction and internal fixation of the glenoid neck fracture through a posterior approach, as described by Brodsky et al. (1987), with the patient in the lateral decubitus position, may also be required.

The **acromion** is fractured by a direct blow from the superior aspect or by superior displacement of the humeral head. Stress fracture results from superior migration of the humeral head due to a long-standing rotator cuff tear. A stress fracture, therefore, is an indication for an arthrogram or MRI to evaluate the rotator cuff. Depression of the acromion is associated with traction injury of the brachial plexus.

Minimally displaced fractures of the acromion are treated conservatively. These are followed closely for the first 3 weeks because they may displace. Significant displacement impairs glenohumeral motion because of impingement on the rotator cuff. Displaced fractures are managed with open reduction and internal fixation with a screw or tension band wire.

Isolated **fracture of the coracoid process** results from a direct blow, avulsion by muscle pull, or is a stress fracture (i.e., "trap shooter's shoulder"). Fractures occur through the base or the tip. When minimally displaced, they heal uneventfully.

Displaced coracoid fractures occur in combination with an acromioclavicular dislocation. The coracoid is avulsed from the scapula by the coracoclavicular ligaments. Management is open reduction and fixation of the coracoid with a single screw and temporary transarticular fixation of the acromioclavicular dislocation. Displacement of the coracoid can cause compression of the suprascapular nerve and paralysis of the external rotators of the shoulder (i.e., the supraspinatus and infraspinatus). When this occurs, open reduction and fixation of the coracoid and decompression of the nerve are indicated.

The management of **intraarticular fractures of the glenoid** is based on the amount of displacement, the type of fracture, and the presence of glenohumeral instability.

Undisplaced fractures are managed with a sling and immobilization as described for fractures of the body of the scapula. Displaced simple fractures (3 mm or more) are managed with open reduction and internal fixation. The degree of congruity of the articular surface is determined by anteroposterior, glenoid tangential, and axillary radiographs and CT. Instability of the glenohumeral articulation is expected when the fragment is displaced 1 cm and when the fragment comprises one-fourth of the articular surface. Frequently, subluxation will be evident on the initial radiographs. An anterior approach through the deltopectoral interval is used to expose fractures of the anterior glenoid rim only. Transverse, vertical, and minimally comminuted fractures where reduction and fixation can be obtained should be approached posteriorly, as described by Brodsky et al. (1987) and Kavanagh et al. (1993). Posterior exposure is accomplished with the patient prone or in the lateral decubitus position. Through a vertical incision, the posterior deltoid is mobilized either by abducting the arm or by a limited release from the scapular spine, and the interval between the infraspinatus and teres minor is developed to expose the fracture and posterior capsule. The axillary nerve and posterior circumflex humeral vessels are identified and protected, as is the suprascapular nerve. Additional exposure may be obtained with a vertical incision through the tendinous portion of the infraspinatus muscle. Large fragments are reduced and stabilized with screws or plates. Kirschner wires and cerclage wires may break or migrate and are not used. In severely comminuted fractures, the fragments are excised and replaced with an iliac crest bone graft contoured to the shape of the osseous defect and fixed to the glenoid with screws. Alternatively, if the fracture involves the anterior rim, the coracoid process is osteotomized and transferred to the defect.

Complex fractures of the glenoid pose special problems. The surgeon must decide whether an extensive surgical procedure will result in a reduced stable glenoid; if not, closed management is indicated. These fractures can be difficult to manage surgically because the necessary exposure is extensive. Postoperative management depends on the stability of fixation and the surgical approach. Ideally, early passive motion is possible.

Closed management consists of an initial period of immobilization followed by early range of motion to mold the articular fragments into as normal a position as possible. The optimal position and type of immobilization are determined by comparing anteroposterior and axillary radiographs of the glenohumeral joint with the arm at the side and in various positions of elevation and rotation. Immobilization may be in the form of a sling and swathe, traction, or an airplane splint. At 3 to 4 weeks, healing has progressed to the point that immobilization can be discontinued. Range of motion is continued in a sling for an additional 3 to 6 weeks. Between 6 and 9 weeks, the sling is discontinued and active range of motion is initiated.

Complications

Complications of scapular fractures include chronic glenohumeral instability, posttraumatic glenohumeral arthrosis, rotator cuff injury, and impingement.

When these complications occur, conservative management with nonsteroidal anti-inflammatory medication, physical therapy, intraarticular steroid injection, or a surgical procedure to address the most important pathology can be considered.

MRI with intraarticular contrast and CT can be used to substantiate a clinical diagnosis of rotator cuff tear, impingement syndrome, or glenohumeral arthrosis. Rotator cuff repair, decompression of impingement on the rotator cuff, and replacement arthroplasty would be the major surgical options for usual complications. Arthrodesis would be indicated rarely in those instances when posttraumatic glenohumeral arthrosis is associated with neurological deficit from axillary nerve or brachial plexus injury.

STERNOCLAVICULAR JOINT INJURIES

Classification

Injuries of the sternoclavicular joint are classified as sprains or dislocations. Sprains are undisplaced. Dislocations are anterior or retrosternal.

Diagnosis and Initial Management

History and Physical Examination

A history of injury, pain, and asymmetry of the sternoclavicular joints are the cardinal signs of this injury. The patient supports the injured extremity and tilts the head toward the affected side. Pain and swelling without injury may be signs of septic arthritis or condensing osteitis of the distal end of the clavicle. Spontaneous atraumatic anterior subluxation occurs in young patients with ligamentous laxity and is managed conservatively. In patients younger than 25 years of age, epiphyseal separation must be differentiated from dislocation.

Radiographic Examination

Routine anteroposterior radiographs of the sternoclavicular joint are not diagnostic. Two projections designed to show sternoclavicular joint dislocation are the Hobbs view and the Rockwood view. In the Hobbs view, the seated patient leans forward over a cassette so that the back of the neck is parallel to the table. The beam is directed through the neck onto the cassette. In the Rockwood view, the patient is supine. The beam is tilted 40° cephalad and aimed at the sternum. A cassette is placed on the table so that the beam will project both clavicles onto the plate. In an anterior sternoclavicular dislocation, the clavicle appears to

FIG. 8-3   Rockwood view of a right anterior sternoclavicular dislocation.

be anterior and riding higher than the uninjured side (Fig. 8-3). In a retrosternal dislocation, the clavicle appears to be posterior and is lower than the uninjured side. CT scans differentiate sternoclavicular dislocation from fracture of the medial end of the clavicle and assess the adequacy of reduction (Fig. 8-4).

Initial Management

Initial management consists of a sling. The patient is observed for respiratory and circulatory problems.

Associated Injuries

Compression of the structures of the thoracic inlet may occur with posterior dislocation and should be specifically ruled out. Acutely, this may

FIG. 8-4   Computed tomographic scan showing anterior displacement of the right clavicle in relation to the sternum and the left sternoclavicular joint.

become life threatening; subacutely, it is an indication for surgery. Symptoms of compression of these structures include shortness of breath and hoarseness, dysphasia, paresthesia, or weakness of the upper extremity.

Definitive Management

Sprains of the sternoclavicular joint are treated symptomatically. Anterior dislocations become asymptomatic, and reduction (which is usually unstable) is rarely indicated. When reduction is attempted, it is performed in the following fashion. The patient is supine with a bolster between the shoulder blades. A posteriorly directed force is placed on the anterior aspect of both shoulders, and the medial end of the clavicle is pressed inferiorly and posteriorly. The shoulders are then held retracted with a figure-of-eight clavicle strap.

Treatment of a retrosternal dislocation of the clavicle is more important. A thoracic surgeon is consulted if the patient has compression of the structures of the thoracic inlet. The technique of manipulative reduction has been described by Buckerfield and Castle (1984). A bolster is placed between the shoulders. The bolster should be thick enough to elevate both shoulders from the table. With the arm adducted to the trunk, caudal traction is applied to the arm while both shoulders are forced posteriorly by direct pressure. Percutaneous manipulation with a towel clip may be required. Reduction is confirmed by lordotic radiographs. Once reduced, the retrosternal dislocation is usually stable. A figure-of-eight clavicle strap is used to hold the shoulders retracted for 4 to 6 weeks.

If closed reduction fails, open reduction is indicated when there are symptoms of mediastinal compression or to prevent subsequent damage to retrosternal structures on the medial end of the clavicle. Metallic internal fixation is dangerous and should not be used.

Complications

The incidence of complications from retrosternal dislocation of the clavicle is 25%. The symptoms associated with these complications are usually corrected with reduction; however, pneumothorax, laceration of the great vessels, and rupture of the trachea and esophagus require emergency intervention. The most serious long-term complications are the result of migration of metallic fixation devices.

Most patients with persistent traumatic anterior displacement of the medial end of the clavicle do not require operative treatment. Resection arthroplasty of the sternoclavicular joint with repair or reconstruction of the costoclavicular ligament to stabilize the medial portion of the clavicle to the first rib may be indicated for severe pain in chronic traumatic anterior dislocations of the sternoclavicular joint and to prevent damage to retrosternal structures with chronic unreduced posterior dislocation.

ACROMIOCLAVICULAR JOINT INJURIES

Classification

Acromioclavicular joint injuries are classified according to the amount and direction of displacement into seven groups (Fig. 8-5). In type I injuries, the acromioclavicular capsule is stretched, but the coracoclavicular ligaments remain intact. The clavicle is undisplaced. In type II injuries, the acromioclavicular capsule is torn, and the coracoclavicular ligaments are stretched or partly torn. The clavicle is displaced less than one-half of its width. In type III injuries, both the acromioclavicular capsule and coracoclavicular ligaments are torn, the coracoclavicular distance is increased, and the clavicle is completely dislocated from the acromioclavicular joint. The deltoid and trapezius muscles are intact and remain attached to the clavicle. In type IV injuries, the clavicle is displaced posteriorly and is buttonholed through the trapezius, blocking closed reduction. In type V injuries, the trapezius and deltoid are torn, and the distal clavicle is displaced superiorly and is covered only by skin and subcutaneous tissue. In type VI injuries, the distal clavicle is dislocated inferiorly and is locked below the coracoid and conjoined tendon. Type VII injuries are panclavicular dislocations.

Diagnosis and Initial Management

History and Physical Examination

There is a history of an axial-loading injury to the lateral aspect of the shoulder, with pain, swelling, and tenderness increasing around the acromioclavicular joint. Prominence of the distal end of the clavicle is present on inspection, with the patient sitting and the weight of the arm unsupported, in type III injuries. When the amount of displacement is in

A

FIG. 8-5   The seven types of acromioclavicular injuries: (*A*) type I, (*B*) type II, (*C*) type III, (*D*) type IV, (*E*) type V, (*F*) type VI, and (*G*) type VII.

FIG. 8-5   *Continued.*

FIG. 8-5   *Continued.*

question, the integrity of the coracoclavicular ligaments is determined by the patient flexing the elbow against resistance, with the arm at the side. When the coracoclavicular ligaments are disrupted, the distal end of the clavicle will seem to rise superiorly as the acromion is pulled distally.

Radiographic Examination

Radiographic confirmation of the acromioclavicular injury and the degree of displacement is obtained with the patient upright and the weight of the arm unsupported. Radiographs taken with the patient supine or with techniques that overpenetrate the acromioclavicular joint obscure displacement. Stress films with the patient holding 5 to 10 lbs. and comparison films with the opposite side are helpful. An axillary view of the shoulder is obtained to assess displacement in the anteroposterior plane. In type I injuries, there is no displacement of the distal end of the clavicle. In type II injuries, the distal end of the clavicle is slightly elevated but not completely displaced from its articulation with the acromioclavicular. In type III injuries, the distal end of the clavicle is displaced superiorly and the coracoclavicular distance is increased. The distance between the coracoid process and the clavicle differs; therefore, it is important to obtain comparison views of the other shoulder. In type IV injuries, the distal end of the clavicle is displaced posteriorly. Displacement is best visualized on the axillary view. In type V, VI, and VII injuries, the amount and direction of displacement are indicated the type of injury.

Initial Management

Initial management is a sling.

Definitive Management

Type I and II injuries are treated symptomatically with a sling and ice. The sling is removed daily for range-of-motion exercises of the shoulder.

The treatment of type III injuries is controversial. The natural history of unreduced type III dislocations is that the pain diminishes and disappears and the deformity persists but improves. Nonoperative management is recommended. This consists of the use of a sling and early range-of-motion exercises. The use of a shoulder harness to maintain reduction of the acromioclavicular joint is not recommended because it is poorly tolerated and has no effect on ultimate displacement.

If open reduction and internal fixation is attempted, the distal clavicle, acromion, and coracoid are exposed. The joint is debrided, reduced, and stabilized with a large, smooth Steinman pin. The pin is left protruding through the skin laterally and bent to prevent migration. The capsule of acromioclavicular joint is repaired with the coracoclavicular ligaments. Postoperatively, the arm is maintained in a sling. The pins are removed at 6 weeks. Physical therapy is not started until the pins have been removed to prevent breakage. Another surgical option in the acute dislocation is resection of the distal 2 cm of the clavicle and transfer of the coracoclavicular ligament from its acromial attachment into the distal end of the clavicle, as described by Weaver and Dunn (1972). Procedures that use a Bosworth screw passed through the clavicle into the coracoid and heavy nonabsorbable suture looped under the coracoid process and around the clavicle to tether the clavicle to the coracoid are associated with frequent material complications.

Type IV, V, and VI injuries are treated with open reduction and internal fixation of the acromioclavicular joint. Type VII injuries are managed with open reduction and stabilization of the acromioclavicular joint and closed reduction of the sternoclavicular joint. Reduction of the sternoclavicular joint is maintained with a figure-of-eight splint.

Complications

Complications include shoulder stiffness, deformity, chronic dislocation, and posttraumatic arthritis. Shoulder stiffness is prevented with early range-of-motion exercises. The deformity diminishes but does not disappear. Symptomatic chronic dislocation and posttraumatic arthritis are managed with resection of the distal 2 cm of the clavicle and transfer of the coracoclavicular ligament from its acromial attachment to the distal end of the clavicle.

Complications following open management are more significant. The most frequent is loss of reduction. The most significant is breakage and migration of a pin, which is potentially fatal if the pin migrates to the heart or great vessels.

SELECTED READINGS

Fractures of the Clavicle

Hill JM, McGuire MH, Crosby LA: Closed treatment of displaced middle third fractures of the clavicle gives poor results. *J Bone Joint Surg* 79B:537–539, 1997.

Kona J, Bosse MJ, Staeheli JW, Rosseau RL: Type II distal clavicle fractures: a retrospective review of surgical treatment. *J Orthop Trauma* 4:115–120, 1990.

Fractures of the Scapula

Brodsky JW, Tullos HS, Gartsman GM: Simplified posterior approach to the shoulder joint. *J Bone Joint Surg* 69A:773–774, 1987.

Goss TP: Fractures of the glenoid cavity. Current concepts review. *J Bone Joint Surg* 74A:299–305, 1992.

Hardegger FA, Simpson LA, Weber BG: The operative treatment of scapular fractures. *J Bone Joint Surg* 66B:725–731, 1984.

Harris RD, Harris JH Jr: The prevalence and significance of missed scapular fractures in blunt chest trauma. *Am J Rheum* 151:747–750, 1988.

Herscovici D Jr, Fiennes AG, Allgower M, Ruedi TP: The floating shoulder: Ipsilateral, clavicle and scapular neck fractures. *J Bone Joint Surg* 74B:362–364, 1992.

Kavanagh BR, Bradway JK, Cofield RH: Open reduction and internal fixation of displaced intra-articular fractures of the glenoid fossa. *J Bone Joint Surg* 75A:479–484, 1993.

Leung KS, Lam TP: Open reduction and internal fixation of ipsilateral fractures of the scapular neck and clavicle. *J Bone Joint Surg* 75A:1015–1018, 1993.

Sternoclavicular Joint Injuries

Buckerfield CT, Castle ME: Acute traumatic retrosternal dislocation of the clavicle. *J Bone Joint Surg* 66A:379–385, 1984.

Eskola A: Sternoclavicular dislocation: A plea for open treatment. *Acta Orthop Scand* 57:227–228, 1986.

Rockwood CA, Groh GI, Wirth MA, Grassi FA: Resection arthroplasty of the sternoclavicular joint. *J Bone Joint Surg* 79A:387–393, 1997.

Acromioclavicular Joint Injuries

Bannister GC, Wallace WA, Stableforth PG, Hutson MA: The management of acute acromioclavicular dislocation. A randomised prospective controlled trial. *J Bone Joint Surg* 71B:848–850, 1989.

Tibone J, Sellers R, Tonino P: Strength testing after third degree acromioclavicular dislocations. *Am J Sports Med* 20:328–331, 1992.

Weaver JK, Dunn HK: Treatment of acromioclavicular injuries, especially complete acromioclavicular separation. *J Bone Joint Surg* 54A:1187–1194, 1972.

9 | Fractures of the Humeral Shaft

John A. Elstrom

The humeral shaft is the diaphyseal portion of the bone. This excludes the metaphysis proximal to the pectoralis major insertion and distal to the brachialis origin.

ANATOMY

Important anatomic considerations include the deforming forces following fracture and the relation between the humeral shaft and surrounding neurovascular structures.

The two forces that displace and angulate the fragments following fracture are gravity and unopposed muscle pull. Thin patients' arms hang vertically at their sides, and gravity exerts axial traction. Obese patients' fractures develop varus (apex lateral) angulation.

Contraction of the muscles inserting on and originating from the humerus results in deforming forces at different levels of fracture. When fractures occur between the pectoralis major and the deltoid insertions, the proximal fragment is adducted by the pectoralis. The distal fragment is shortened, pulled laterally, and abducted by the deltoid muscle. When the fracture is distal to the deltoid insertion, the proximal fragment is abducted. Contraction of the triceps overcomes that of the biceps and brachialis and results in apex anterior angulation at the fracture site.

The radial nerve is the neurovascular structure most frequently injured when the humeral shaft is fractured because of its close proximity to the shaft of the humerus. As the radial nerve runs distally around the humerus, it lies in the musculoskeletal groove formed by the origin of the brachialis muscle and the cortex of the humerus. Proximally, the radial nerve is cushioned from the humerus by a layer of the medial head of the triceps. Distally, the nerve lies directly on the posterior and lateral cortex of the humerus, making its injury much more likely with fractures at this level (Fig. 9-1).

The radial nerve begins to cross the posterior aspect of the humerus approximately 20 cm proximal to the medial epicondyle and leaves the posterior aspect of the humerus approximately 14 cm proximal to the lateral epicondyle (just above the distal half of the humeral shaft). At this point, the nerve trifurcates into a branch to the medial head of the triceps, the lower lateral brachial cutaneous nerve, and the continuation of the nerve into the forearm as it pierces the intermuscular septum approximately 10 cm proximal to the lateral epicondyle. The position of the radial nerve makes the usual posterior triceps-splitting approach unsatisfactory for plate application in fractures above the distal third of the humerus.

FIG. 9-1   The radial nerve is frequently trapped between the fragments of an oblique fracture of the distal third of the humerus.

The brachial artery runs along the medial border of the biceps, giving off nutrient arteries and small arteries supplying the periosteum. Application of a plate disrupts the periosteal circulation. Insertion of an intramedullary nail disrupts the endosteal circulation.

Classification

Humeral shaft fractures are classified according to their location and according to the fracture pattern. Thus, the fracture is described as proximal, midshaft, or distal and as transverse, oblique, segmental, or comminuted (Fig. 9-2).

Diagnosis and Initial Management

History and Physical Examination

There is evidence of injury, pain, and deformity. The skin is inspected for puncture wounds or lacerations.

Radiographic Examination

The radiographic examination consists of two radiographs of the humerus at right angles. Care is taken not to rotate the extremity but to rotate the patient to obtain true anteroposterior and lateral views. Radiographs of the shoulder and elbow are obtained.

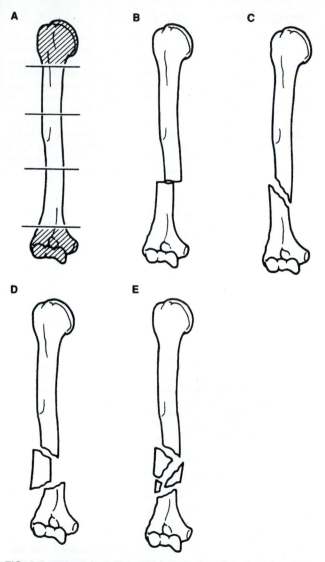

FIG. 9-2 Fractures of the humerus are classified as involving (*A*) the proximal, middle, or distal third and as (*B*) transverse, (*C*) oblique, (*D*) segmental, or (*E*) comminuted.

Initial Management

Initial management consists of splinting the fracture and supporting the arm, which is done as part of the closed management or to temporize until surgery. Hanging the arm at the side reduces oblique and comminuted fractures. A transverse fracture that is displaced and shortened is reduced by gentle axial traction and manipulation. Segmental fractures cannot be adequately reduced by closed methods and are aligned. Once reduction or satisfactory alignment has been achieved, a coaptation splint is applied. The splint starts in the axilla, runs distally along the medial side of the arm around the elbow, and continues up the lateral side of the arm to the acromion. The splint is held to the arm with a loosely applied elastic bandage. The elbow is flexed to 90°, and the forearm is supported from the neck by a collar and cuff.

Associated Injuries

The injury most frequently associated with a humeral shaft fracture is a radial neuropraxia. Radial nerve injury, indicated by loss of sensation on the dorsum of the thumb and inability to extend the wrist and metacarpophalangeal joints, is associated with 10–20% of all humeral shaft fractures. When a radial nerve palsy is identified after a closed fracture, the wrist and dorsum of the thumb are examined at intervals for return of function. If at 3 months there is no sign of return, an electromyograph is obtained. If there are no reinnervation potentials, the nerve is assumed to be disrupted or entrapped in callus and is explored. Laceration or entrapment in callus is found in approximately 25% of radial nerves explored for failure to show signs of recovery after 3 months. If reinnervation potentials are present, the radial nerve is in continuity, and exploration is pointless. Early exploration of the radial nerve should be performed when there is a radial nerve palsy associated with an open fracture, when open reduction and internal fixation is to be performed for indications listed below, in instances when the nerve may be caught in the fracture site such as the oblique fracture of the distal humerus (Holstein–Lewis fracture), and when neuropraxia occurs at the time of manipulative reduction. Radial nerve palsy may also develop in association with swelling of the arm after fracture reduction, but these palsies usually resolve.

Associated injuries of the brachial artery, ulnar nerve, median nerve, and musculocutaneous nerve are ruled out by the focused neurovascular examination of the forearm and hand. Associated fractures of the proximal and distal humerus, scapula, clavicle, ulna, and radius are ruled out by radiographs of the shoulder and elbow.

Definitive Management

The most important aspect of the management of humeral shaft fractures is to identify and understand when operative treatment is necessary. Most fractures of the humeral shaft are managed nonoperatively. Relative indications for open management include open fractures; segmental fractures; multiple trauma; injury of the brachial artery; ipsilateral fractures and dislocations of the elbow, shoulder, and forearm; bilateral humeral shaft fractures; obese or uncooperative patients; pathologic fracture; and failed closed reduction.

Closed Management

The goal of closed management is a united fracture without deformity. Up to 20° of varus angulation and 2 cm of shortening result in minimal functional loss and is acceptable cosmetically. There are four methods of closed management: hanging arm cast, Velpeau dressing, coaptation splint, and functional brace.

The **hanging arm cast** is basically a way to apply traction. Its disadvantage is that it must be closely monitored, and a high degree of patient cooperation is required. Its advantage is that it can be adjusted frequently to improve alignment. Hanging arm cast is contraindicated for obese patients because the arm will not hang vertically at the side and for transverse fractures because of overdistraction. The fracture is not immobilized, and for the first 2 weeks there is discomfort at the fracture site. The cast is applied so that the proximal end is at the fracture site or slightly higher. The elbow is flexed to 90°, with the forearm in neutral rotation. The cast is suspended from the wrist by a cuff around the neck. Posterior angulation is corrected with a longer cuff and anterior angulation with a shorter cuff. Lateral angulation (varus) is corrected by attaching the cuff to the dorsum of the wrist; medial angulation (valgus) is corrected by attaching the cuff to the volar side of the wrist. The patient must sleep in a sitting position to maintain alignment. Radiographs are obtained weekly for 4 to 6 weeks. When there is callus on the radiographs, the cast is removed, and the arm is examined. If there is clinical union (i.e., no motion or pain at the fracture site with gentle stressing), the hanging cast is discontinued, and the arm is protected in a sling. If clinical union is not present, a functional brace is applied for an additional 2 to 6 weeks and active forearm rotation and elbow flexion exercises are initiated.

The **Velpeau dressing** immobilizes the arm by holding it to the chest. This method is helpful for minimally displaced fractures in elderly patients. The Velpeau dressing is a collar and cuff that suspends the wrist from the neck, and plaster or 6-inch Ace wraps hold the humerus to the chest. It is maintained for 4 to 6 weeks, at which time the arm is protected in a sling and active range-of-motion exercises of the elbow are initiated.

The **coaptation splint** is useful for fractures that are angulated because the plaster can be molded to correct varus or valgus deformity. Application of the splint is described in the "Initial Management" section. Three to four weeks postinjury, active forearm rotation and elbow flexion in the splint are initiated. The external support is discontinued when there is clinical union.

The **functional brace** is a prefabricated polypropylene sleeve that extends from the shoulder to just above the elbow. The fracture is managed initially with a coaptation splint. The functional brace is applied 1 to 2 weeks postinjury. Physical therapy is started at 2 weeks and advanced as tolerated. The brace is discontinued when there is clinical union, usually at 4 to 8 weeks.

Open Management

There are three methods of stabilizing the fracture once it is opened and reduced: external fixation, compression plate fixation, and intramedullary fixation.

External fixation can be used for severely contaminated open fractures with extensive soft tissue damage. The pins in the middle and distal thirds of the humerus are placed under direct vision to avoid radial nerve injury. Early bone grafting and conversion to another type of fixation can be done when wound healing is progressing satisfactorily to minimize the incidence of nonunion and pin tract infection.

Compression plate fixation of the humeral shaft allows rapid return of shoulder and elbow motion, and union rates approach 97%. An anterolateral approach along the lateral border of the biceps that splits the brachialis muscle is used to expose the fracture. Alternatively, a modified posterior approach that retracts the entire triceps medially, as described by Gerwin et al. (1996), can be used to obtain more adequate exposure of the humeral shaft than is obtained with the direct posterior triceps-splitting approach. A broad 4.5-mm dynamic compression plate (DCP) or the new narrow 4.5-mm limited-contact DCP can be used with a minimum of six cortices above and below the fracture. Bone defects are grafted with autogenous cancellous bone.

Intramedullary fixation of humeral shaft fractures has several advantages including a decreased risk of infection and nerve injury, a higher rate of union, and a lower incidence of implant failure. The primary disadvantage of intramedullary nailing of humeral shaft fractures is insertion site symptoms. The two types of intramedullary nails are flexible (i.e., Ender's nails and Rush rods) and rigid (e.g., the interlocking nail).

Flexible intramedullary nails are inserted antegrade or retrograde. Antegrade insertion is performed through a deltoid-splitting approach. The insertion portal is just distal to the greater tuberosity to minimize rotator cuff symptoms. Retrograde insertion is performed through a triceps-splitting approach. The insertion portal is 2 cm proximal to the olecranon fossa in the midline of the distal humerus. Whether the flexible intramedullary nails are inserted antegrade or retrograde, they are yoked together at the insertional portal with a wire passed through the eyelets to prevent back out. The leading ends are flared to provide rotational control.

Rigid intramedullary nails must be locked proximally and distally to prevent shortening and rotation through the fracture (Fig. 9-3). Nail insertion is antegrade via a deltoid-splitting approach. The insertion portal is through the supraspinatus tendon about 1.5 cm medial to the greater tuberosity, in line with the medullary canal. When necessary, the medullary canal is enlarged by reaming. Proximal locking is mandatory to prevent proximal nail migration with impingement against the acromion or damage to the rotator cuff. Distal locking is done by an open technique to ensure that the drill guide maintains contact with bone to avoid neurovascular injury. Locked intramedullary nailing is especially beneficial for pathologic fractures of the humerus associated with metastatic disease. Nonoperative treatment of these particular

A

FIG. 9-3 *A, B:* A transverse midshaft fracture managed with locked intramedullary nailing. Important features to note: the proximal end is countersunk to prevent impingement, the fracture is impacted, and the nail is locked proximally and distally. Courtesy of Dr. Robert F. Hall, Jr.

B

FIG. 9-3   *Continued.*

humeral fractures is remarkably unsuccessful in achieving fracture healing and restoration of function.

Complications

The most significant complication of humeral shaft fracture is nonunion. The diagnosis of nonunion is made at 6 months if there has been no progression of clinical or radiographic healing in the prior 3 months. Methods of management are electrical stimulation, reamed intramedullary nailing, plating and bone grafting, and dynamic external fixation. Electrical stimulation is less successful for humeral nonunions than for nonunions of other bones; however, it can be successful and has no surgical risk. Reamed nailing of humeral nonunions is less successful in the management of humeral nonunions than in tibial or femoral nonunions. Plating *with* autogenous bone grafting has the best chance of success but also exposes the patient to the risk of infection and implant failure. Dynamic external fixation done *with* bone grafting uses a fixator to compress or distract the nonunion site.

SELECTED READINGS

Bell MJ, Beauchamp CG, Kellam JK, McMurty RY: The results of plating humeral shaft fractures in patients with multiple injuries. *J Bone Joint Surg* 67B:293–296, 1985.

Gerwin M, Hotchkiss RN, Weiland AJ: Alternative operative exposures of the posterior aspect of the humeral diaphysis. *J Bone Joint Surg* 78A:1690–1695, 1996.

Hall RF, Pankovich AM: Enders nailing of acute fractures of the humerus. *J Bone Joint Surg* 69A:558–567, 1987.

Packer JW, Foster RR, Garcia A, Grantham SA: The humeral fracture with radial nerve palsy: is exploration warranted? *Clin Orthop* 92:34–88, 1972.

Pollock FH, Drake D, Bovill EG, Day L, Trafton PG: Treatment of radial neuropathy associated with fractures of the humerus. *J Bone Joint Surg* 60A:239–243, 1981.

Redmond BJ, Biermann JS, Blasier RB: Interlocking intramedullary nailing of pathologic fractures of the shaft of the humerus. *J Bone Joint Surg* 78A:891–896, 1996.

Sarmiento A, Kinman PB, Galvin E, Schmitt RH, Phillips JG: Functional bracing of fractures of the shaft of the humerus. *J Bone Joint Surg* 59A:596–601, 1977.

10 | Fractures and Dislocations of the Elbow

Edward R. Abraham   Mark Gonzalez
Clayton R. Perry

This chapter reviews fractures and dislocations of the elbow or cubital articulation. These injuries include fractures of the distal humerus (i.e., isolated medial and lateral condylar fractures, transcondylar fractures, supracondylar fractures, and intercondylar fractures), fractures of the radial head and neck, fractures of the olecranon, fractures of the ulna and radius associated with a dislocation, and dislocations of the humeroulnar articulation.

ANATOMY

The elbow is the articulation of the humerus of the arm to the radius and ulna of the forearm. The **distal humerus** consists of the extraarticular medial and lateral epicondyles, which are diverging columns separated by the intraarticular trochlea and capitellum (Fig. 10-1). The distal humerus is angled anteriorly at approximately 30°. The humerus widens and flattens as it bends forward. The trochlea articulates with the trochlear notch of the proximal ulna. The trochlea articular surfaces extend from the coronoid fossa anteriorly to the olecranon fossa posteriorly. The anterior and posterior fossae provide space for the coronoid and the olecranon, respectively, at the extremes of motion. The capitellum is a spherical structure that articulates with the concave radial head.

The proximal radius consists of a head and neck that form a 15° angle with the radial diaphysis. The radial head is dish shaped. The outer circumference articulates with the radial notch of the ulna.

The radial notch of the olecranon forms an arc of 40–70°. The trochlear notch forms an arc of 180°.

The prominent medial epicondyle is the origin for the flexor-pronator muscles and the ulnar collateral ligaments. The epicondyle protects the ulnar nerve that runs in its sulcus. Attached to the smaller lateral epicondyle are the supinator–extensor muscle group and lateral collateral ligament.

The distal articular surface of the humerus is oriented in 7° of valgus in relation to the long axis. The valgus orientation of the distal humerus combines with the ulnar angulation of the olecranon to produce a carrying angle of up to 20° with the elbow in full extension. When viewed from the side, the capitellum and trochlea are translated anterior to the long axis of the humerus, and a line drawn along the anterior cortex of the humerus shaft transects the center of the capitellum.

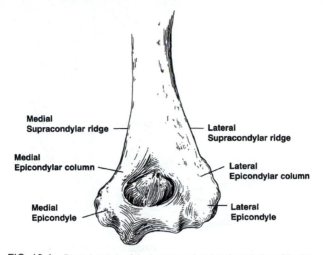

FIG. 10-1   Posterior view of the humerus showing the relation of the lateral and medial columns to the olecranon fossa.

The medial collateral ligament of the elbow originates on the medial epicondyle and consists of two portions. The anterior portion inserts on the medial aspect of the coronoid process. The posterior portion attaches to the medial aspect of the olecranon. The radial collateral ligament originates on the lateral epicondyle and has insertions on the annular ligament and on the olecranon. The annular ligament surrounds the radial neck and stabilizes the radial ulnar articulation. Anteriorly, the annular ligament is attached to the anterior margin of the radial notch. Posteriorly, it is broader and attached to a ridge posterior to the radial notch (Fig. 10-2).

The capsule of the elbow joint attaches to the humerus anteriorly above the coronoid and radial fossae and posteriorly above the olecranon fossa. Distally, it attaches to the coronoid process of the ulna and the annular ligament and is continuous with the radial and ulnar collateral ligaments.

The principal muscles responsible for active elbow motion are divided into four groups. The extensors are the triceps brachii and anconeus. The triceps muscle inserts into the posterior surface of the olecranon process and along the proximal ulna, where it is referred to as the *extensor expansion*. The flexors comprise the brachialis, biceps, and brachioradialis. Anteriorly, the brachialis muscle attaches to the coronoid process. The biceps tendon attaches to the radial tuberosity. Forearm supination is the function of the biceps and supinator, and forearm pronation is produced by the pronator teres and pronator quadratus.

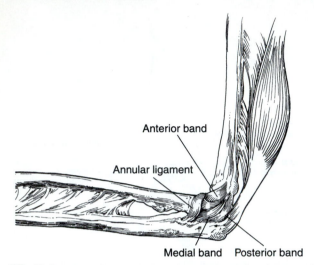

FIG. 10-2 Lateral view of the elbow showing the relation of the lateral collateral ligament to the annular ligament and the attachment of the anterior band on the annular ligament and the posterior band on the olecranon.

BIOMECHANICS

The humeral ulnar and humeral radial articulations function as a hinge. The joint permits flexion to 160° and extension to 0°. Valgus stability is provided primarily by the anterior fibers of the medial collateral ligament and secondarily by the radiocapitellar articulation. Varus stability is provided by the band of the lateral collateral ligament that inserts on the ulna. Motion from 30° to 130° is the range most important for activities of daily living.

The radiocapitellar articulation is a pivot or trochoid joint and allows for both flexion and extension of the ulnohumeral joint and forearm rotation of approximately 165°. It permits 80° of forearm pronation and 85° of supination. The anterolateral quadrant of the radial head does not articulate with the radial notch, even in the extremes of pronation and supination, and is a portal for screw or Kirschner wire fixation. An important relation between the radius and capitellum is the constant axis of rotation. A line is drawn along the long axis of the radius and transects the center of the capitellum regardless of the degree of elbow flexion (Fig. 10-3). The longitudinal relation of the radius and the ulna is maintained by the forearm interosseous membrane, the triangular fibrocartilage complex distally, and the radiocapitellar articulation proximally.

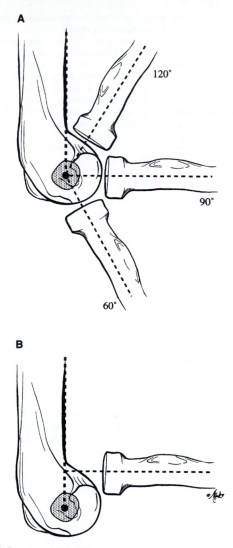

FIG. 10-3   (*A*) Normal relation of the radial shaft and radial head to the center of the capitellum. (*B*) Anterior radial head dislocation.

Excision of a fractured radial head when the interosseous ligament is torn will lead to proximal migration of the radius.

The radial head serves as a restraint to valgus stresses across the elbow joint by acting as a fulcrum for the medial collateral ligament. It also transfers stresses from the hand and wrist to the distal humerus. Forces applied in a proximal direction axially along the shaft of the radius result in tightening of the central tendinous portion of the interosseous membrane. These forces are then transmitted from the radius through the interosseous membrane to the ulna and eventually to the trochlea. When the radial head has been removed, proximally directed stresses result in ulnar shift of the radius as opposed to tightening of the interosseous membrane, thereby altering stress transmission to the ulna and the mechanics of the distal radioulnar joint.

DISTAL HUMERUS FRACTURES

The complex anatomy of the distal humerus makes fracture management very challenging. The goals of surgery are to restore the anatomy of the joint surface and provide stable fixation that will allow early joint mobilization.

Classification

Fractures of the distal humerus are divided into supracondylar fractures, transcondylar fractures, intercondylar fractures, condylar fractures, trochlear fractures, capitellar fractures, and fractures of the epicondyles.

SUPRACONDYLAR FRACTURES OF THE HUMERUS

Supracondylar fractures are characterized by dissociation between the diaphysis and the condyles of the distal humerus. The fracture may extend distally and involve the articular surface.

Classification

The classification is based on the presence of supracondylar comminution, intercondylar extension, and intercondylar comminution. There are four types of supracondylar fractures: fractures without intercondylar extension (type I), fractures with intercondylar extension but no comminution (type II), fractures with intercondylar extension and supracondylar comminution (type III), and fractures with intercondylar comminution (type IV; Fig. 10-4). Type IV fractures frequently have supracondylar comminution.

Diagnosis and Initial Management

History and Physical Examination

There is pain and instability of the elbow. The fracture may have been caused by a fall on the outstretched hand or by a direct blow. On physi-

FIG. 10-4   The classification system of supracondylar fractures of the distal humerus: (A) type I fracture, (B) type II fracture, (C) type III fracture, and (D) type IV fracture.

FIG. 10-4   *Continued.*

cal examination there is deformity, instability, and crepitation. The normal relation of the epicondyles to the tip of the olecranon is not present in fractures with intercondylar involvement (types II, III, and IV).

Radiographic Examination

Anteroposterior, lateral, and oblique radiographs determine the extent of injury. Computed tomography (CT) and special views are usually not necessary.

Initial Management

Initial management consists of alignment, immobilization in a long arm splint, and application of ice. The reduction may be unstable; therefore, repeated alignment attempts are not indicated. The fracture is aligned by hanging the arm at the side with the elbow flexed at 90°. The fracture is splinted with a single posterior slab of plaster extending from the shoulder to the wrist. The upper part of the splint is reinforced with a sugar tongs splint, but a circumferential cast is not used because there may be significant swelling.

Associated Injuries

Associated injuries of the brachial artery and of the median, ulnar, and radial nerves can be associated with these fractures. The patient must be examined specifically for these injuries. In addition, compartment syndrome of the forearm may develop and is considered a surgical emergency. The physical signs of compartment syndrome include pain at rest, pain with passive stretch of the muscles in the compartment, palpably tense compartments, and paresthesias. Radiographs of the shoulder, humeral diaphysis, forearm, and wrist are obtained, although there are no specific associated bony injuries.

Definitive Management

The goal of management is a healed fracture with a functional range of motion in the elbow. Usually, the best way to achieve this goal is anatomic reduction of the fracture, stabilization of the fragments with plates and screws, and early motion of the elbow. Extensive comminution, loss of the humeral condyles, massive soft tissue injury, or an injury of the brachial artery that requires rapid stabilization may preclude plate fixation. In these cases, the fracture is managed with an external fixator.

External fixator half-pins are inserted laterally in the humerus and, if the elbow is spanned, dorsally in the ulna. Pin insertion in the humerus occurs through incisions that are adequate to visualize the humerus and avoid the radial nerve. To prevent the ulnar pins from blocking forearm rotation, they are inserted with the forearm in 30° of supination. The postoperative management is tailored to suit each patient. Consideration must be given to repeat debridements, delayed closure, bone grafting, free tissue transfer, delayed internal fixation, and arthrodesis.

Open reduction, stabilization, and early motion result in the greatest return of function. The surgical approach and technique of fixation depend on the type of fracture.

Supracondylar fractures without intercondylar extension (type I) may be exposed through a medial or lateral approach. A pure posterior approach allows stabilization with posterior plates placed along the lateral column and medial column. The plates should be placed orthogonally to maximize stability.

Fractures with involvement of the distal articular surface of the humerus (types II, III, and IV) are exposed through the transolecranon approach. The articular surface of the distal humerus is exposed by osteotomizing the olecranon and reflecting it with the attached triceps tendon proximally. The olecranon is osteotomized transversely to create a fragment approximately 2.5 cm in length. It is subsequently reattached in a tension band construct with two K-wires and a figure 8 wire passed transversely through a drill hole distal to the osteotomy site. After the fracture is adequately exposed, the intercondylar component is reduced and then stabilized with screws and Kirschner wires. In fractures with intercondylar comminution (type IV), it is important not to lag the fragments together because this will decrease the medial–lateral diameter of the articular surface, resulting in joint incongruity. After the intercondylar fracture is reduced and stabilized, the supracondylar component is reduced and stabilized with medial and lateral plates. If there is supracondylar comminution (all type III and most type IV fractures), autogenous cancellous bone graft is used.

Postoperatively, the elbow is immobilized at 90° in a splint extending from the wrist to the shoulder. When incisional pain becomes tolerable, active range of motion is initiated. This is done several times a day. At all other times, the splint is worn. At 4 to 6 weeks, the splint is discontinued and a sling is worn. At 8 to 10 weeks, all immobilization is discontinued, and passive range of motion and strengthening are initiated.

Occasionally in fractures with extreme comminution, where stable internal fixation cannot be anticipated, lateral skeletal traction through the olecranon, with the forearm supported in a vertical position with skin traction, may be required (see Chap. 3).

Complications

Complications of supracondylar fractures of the humerus include loss of fixation, nonunion, and posttraumatic arthritis.

Loss of fixation occurs because of inadequate stabilization, extreme comminution, or overenthusiastic physical therapy. Once fixation has been lost, revision and bone grafting are necessary. Immobilization is not used when fixation has been lost because it results in loss of motion of the elbow.

Nonunion usually involves the supracondylar component of the fracture as the intercondylar component readily heals. If elbow motion is severely restricted, the prognosis is poor. Management is rigid stabilization and bone grafting.

Posttraumatic arthritis is more common in fractures with intercondylar comminution (type IV). Management options range from conservative therapy with nonsteroidal antiinflammatory medication and steroid injections to surgical debridement with radial head resection to improve motion. Arthrodesis or arthroplasty are rarely required.

TRANSCONDYLAR FRACTURES

The primary fracture line of a transcondylar fracture is intracapsular and transverse; the line passes through the epicondyles, olecranon, and coronoid fossae. These low-energy fractures occur in older, more osteopenic patients than do supracondylar fractures.

Classification

Classification is based on the presence and direction of displacement. Most displaced fractures are of the extension type in which the distal fragment is displaced posteriorly in relation to the humeral shaft. Occasionally there is a T-type fracture with a vertical fracture line or dislocation of the humeral condyles from the trochlear notch (a Posada fracture; Fig. 10-5). Based on these parameters, transcondylar fractures are classified into one of four basic patterns.

The transverse fracture line is the only fracture line present in undisplaced type I fractures and simple displaced fractures (type II). T-type fractures (type III) have, in addition to the transverse fracture line, a vertical fracture line separating the capitellum from the trochlea. In fracture–dislocations (type IV), the humeral condyles are dislocated anteriorly from the trochlear notch and the distal metaphysis of the humerus articulates with the trochlear notch. Fracture–dislocations may be a T-type.

Diagnosis and Initial Management

History and Physical Examination

Physical findings other than pain are not remarkable. The epicondyles and the tip of the olecranon can be palpated, and their relation is normal in all but fracture–dislocations (type IV). When this relation is normal, it distinguishes a transcondylar fracture from an elbow dislocation, an isolated fracture of an epicondyle, an olecranon fracture, and a displaced supracondylar-intercondylar fracture.

A

B

C

D

FIG. 10-5 The classification system for transcondylar fractures of the distal humerus: (A) type I fracture, (B) type II fracture, (C) type III fracture, and (D) type IV fracture.

Radiographic Examination

The diagnosis is confirmed by anteroposterior lateral and oblique radiographs.

Initial Management

Initial management is immobilization in a long arm splint and sling.

Associated Injuries

Associated injuries are uncommon. The routine, focused neurovascular examination is performed, and radiographs of the shoulder, humerus, forearm, and wrist are obtained.

Definitive Management

Undisplaced fractures are managed with a long arm cast and a sling. The cast is removed at 3 to 4 weeks, and gentle range-of-motion exercises are initiated. The arm is protected in a splint for 6 to 8 weeks. In simple displaced fractures, closed reduction and casting will not be successful because of fracture instability. Reduction and stabilization are carried out by the transolecranon approach. Stable fixation is difficult to achieve because the distal fragments are small, and a large percentage of the fragment surface is covered with articular cartilage. Ulnar nerve transposition allows the cubital tunnel to be used as an additional point of fixation. Laterally, the posterior distal extraarticular portion of the capitellum is the preferred point of fixation. Simple displaced fractures are stabilized with reconstruction plates which are more easily contoured to the curvature of the medial epicondyle when the cubital tunnel is used as an additional point of fixation. Fixation with a reconstruction plate may also be attempted laterally if the remaining distal fragment on that side is large enough but frequently all that can be accomplished is cancellous screw fixation from the distal capitellum up the lateral column. In T-type fractures, the distal fragments are first lagged together and then fixed to the proximal humerus. Because there is no bone loss, lagging the distal fragments will not result in a congruous joint.

Postoperatively, supervised active motion is started when incisional pain allows. When the patient is not undergoing physical therapy, the fixation is protected in a long arm splint. At 6 to 8 weeks, the splint is discontinued.

Complications

All patients lose elbow motion, particularly extension. Loss of motion is less in undisplaced fractures than it is in T-type and fracture–dislocations.

The complication unique to transcondylar fractures is loss of fixation due to the small size of the distal fragments and their osteopenia. Patients are followed at biweekly intervals with radiographs. If loss of fixation has already occurred, either the fixation can be revised or active range of motion exercises can be continued. Revision of the fixation is difficult, and stabilization of the fracture may not be possible. Active range of motion is encouraged with the expectation that the fracture will go on to nonunion, but a functional range of motion can be obtained through the nonunion site. Total elbow arthroplasty has been described as primary treatment for distal humeral fractures in elderly patients, in particular those with rheumatoid arthritis with poor bone stock.

FRACTURES OF MEDIAL AND LATERAL CONDYLES OF THE HUMERUS

Isolated fractures of the medial or lateral condyle of the humerus are rare. The fragment includes the entire condyle (the epicondyle and either the capitellum or trochlea) or just the articular portion of the condyle (capitellum or trochlea).

Classification

Isolated fractures of the medial or lateral condyle of the humerus are first classified according to whether they involve the entire condyle or just the articular portion of the condyle. The distinction between these two types of fractures is important because fractures involving only the trochlea or capitellum are avascular, with no soft tissue attachments. Fractures of the entire condyle occur in a younger age group than do fractures of the capitellum and trochlea.

Milch divided **fractures of the entire condyle** into two groups: avulsion fractures and compression fractures (Fig. 10-6).

Avulsion fractures are the result of a varus (lateral condyle fracture) or valgus (medial condyle fracture) stress across the elbow. Radiographically, they are recognized by distal displacement of the fracture fragment. **Compression fractures** are produced by impaction of the trochlea or radial head into the distal humerus. This impaction can be the result of a longitudinal force or a varus (fracture of the medial condyle) or valgus (fracture of the lateral condyle) force across the elbow. Radiographically, compression fractures are recognized by proximal displacement of the fragment.

Compression fractures are further divided into stable fractures and fracture–dislocations. The key to stability is the status of the trochlea. In the case of the lateral condylar fractures, if the lateral wall of the trochlea is disrupted, the fracture is unstable; if it is intact, the fracture is stable. In the case of medial condylar fractures, if the medial wall of the trochlea is disrupted, the fracture is unstable; if it is intact, the fracture is stable. The olecranon subluxes laterally or medially if the fracture is unstable.

Fractures involving only the articular portion of the condyle are the result of the radial head or coronoid process impacting the **capitellum** or **trochlea**.

FIG. 10-6 The classification of isolated fractures of the humeral condyles: (A) avulsion fracture of the medial condyle, (B) avulsion fracture of the lateral condyle, (C) unstable compression fracture of the medial condyle, and (D) stable compression fracture of the lateral condyle.

FIG. 10-6   *Continued.*

Fractures of the capitellum are divided into three groups (Fig. 10-7): the **Hahn–Steinthal fracture**, in which the fragment includes the entire capitellum (Fig. 10-8); the **Kocher–Lorenz fracture**, in which the fragment includes only subchondral bone and the articular surface; and the **compression** fracture of the capitellum, with comminution of the articular surface. Isolated fractures of the trochlea are rare and are usually associated with a fracture of the capitellum. These are coronal shear fractures of the distal end of the humerus and are characterized by a double-arc sign, with one arc representing the subchondral bone of the capitellum and the other the lateral ridge of the trochlea.

Diagnosis and Initial Management

History and Physical Examination

The physical findings other than pain and limitation of motion are not remarkable, unless there is an associated dislocation. Occasionally, when the capitellum is fractured, the fragment can be palpated laterally.

Radiographic Examination

Anteroposterior and lateral radiographs confirm the diagnosis.

Initial Management

The elbow is splinted at 90° and iced.

Associated Injuries

Other than sprain of the contralateral collateral ligament, there are no specific injuries associated with fractures of the humeral condyles. The

FIG. 10-7 The classification of isolated fractures of the capitellum: (A) Hahn–Steinthal fracture, (B) Kocher–Lorenz fracture, and (C) compression fracture of the capitellum.

FIG. 10-8 Lateral radiograph of the elbow. This is a Hahn–Steinthal fracture of the capitellum.

focused neurovascular examination is performed, and radiographs of the shoulder, humerus, forearm, and wrist should be obtained.

Definitive Management

Definitive management of displaced fractures of the humeral condyles is operative. The two options are reduction and stabilization and excision of the fragments. Excision is an option only for fractures of the capitellum.

Open Reduction and Internal Fixation

Fractures of the entire lateral condyle are approached through the interval between the extensor carpiulnaris and the anconeus (the Kocher J approach) or through the anconeus approach, as described by Pankovich. Flexion of the elbow and extension of the wrist relax the extensor muscles inserting on the fragment, thus aiding reduction. Usually there is a large spike of epicondyle that can be fixed to the distal humeral metaphysis with screws or a plate. Screw placement must avoid the olecranon fossa.

Fractures of the capitellum are exposed through the anconeus approach. The Hahn–Steinthal fracture is stabilized with Herbert screws, small countersunk bone screws, or with threaded Kirschner wires directed anterior to posterior and buried below the articular surface. In Kocher–Lorenz and compression fractures, the fragment may be excised.

Fractures of the medial condyle are approached through a straight medial incision while taking care to protect the ulnar nerve. Like fractures of the lateral condyle, these usually are easily reduced and stabilized. Flexion of the elbow and wrist relaxes the flexor muscle mass attached to the fragment.

Coronal shear fractures of the distal end of the humerus are approached through an extended lateral Kocher approach. The operative exposure must be extensive enough so that elevation of the anterior elbow capsule, thereby permitting retractors to be placed over the medial column of the distal end of the humerus, exposes the entire anterior articular surface. After provisional fixation with Kirschner wires, definitive fixation with Herbert screws or cancellous-bone screws is performed.

Postoperatively, the arm is protected in a splint and sling. When incisional pain has decreased, supervised range of motion is begun. At 6 weeks, the fracture is healed enough to discontinue the sling.

Complications

The complications of isolated condylar fractures include arthritis, loss of motion, heterotopic ossification, nonunion, avascular necrosis, and malunion.

Posttraumatic joint stiffness is associated with soft tissue and articular cartilage damage from the original injury. Refractory contractures not responsive to physical therapy and dynamic splinting may require surgical release. An anterior contracture is associated with loss of extension and can be treated by anterior capsulotomy. Loss of flexion is similarly treated by posterior release. Intraarticular contractures require an articular release and a dynamic hinged fixator with distraction. Severe articular involvement may require fascial interposition arthroplasty in conjunction with a dynamic hinged fixator. Arthrotomy and resection of the radial head and release of intraarticular adhesions is another treatment option.

Heterotopic ossification may occur after elbow injury and is associated with loss of joint motion. Excision of heterotopic bone is delayed until a process has matured and is followed by physical therapy, oral Indomethacin, and radiation therapy to prevent recurrence.

RADIAL HEAD FRACTURES

Radial head fractures involve the proximal intraarticular portion of the radius.

Classification

Fractures of the radial head are classified according to displacement, extent of involvement, and associated dislocations (Fig. 10-9). Type I fractures are undisplaced. Type II fractures are displaced fractures involving only part of the head. Type III fractures involve the entire head and are frequently comminuted. Type IV fractures are radial head frac-

FIG. 10-9 The classification of radial head fractures: (*A*) type I, (*B*) type II, (*C*) type III, and (*D*) type IV. In this drawing, a Monteggia fracture–dislocation is illustrated.

tures associated with elbow instability or radioulnar dissociation (i.e., the Essex–Lopresti lesion or Monteggia equivalent).

Diagnosis and Initial Management

History and Physical Examination

There is pain localized to the radial head. The mechanism of injury is usually a fall forward with the elbow extended and the forearm pronated. The necessity for operative or closed management is determined clinically. The two important indications for operative intervention are a block to forearm rotation and ligamentous instability. The hematoma is aspirated, and the elbow is injected with local anesthetic. The forearm is passively rotated with the elbow in different degrees of flexion. Ligamentous instability is due to disruption of the medial collateral ligament. Stability is assessed with the forearm supinated and the elbow flexed at 15°, thus relaxing the anterior capsule and removing the olecranon from the olecranon fossae. A gentle valgus stress is applied to the elbow. If the elbow "books" open, the medial collateral ligament is torn.

Radiographic Examination

Anteroposterior and lateral views confirm the diagnosis. The radiocapitellar view may provide additional information. The forearm is placed in neutral rotation, and the elbow is flexed and positioned on the cassette as for a routine lateral. The x-ray tube is angulated 45° toward the humeral head.

Initial Management

The elbow is splinted at 90° and placed in a sling. In cases in which the radial head is dislocated, open reduction is performed emergently.

Associated Injuries

Associated neurovascular injuries are uncommon but must be ruled out. Radiographs of the humerus, shoulder, and wrist are obtained. The distal radioulnar joint is examined for tenderness, instability, and prominence of the distal ulna. If these are present, there may be an associated Essex–Lopresti lesion. The distal humerus is examined for associated fractures of the capitellum and avulsion fractures of the medial epicondyle (indicative of a medial-collateral ligament avulsion).

Definitive Management

Management is based on the type of fracture. Type I fractures (undisplaced) and type II and III fractures without a mechanical block are managed nonoperatively. The patient is placed in a sling for 3 weeks, and gentle active range of motion is encouraged. At 3 weeks, the sling is discontinued, and more aggressive physical therapy is initiated.

Fractures associated with elbow instability or with a mechanical block to elbow motion are managed operatively. The decision to reduce and internally fix the fracture or to excise the radial head, with or without prosthetic replacement, is made once the fracture is exposed. Circumstances that mitigate against fixation of the radial head are an elderly patient, injury of the capitellum, and preexisting osteoarthritis. Circumstances that mitigate for fixation include a young patient, involvement of only part of the radial head (i.e., type II), and associated dislocation of the radial head (i.e., type IV). In cases with associated ligamentous injuries, there are two alternatives: reduction and fixation of the radial head or excision and replacement of the head with a metallic prosthetic spacer, and ligament repair.

Exposure is done by the anconeus approach. The interval between the anconeus and flexor carpi ulnaris is developed. The insertion of the anconeus is reflected from the ulna and joint capsule by blunt dissection. If the capsule and synovium are not torn, they are incised longitudinally. One should not hesitate to incise the annular ligament to obtain wider exposure. In addition, the proximal or distal portion of the capsular incision can be made in the shape of a T. As the forearm is pronated and supinated, the entire radial head is visualized. Associated fractures of the ulna are reduced and stabilized through the same approach.

Fragments are reduced and fixed with cortical screws, Herbert screws, or Kirschner wires. Ideally, the implants are buried below the articular cartilage. It is important to remember that the anterolateral quadrant of the radial head does not articulate with the ulna and is, therefore, the optimum portal for fixation (Fig. 10-10). If depression of the articular surface is present, reduction and bone grafting are performed. If the radial head is resected, the neck is preserved. The edges of the metaphysis are smoothed, and any bony spikes are removed. If a metallic prosthesis is inserted, the size should match that of the radial head excised. A metal prosthesis, made with vitallium or titanium, is preferred over the once popular silastic implant (Fig. 10-11). Silicone synovitis and poor force-bearing properties have decreased the usefulness of the silicone prosthesis.

Prior to fixation or radial head replacement, the elbow and forearm are put through a range of motion. If the elbow subluxates, the anterior capsular or coronoid process fracture should be repaired to the bed of the coronoid process prior to fixation or replacement of the radial head, if possible through the lateral incision or through a medial incision to repair the medial collateral ligament or anterior capsule if repair through the lateral incision is not possible. In addition to elbow stability, the stability of the distal radioulnar joint is assessed. If radioulnar dissociation is present, the distal ulna will sublux dorsally with pronation of the forearm.

FIG. 10-10   Fracture of the radial head treated by open reduction and internal fixation (*A*) and with a mini plate and screws (*B*).

FIG. 10-11   Fracture of the radial head treated with metallic prosthetic replacement.

Postoperatively, the arm is placed in a sling. A splint is added if there is associated ligamentous injury. The sling or splint is removed three times a day for supervised active range-of-motion exercises. At 3 to 4 weeks, the sling and splint are discontinued. Patients with associated radioulnar dissociation present a unique set of problems. In these injuries, the interosseous membrane and distal radial ulnar joint capsule are disrupted, and the pronation and supination exercises may result in displacement. Therefore, after open reduction and internal fixation of the radial head, the distal radioulnar joint is pinned with the forearm in neutral rotation. Four weeks postinjury, the pin is removed. The splint is continued but is removed three times a day for active range of motion. At 6 weeks, the splint is discontinued. In cases in which a prosthesis has been used, consideration can be given to removal of the prosthesis 1 year postinjury in young patients. After this time, the radius should not migrate proximally.

Complications

The complications following radial head fracture include loss of motion, posttraumatic arthritis, and shortening of the radius with resultant wrist pain.

Loss of motion is the most common complication seen with either nonoperative or operative management. Surgical removal of displaced or angulated small fragments or radial head excision for an incongruous radial capitellar joint can be attempted to improve joint motion.

Posttraumatic arthritis is managed with nonsteroidal antiinflammatory medication and local steroid injection; occasionally, excision of the radial head is required.

Radial shortening can follow excision of the radial head. The patient complains of pain at the distal radioulnar joint, made worse by grip and attempting to rotate the forearm. In many cases, there is obvious proximal migration of the radius in relation to the ulna. Magnetic resonance imaging (MRI) may be required to demonstrate disruption of the ligamentous portion of the interosseous membrane. In symptomatic patients, when conservative treatment has failed, ulnar shortening has been shown to be ineffective, as have most other methods of surgical reconstruction, in leveling the distal radioulnar joint. In instances in which damage to the interosseous membrane is suspected, radial head resection must be avoided. When the fracture is too comminuted to achieve internal fixation, a delayed radial head excision, the use of a radial head prosthesis or allograft, and repair or reconstruction of the central band of the interosseous membrane need to be considered.

OLECRANON FRACTURES

Olecranon fractures involve the ulna proximal to the coronoid process. The majority of olecranon fractures are intraarticular. There may be an associated fracture of the radial head or displacement of the ulna with a dislocation of the radiocapitellar articulation. The absence of a diastasis distinguishes olecranon fractures from other injuries (e.g., Monteggia fracture) that also involve the proximal ulna.

Classification

Olecranon fractures are classified into six types based on the presence of displacement, intraarticular involvement, comminution, radial head fracture, and radiocapitellar dislocation (Fig. 10-12). Type I fractures are displaced less than 2 mm, without an intraarticular stepoff. Type II fractures are extraarticular and involve the proximal portion of the olecranon. These fractures are an avulsion of the triceps from the proximal ulna. Type III fractures are simple intraarticular fractures with a transverse or oblique pattern. Type IV fractures are comminuted. The fracture lines may extend distal to the olecranon, and there may be depression of an intraarticular segment. Type V and VI fractures are an olecranon fracture with either an associated anterior dislocation of the radiocapitellar articulation or an associated radial head fracture. The olecranon fracture in a type V or VI fracture is invariably displaced and intraarticular (i.e., a type III or IV fracture).

Diagnosis and Initial Management

History and Physical Examination

There is pain localized to the elbow and a history of trauma. Type II fractures are caused by indirect trauma, whereas type III and IV frac-

FIG. 10-12 The classification of olecranon fractures: (A) type I, (B) type II, (C) type III, (D) type IV, (E) type V, and (F) type VI.

tures are caused by direct trauma. Type V and VI fractures are high-energy injuries caused by a combination of direct and indirect forces. The physical findings are ecchymosis swelling and, if the fracture is displaced, a palpable gap at the fracture site. A break in the skin is assumed to communicate with the fracture.

FIG. 10-12 *Continued.*

Radiographic Examination

Lateral and anteroposterior views of the elbow are obtained. The lateral view shows the location and direction of the fracture line, the degree of comminution, and whether there is an associated radiocapitellar dislocation. The anteroposterior view shows the presence of an associated radial head fracture.

Initial Management

The arm is placed in a sling for comfort. A splint is not required. If there is an associated anterior subluxation, a closed reduction will not be successful because of instability, and the fracture should be stabilized as soon as possible.

Associated Injuries

Associated neurovascular injuries are rare but must be ruled out. Radiographs of the humerus, shoulder, forearm, and wrist are obtained.

Definitive Management

The goal of management is an elbow with a functional, painless range of flexion and extension. It is important to preserve flexion even at the cost of losing extension; therefore, prolonged splinting of the elbow in extension is seldom indicated. The articular surface should be anatomically reduced to minimize the incidence of posttraumatic arthritis.

Undisplaced fractures (type I) are managed by splinting the elbow at 90° for 3 weeks. The splint is removed once a day for active range of motion. Radiographs are obtained at weekly intervals to confirm that the fragments have not displaced. At 3 weeks, the splint is discontinued, and a sling is used for the next 3 weeks.

Type II, III, IV, V, and VI fractures are managed surgically. Type II–V fractures are approached by way of a straight posterior incision over the subcutaneous border of the olecranon. Type II and transverse type III fractures can be stabilized by using the tension band technique with 2.0-mm Kirschner wires and an 18-gauge wire. A 6.5-mm cancellous screw and washer can be substituted for the Kirschner wires. Oblique type III fractures and all type IV and V fractures are stabilized with a plate and screws. A one-third semitubular plate or 3.5-mm reconstruction plate may be used. Fixation with a plate as opposed to a tension band wire is indicated for two reasons: first, to prevent shortening of axially unstable fractures (i.e., oblique type III fractures and type IV fractures); and second, to provide rigid stabilization of the olecranon and prevent anterior subluxation of the radial head in patients with type V fractures. Type VI fractures have an associated fracture of the radial head. The radial head fracture is reduced and stabilized.

Postoperatively, early active motion is encouraged after incisional pain has become tolerable (usually by the third postoperative day).

Complications

Complications include loss of fixation, nonunion, infection, posttraumatic arthritis, and radioulnar synostosis.

Loss of fixation is managed by either revising the fixation or excising the proximal fragment and attaching the triceps tendon to the remaining olecranon. Before the fragment is excised, it must be confirmed that the elbow is stable without the fragment (i.e., that the radial head and remaining olecranon will not sublux anteriorly once the fragment is removed). If a minimum of 30° of the trochlear notch remains, the elbow will probably be stable, but this must be confirmed intraoperatively by removing all fixation, flexing the elbow to 90°, and gently stressing the elbow.

Nonunion may be asymptomatic due to fibrous tissue between the fragments. Symptomatic nonunions are managed with reduction, plate fixation, and autogenous cancellous bone grafting.

Infection occurs occasionally because of the subcutaneous location of the fracture. It is managed aggressively because of elbow joint proximity. Fixation is removed to gain access to the joint for debridement and irrigation. Necrotic bone is debrided, and the fracture is stabilized. Systemic antibiotics are continued a minimum of 6 weeks.

Posttraumatic arthritis is managed conservatively with nonsteroidal antiinflammatory medication or steroid injection. Surgical alternatives include arthroplasty and, rarely, arthrodesis.

Radioulnar synostosis occurs most frequently after type IV, V, or VI fractures. Management alternatives include doing nothing, resection of an osseous bridge, or osteotomy to place the hand in a more functional position.

ELBOW DISLOCATIONS

This section reviews elbow dislocations, excluding Monteggia fractures and isolated dislocations of the radial head.

Classification

Elbow dislocations are classified according to the position of the radius and ulna in relation to the distal humerus. The types of elbow dislocations are posterior, medial, lateral, anterior, and divergent.

Posterior dislocations are by the far the most common type of elbow dislocation. In addition to being posteriorly displaced, the radius and ulna may be displaced slightly laterally or medially. The presence of medial or lateral displacement does not affect the management or the prognosis.

The presence of a fracture of the radial head or coronoid process will frequently render any attempt at reduction unstable and will usually require that open management of these fractures be undertaken.

Medial and lateral dislocations are rare injuries. These have a poorer prognosis than the more common posterior dislocation. Frequently, a medial or lateral dislocation is, in reality, a subluxation (i.e., in a medial dislocation, the trochlear notch articulates with the medial epicondyle, and the radial head articulates with the trochlea; in a lateral dislocation, the trochlear notch articulates with the capitellum; Fig. 10-13).

Anterior dislocations of the elbow are extremely rare injuries. The mechanism of injury is either traction on the forearm with the elbow extended or a blow to the posterior aspect of the flexed elbow.

Divergent dislocations are also rare injuries. They are distinct from other types of elbow dislocations because there is dissociation of the radius and ulna. The annular ligament and interosseous membrane must be torn for a divergent dislocation to occur. There are two varieties, anteroposterior and medial–lateral. In anteroposterior divergent dislocations, the radial head is dislocated anteriorly into the coronoid fossa, and

FIG. 10-13   Lateral dislocation of the elbow. On the lateral projection (not shown), the olecranon articulates with the capitellum.

the ulna is dislocated posteriorly, with the coronoid process in the olecranon fossa. In medial–lateral divergent dislocations, the radial head articulates with the trochlea, and the trochlear notch articulates with the capitellum.

Diagnosis and Initial Management

History and Physical Examination

The patient presents with pain and swelling of the elbow. All elbow dislocations are characterized by loss of the normal relation of the epicondyles to the tip of the olecranon. This physical finding may be obscured by swelling. However, if present, it distinguishes elbow dislocation from other injuries such as extraarticular supracondylar and transcondylar fracture of the humerus. Posterior dislocations are further characterized by apparent shortening of the forearm and the elbow's being fixed in 45° of flexion. In medial and lateral dislocations, the elbow appears wider than normal, and there may be some active and passive motion of the elbow. In anterior dislocations, the elbow is fixed in extension, the forearm is usually supinated, and the capitellum and trochlea are palpable posteriorly. In divergent dislocations, the forearm appears shortened, and the elbow is fixed in different amounts of flexion.

Radiographic Examination

The diagnosis of elbow dislocation is confirmed by anteroposterior and lateral radiographs. Oblique views are helpful to define further the relation between the distal humerus and the radius and ulna. Special views and CT scans usually do not define the injury further.

Initial Management

The elbow is splinted or held in a sling until radiographs are obtained and a closed reduction can be performed.

Associated Injuries

Associated injuries of the surrounding neurovascular structures occur. The most clinically significant injury involves the brachial artery. Associated injuries of the median, ulnar, and radial nerves occur with relative frequency. Therefore, a careful neurologic examination is performed. Associated bony injuries are also common. The most clinically significant are fractures of the coronoid process and the radial head or neck. The combination of a coronoid process fracture and radial head fracture will require open reduction and reattachment of the coronoid process fracture and open reduction and internal fixation or replacement of the radial head fracture to achieve stability. An undisplaced fracture of the radial head or neck may displace during closed reduction. In addition to radial head and neck fractures, there are frequently fractures of the medial or lateral epicondyles. These fractures become clinically significant when they prevent a concentric reduction; if they remain displaced, nonunion is likely. The distal humerus is examined for evidence of osteochondral fractures that increase the likelihood of posttraumatic arthritis and prevent concentric reduction.

Definitive Management

In most cases, management is closed reduction under local anesthesia followed by splinting. Regional or general anesthesia with fluoroscopic monitoring is indicated if there is an associated undisplaced radial head or neck fracture. Open reduction is indicated if there are any of the following: interposed osteochondral fragment preventing concentric reduction, irreducible dislocation, operative displacement of a fracture of the radial head or neck, or ligamentous instability.

Closed reduction is performed as atraumatically as possible. This requires adequate analgesia and muscle relaxation. The specific reduction maneuver depends on the type of dislocation.

Posterior dislocation is reduced by traction in line with the deformity after correcting any medial or lateral displacement of the forearm to align the olecranon with the distal humerus. This method allows the coronoid process to slip distally past the humerus, and the elbow is flexed to 90°. There should be immediate relief of pain and increased motion. If this maneuver fails, the patient is placed prone on a stretcher, with the arm and forearm hanging over the edge. Five to ten pounds of weight are suspended from the wrist. After 5 min, the arm is lifted while flexing and reducing the elbow. Failure to adequately reduce the fracture in the emergency room requires repeating the process in the operating room under general or regional anesthesia with complete anesthesia and muscle relaxation. Incarcerated loose fragments, soft tissue, or an incarcerated medial epicondyle may block reduction, necessitating an arthrotomy. Dislocations older than 10 days are better treated by open reduction. The Kocher incision will provide access to the radial capitellar joint, and a medial approach will provide access to the medial epicondyle and the ulnar humeral joint. Fracture of the radial head can be associated with an elbow dislocation and medial collateral ligament disruption. A displaced radial head can block pronation and supination. Because the radial capitellar articulation is a secondary stabilizer to valgus stress, it is preferable to repair the radial head to avoid valgus instability. If repair is not possible, medial collateral ligament repair with radial head replacement or allograft should be considered. Large displaced fractures of the coronoid process have been associated with recurrent dislocation and should be repaired.

Medial and lateral dislocations are reduced by traction and medial or lateral pressure.

Anterior dislocations are reduced by applying longitudinal traction to the forearm. Pressure is applied to the anterior aspect of the forearm, while couterpressure is applied to the posterior aspect of the humerus.

Anteroposterior divergent dislocations are reduced by reducing first the ulna and then the radius. The ulna is reduced as if it were a posterior dislocation. The radial head is reduced by direct pressure and supination of the forearm. Medial–lateral dislocations are reduced with traction and by pressing the radius and ulna together.

Complications

Complications of elbow dislocations include posttraumatic arthritis, loss of motion, chronic instability, and heterotopic ossification.

Chronic instability after elbow dislocation can cause chronic subluxation, redislocation, valgus instability, or rotatory instability. Chronic subluxation and redislocation should be managed with repair or reattachment of the anterior capsule and coronoid process, repair or prosthetic replacement of a fractured radial head, and repair or tendon reconstruction of the medial and/or lateral (ulnohumeral) ligaments in conjunction with a hinged brace or hinged external fixator. Valgus instability is managed by repair or reconstruction of the anterior portion of the medial collateral ligament, and posterolateral instability is managed by repair or reconstruction of the lateral (ulnohumeral) ligaments.

Heterotopic ossification usually involves the collateral ligaments, capsule, or brachialis. Initially, it is managed by discontinuing all passive motion exercises and administering indomethacin. After the heterotopic bone has matured, as indicated by a cold bone scan and normal serum alkaline phosphatase levels, it can be excised. Preoperatively, CT or MRI helps to delineate the relation of the heterotopic ossification to surrounding nerves and arteries.

SELECTED READINGS

General

Hotchkiss RN, Green DP: Fractures and dislocations of the elbow, *In* Rockwood CA Jr, Green DP and Bucholz RW (eds). *Fractures in adults. vol. 1*, 4th ed. Philadelphia, JB Lippincott, 1996, pp. 929–1024.

Jupiter JB: Trauma of the adult elbow. *In* Browner B, Levine A, and Trafton P (eds). *Skeletal trauma, vol. II*, 2nd ed. Philadelphia, WB Saunders, 1997.

Morrey BF: Current concepts in the treatment of fractures of the radial head, the olecranon, and the coronoid. *J Bone Joint Surg* 77A:316–317, 1995.

Morrey BF: *The elbow and its disorders*, 2nd ed. Philadelphia, WB Saunders, 1993.

Pankovich AM: Anconeus approach to the elbow joint and the proximal part of the radius and ulna. *J Bone Joint Surg* 59A:124–126, 1977.

Distal Humerus Fractures

Cobb TK, Morrey BF: Total elbow arthroplasty as primary treatment for distal humeral fractures in elderly patients. *J Bone Joint Surg* 79A:826–832, 1997.

Gabel GT, Hanson G, Bennett JB, Noble PC, Tullos HS: Intraarticular fractures of the distal humerus in the adult. *Clin Orthop* 216:99–108, 1987.

Grantham SA, Noms TR, Bush DC: Isolated fracture of the humeral capitellum. *Clin Orthop* 161:262–269, 1981.

Helfet DL, Hotchkiss RN: Internal fixation of the distal humerus:a biomechanical comparison of methods. *J Orthop Trauma* 4:260–264, 1990.

Henley MB, Bone CB, Parker B: Operative management of intraarticular fractures of the distal humerus. *J Orthop Trauma* 1:24–35, 1987.

Holdsworth BJ, Mossad MM: Fractures of the adult distal humerus. Elbow function after internal fixation. *J Bone Joint Surg* 72B:362–365, 1990.

McKee MD, Jupiter JB, Bamberger HB: Coronal shear fractures of the distal end of the humerus. *J Bone Joint Surg* 78A:49–54, 1996.

Milch H: Fractures and fracture–dislocations of the humeral condyles. *J Trauma* 4:592–607, 1964.

Perry CR, Gibson CT, Kowalski MF: Transcondylar fractures of the distal humerus. *J Orthop Trauma* 3:98–106, 1989.

Simpson LA, Richards RR: Internal fixation of a capitellar fracture using Herbert screws. *Clin Orthop* 209:166–168, 1986.

Radial Head Fractures

Broberg MA, Moncy BF: Results of delayed excision of the radial head after fracture. *J Bone Joint Surg* 68A:669–674, 1986.

Coleman DA, Blair WF, Shurr D: Resection of the radial head for fractures of the radial head. Long-term follow-up of seventeen cases. *J Bone Joint Surg [Am]* 69:385–392, 1987.

Esser RD, Davis S, Taavao T: Fractures of the radial head treated by internal fixation: late results in 26 cases. *J Orthop Trauma* 9:318–323, 1995.

Hotchkiss RN: Displaced fractures of the radial head. Internal fixation or excision? *J Am Acad Orthop Surg* 5:1–10, 1997.

Hotchkiss RN: Fractures of the radial head and related instability and contracture of the forearm. Instructional Course Lectures, Rosemont, IL, American Academy of Orthopaedic Surgeons, 47:173–177, 1998.

Mason ML: Some observations of fractures of the head of the radius with review of one hundred cases. *Br J Surg* 42:123–132, 1954.

Olecranon Fracture

Colton CL: Fractures of the olecranon in adults. *Injury* 5:121–129, 1973.

Hume MC, Wiss DA: Olecranon fractures: a clinical and radiographic comparison of tension band wiring and plate fixation. *Clin Orthop* 285:229–235, 1992.

Ring D, Jupiter JB, Sanders RW, Mast J, Simpson NS: Transolecranon fracture dislocation of the elbow. *J Orthop Trauma* 11:545–550, 1997.

Dislocations

Mantle JA: Recurrent posterior dislocation of the elbow. *J Bone Joint Surg* 48B:590, 1966.

Mehloff TL, Noble PC, Bennett JB, Tullos HS: Simple dislocation of the elbow in the adult. *J Bone Joint Surg* 70A:244–249, 1988.

Complications

Birghton CT: Current concepts review: treatment of nonunions with electricity. *J Bone Joint Surg* 53B:425, 1971.

Galbraith KA, McCullough CJ: Acute nerve injury as a complication of closed fractures or dislocation of the elbow. *Injury* 11(2):159, 1979.

Gelberman RH, Garfin SR, Hergenroeder PJ, Mubarek SJ, Menon J: Compartment syndromes of the forearm: diagnosis and treatment. *Clin Orthop* 161:252–261, 1981.

Morrey BF: Complex instability of the elbow. Instructional Course Lectures, Rosemont, IL, American Academy of Orthopaedic Surgeons, 47:157–164, 1998.

O'Driscoll SW, Bell DF, Morrey BF: Posterolateral rotatory instability of the elbow. *J Bone Joint Surg* 73A:440–446, 1991.

Sowa DT, Hotchkiss RN, Weiland AJ: Symptomatic proximal translation of the radius following radial head resection. *Clin Orthop* 317:106–113, 1995.

Thompson HC III, Garcia A: Myositis ossificans: aftermath of elbow injuries. *Clin Orthop* 50:129–134, 1967.

Urbaniak JF, Hansen PE, Beissinger SF, Aitken MS: Correction of posttraumatic flexion contracture of the elbow by anterior capsulotomy. *J Bone Joint Surg* 67A:1160–1164, 1985.

11 | Fractures of the Forearm

John A. Elstrom   Clayton R. Perry

The fractures of the forearm discussed in this chapter include fractures of both the radius and ulna, isolated fractures of the radius and ulna, the Monteggia fracture (fracture of the ulna with dislocation of the radial head), the Galeazzi fracture (fractures of the distal radius with displacement of the distal radioulnar joint), and the Essex–Lopresti injury (radioulnar dissociation with injury at the radial capitellar joint).

ANATOMY

Important anatomic features of the forearm include: the radius, the ulna, the proximal and distal radioulnar articulations, the interosseous membrane, muscles, nerves, and arteries. The proximal and distal radioulnar articulations are described in Chapters 10 and 12.

The **radius** is an extension of the hand. Straightening of its apex lateral bow results in loss of forearm rotation. The shaft of the radius is triangular in cross section with its ulnar corner, serving as the attachment of the interosseous membrane. The blood supply of the diaphyseal cortex of the radius is through periosteal and intramedullary vessels. The intramedullary vessels originate from a single nutrient artery that enters the radius through a foramina on the anterior surface of the radius in its proximal third.

The **ulna** is an extension of the arm; it has a slight apex posterior curve. The proximal half of the ulna has an apex lateral curve, and the distal half has an apex medial curve. The radial border of the ulna serves as the attachment of the interosseous membrane. The posterior, or subcutaneous, surface is the origin of the deep fascia of the forearm. The blood supply of the ulna is through periosteal and intramedullary vessels. The intramedullary vessels originate from a single nutrient artery that enters the ulna through a foramina located on the anterior surface of the ulna just proximal to its midpoint.

The **interosseous membrane** is a fascial sheet whose fibers are directed fanwise from the radius to the ulna. A condensation of fibers in its midsubstance is termed the **interosseous ligament**. Gaps in the interosseous membrane transmit the anterior and posterior interosseous vessels. The interosseous membrane separates the flexor and extensor compartments and serves as the origin of both flexor and extensor muscles. It also dampens the transmission of proximally directed forces along the radius to the capitellum. An intact interosseous membrane is strong enough to resist proximal migration of the radius, making possible resection of the radial head.

The **muscles** of the forearm are divided into flexor and extensor compartments. The flexors are further divided into superficial flexors that

131

originate from the humerus and deep flexors that originate from the radius, ulna, and interosseous membrane. The superficial group includes the pronator teres, flexor carpi radialis, palmaris longus, flexor carpi ulnaris, and flexor digitorum superficialis. The deep flexor group includes the flexor digitorum profundus, the flexor pollicis longus, and the pronator quadratus. All the flexors are innervated by the median nerve or its anterior interosseous branch, except the flexor carpi ulnaris and the ulnar side of the flexor digitorum profundus. These are innervated by the ulnar nerve.

The **anterior interosseous nerve** arises from the posterior aspect of the median nerve in the proximal forearm and supplies the flexor pollicis longus, flexor digitorum profundus, part of the flexor superficialis, and pronator quadratus. It has terminal sensory fibers to the joints that make up the wrist. Injury to the anterior interosseous nerve is usually indicated by weakness or loss of interphalangeal joint flexion of the thumb and index finger.

The **extensor** compartment is divided into superficial and deep groups. The muscles of the superficial group originate from the humerus and common extensor tendon. The superficial group includes the brachioradialis, the extensor carpi radialis longus and brevis, the extensor digitorum, the extensor digiti minimi, and the extensor carpi ulnaris. The deep extensor group includes the supinator, abductor pollicis longus, the extensor pollicis longus and brevis, and the extensor indicis. The muscles of the deep extensor group, with the exception of the supinator, originate from the radius, ulna, and interosseous membrane. The muscles of the extensor compartment are innervated by the radial nerve or its terminal muscular branch, the posterior interosseous nerve.

Three muscles span the radius and ulna: the pronator teres, the pronator quadratus, and the supinator. Following a forearm fracture, they narrow the interosseous space, resulting in loss of forearm rotation.

The **brachial artery** divides into the **radial and ulnar arteries** 1 cm distal to the elbow joint. The radial artery runs along the radial side of the forearm to the wrist, where it lies between the flexor carpi radialis tendon and the radius. It is most easily palpated in this location. The radial artery terminates in the deep palmar arch. The ulnar artery runs along the ulnar side of the forearm until it reaches the wrist. Along the way, it gives off several branches, the most important of which is the common interosseous artery. The common interosseous artery in turn gives off the anterior and posterior interosseous arteries. The anterior interosseous artery runs on the anterior surface of the interosseous membrane with the anterior interosseous branch of the median nerve. It gives off muscular branches and the nutrient arteries supplying the radius and the ulna. The posterior interosseous artery traverses the interosseous membrane proximally to reach the extensor compartment, where it runs between the superficial and deep group of muscles, giving off numerous muscular branches.

Classification

Injuries of the forearm are broadly classified into two groups: simple and complex. **Simple injuries** are fractures without associated ligamentous disruption. Included in this group are isolated fractures of the radius and ulna (the "nightstick" fracture) and fractures of both the radius and the ulna (the "both-bone" fracture; Figs. 11-1 to 11-5). Simple injuries are the result of direct trauma (e.g., a blow to the forearm). They are described as being closed or open, uncomminuted or comminuted, and undisplaced or displaced; if displaced, then shortened or angulated.

Complex injuries are characterized by ligamentous disruption. These injuries disrupt either the proximal, distal, or both radioulnar articulations and part or all of the interosseous membrane. The soft tissue component of these complex injuries, in many cases, is more significant than the fracture.

The **Monteggia fracture** in adults is substantially different than the same injury in children. These injuries are frequently the result of high-energy trauma, and posterior dislocation of the radial head (Bado type II) is more common than anterior dislocation of the radial head (Bado type I; Fig. 11-6). In addition, comminuted fractures of the radial head, fractures of the coronoid process, and a small osteopenic proximal fragment can make the goal of a stable anatomic reduction of all the components of the fracture difficult to achieve. Ipsilateral diaphyseal fracture of the humerus (floating elbow injury) requiring stable plate fixation may be seen with the high-energy Bado type I injuries.

The **Galeazzi fracture and fracture of the distal ulna with ligamentous disruption** are fractures of the distal third of the radius or ulna and a dislocation of the distal radioulnar articulation (Figs. 11-7 to 11-9). Both of these fractures are short oblique fractures occurring at the distal metaphyseal diaphyseal junction. The mechanism of injury of the Galeazzi fracture is forced pronation (usually during a fall on the outstretched hand) or from a direct blow. The mirror injury, fracture of the ulna with dislocation of the distal radioulnar articulation, has been described recently and is not well understood. Both injuries include disruption of the distal radioulnar joint and a tear of the interosseous membrane from its most distal extent to the fracture of the radius or ulna.

FIG. 11-1   Nightstick fracture of the radius.

FIGS. 11-2 and 11-3   Nightstick fractures of the ulna.

FIGS. 11-4 and 11-5   Both-bone fractures.

FIG. 11-6   Monteggia fracture, or a fracture of the ulna, associated with a dislocation of the proximal radius.

FIGS. 11-7 and 11-8   Galeazzi fracture, or a fracture of the distal radius, associated with disruption of the distal radioulnar articulation.

FIG. 11-9   Fracture of the ulna associated with disruption of the distal radioulnar articulation.

Essex–Lopresti injury (radioulnar dissociation) is a fracture or dislocation of the radial head with disruption of the distal radioulnar articulation and tearing of the entire interosseous membrane. Attention may be focused on the injury at the lateral elbow or a Galeazzi-type fracture–dislocation in the distal forearm, but the major component of the injury, radioulnar dissociation, is frequently overlooked. Early diagnosis and appropriate treatment (maintaining a radial capitellar articulation to prevent proximal migration of the radius) is important to obtaining a satisfactory result.

Associated Injuries

Injuries associated with fractures of the forearm include fractures and dislocations of the elbow and wrist, neurovascular injuries, and compartment syndrome.

Radiographs of the wrist and elbow determine whether there are associated fractures or dislocations.

Laceration, compression, or stretching of arteries and nerves frequently occur at the time of the injury. The greater the initial displacement, the greater the chance of an associated neurovascular injury. The presence of pulses distal to the fracture and capillary refill of the nail beds indicates adequate vascularity. In questionable cases, an arteriogram indicates the definitive diagnosis.

The nerve most frequently injured in association with a forearm injury is the posterior interosseous nerve. This is particularly true of Monteggia fractures. Nerve injury is not uncommon in association with forearm fractures and differs greatly with the type of fracture and the forces creating it. Neurologic injury is identified by a focused neurologic examination of the radial ulnar and median nerves.

Compartment syndrome most frequently involves the flexor compartment, but the extensor compartment can also be involved. The patient complains of severe pain. The compartments are tense, and any attempt at passive stretch of the muscles in the compartment exacerbates the pain. Measurement of the compartment pressure produces the definitive diagnosis. The management is emergent surgical decompression, including the bicipital aponeurosis proximally and the carpal tunnel distally.

Diagnosis and Initial Management

History and Physical Examination

There is pain and a history of trauma. There may be obvious deformity. The skin is examined for wounds that may communicate with the fracture. The elbow and distal radioulnar articulation are examined to determine whether they have been injured. Neurological deficit is infrequent except in penetrating injuries and high-energy open fractures.

Radiographic Examination

Radiographs in the anteroposterior and lateral projections of the forearm, wrist, and elbow are adequate to evaluate most injuries of the forearm. Occasionally, comparison views of the opposite wrist or computed tomographic scans of both wrists are helpful in evaluating the relative positions of the distal radius and ulna. Stress views obtained by radially deviating the wrist may be diagnostic of Essex–Lopresti injury.

Initial Management

Initial management is aligning and splinting the forearm. Displaced or angulated fractures are aligned by administering parenteral analgesia and applying traction across the forearm by suspending the hand from fingertraps and hanging 5 to 10 lbs. of weight from the arm. Anatomic alignment of fractures that will be managed operatively is not necessary. Some shortening or angulation is acceptable because it will be corrected at surgery. A splint extending from the proximal humerus across the elbow to the metacarpophalangeal joints is applied. The elbow is flexed to 90°, with the forearm in neutral rotation. If the radial head cannot be reduced with closed methods following a Monteggia fracture, open reduction and stabilization are performed within 24 h of injury to minimize the incidence of neurovascular compromise.

Definitive Management

Simple Injuries of the Forearm

Isolated fractures of the ulna (nightstick fractures) that are displaced less than 50%, angulated less than 15°, and in which the interosseous space is maintained are managed nonoperatively. A splint is applied that extends from the elbow to the metacarpophalangeal joints along the ulnar side of the forearm. At 4 weeks the splint is removed, and the forearm is lightly wrapped in a compression bandage. Radiographs are obtained at 1, 2, 3, and 6 weeks to confirm that alignment has not changed and the fracture is healing.

  Isolated undisplaced fractures of the radius can be managed in a long arm cast but must be carefully followed because they tend to displace. Any displacement or angulation that occurs should be treated by immediate open reduction and internal fixation because it will invariably tend to progress.

Isolated fractures of the radius and ulna that are displaced or angulated or in which the interosseous space is compromised are reduced and stabilized. Fractures of the proximal half of the radius can be approached dorsally, as described by Thompson (1918), or preferably volarly, as described by Henry (1950); fractures of the distal half of the radius are approached volarly. Fractures of the ulna are approached along the subcutaneous border. The fracture is reduced and stabilized with a dynamic compression plate (DCP). If more than half the cortex is comminuted, the fracture is grafted with autogenous cancellous bone.

Intramedullary nailing is indicated for segmental fractures and for fractures of the proximal radius in which the posterior interosseous nerve is vulnerable to injury during the exposure. The nails are inserted ulnar to Lister's tubercle for fractures of the radius and through the olecranon for fractures of the ulna. The nails are bent to restore the normal bow of the radius and ulna, thus reestablishing the interosseous space.

Postoperatively, active range of motion of the forearm, wrist, and elbow is encouraged. If the fracture has been plated, it is assessed as being healed when trabeculae cross the fracture radiographically. This may take up to 6 months. Callus, displacement, or angulation indicate loss of fixation. Healing of fractures that have been stabilized with an intramedullary nail is easier to assess because fixation is not rigid and the patient's symptoms correlate with the amount of healing.

Complex Injuries

An important part of management of complex injuries is adequate treatment of all the components.

Monteggia fracture is managed operatively. The ulnar fracture must be anatomically reduced and plated with a 3.5-mm DCP (tension band fixation and semitubular plates are frequently inadequate). The fracture of the coronoid process and comminuted fracture of the radial head frequently associated with Bado type II fractures require anatomic reduction and stable fixation of the coronoid process and reduction and fixation of the radial head fracture, if possible, or excision of the radial head with or without prosthetic replacement in those fractures that are severely comminuted. Intraoperative radiographs are obtained to confirm that the reduction is anatomic and that the coronoid process and radial head are reduced. Postoperatively, a long arm splint is applied with the elbow in 90° of flexion and the forearm in neutral rotation. Early mobilization of the elbow and forearm within the limits imposed by the soft tissue injury is important to reduce the risk of synostosis.

The less common Bado type I fracture is frequently a high-energy injury with neurovascular damage, compartment syndrome, and ipsilateral fracture of the humerus. Reduction and fixation of the ulnar fracture with a 3.5-mm DCP will usually result in reduction of the radial head dislocation. Any associated fracture of the humerus should be treated with open reduction and internal fixation.

Galeazzi fracture and fracture of the distal ulna with radioulnar disruption are managed with rigid plating of the fracture. The surgical exposure is from a volar approach for the radius and through a skin incision parallel with its subcutaneous border for the ulna. When the ulnar styloid is avulsed by the triangular fibrocartilage, it is reduced and stabilized with Kirschner wires or a screw. The distal radioulnar joint is usually reduced when the radial fracture is plated and radial length is restored. If the distal radioulnar joint is unstable, it can be reduced by supinating the forearm. A short arm splint is applied unless the distal radioulnar joint requires reduction and immobilization in supination.

Radioulnar dissociation (Essex–Lopresti injury) is an injury to the distal radioulnar joint and ipsilateral radiohumeral joint associated with disruption of the interosseous membrane. Excision of the radial head for a comminuted fracture when there is an associated injury at the distal radioulnar joint is contraindicated because proximal migration of the radius may occur. It is recommended that the acute injury be treated with repair of the radiohumeral joint, open reduction and internal fixation of any distal forearm fractures, and immobilization of the distal radioulnar joint in a long arm cast with the forearm in supination. Open reduction with Kirschner wire fixation of the ulna to the radius and repair of the distal radioulnar ligaments should be undertaken if the distal radioulnar joint is unstable.

Open Fractures of the Radius and Ulna

Open fractures of the forearm are classified into three types. Type I is associated with a clean wound and the laceration is shorter than 1 cm. Type II is associated with a laceration longer than 1 cm, without extensive soft tissue damage. The usual cause of type I and type II wounding is penetration from the inside out by one of the fractured bone ends. Type III open fractures are associated with extensive soft tissue damage or a segmental fracture and have been subdivided into type III-A injuries from gunshots with adequate soft tissue coverage and type III-B contaminated environment injuries such as farm or lake injuries with extensive soft tissue damage and significant periosteal stripping associated with significant contamination that is not necessarily visible. There may be foreign material hidden in the depths of the wound, or the environment itself may be associated with large numbers of bacterial organisms such as may be present in a polluted lake or farmyard. Type III-C open fractures are associated with vascular injury necessitating reanastomosis.

The primary consideration in treating these wounds is to prevent soft tissue and bony infection. For this to be accomplished, immediate adequate exploration and debridement of the wound must be performed. Tetanus prophylaxis is assured. The wound should be cleaned and dressed in the emergency room and intravenous antibiotic treatment started. The patient is taken to the operating room, where a general anesthetic or an adequate regional anesthetic that allows the use of the tourniquet is given. After limb preparation, the wounds are extended so that an adequate exploration of the soft tissue and bony injury can be performed. Devitalized skin, fascia, muscle, and bone are removed, and an extensive fasciotomy is performed both proximal and distal to the wound so that devitalized soft tissue and foreign material will not go unnoticed. Neurovascular structures in the vicinity of the wound are exposed so their integrity can be determined. The wound is thoroughly irrigated with an antibiotic solution.

Type I, II, and III-A open fractures can generally be stabilized with primary internal fixation by using a plate and screws, as described for closed fractures; however, the wounds should be left open for delayed wound closure in 3 to 5 days. Intravenous antibiotics are continued for 4 to 5 days unless a wound infection occurs.

Type III-B and type III-C open fractures are generally not suitable for internal fixation. A half-pin external fixator or pins and plaster can be used to maintain reduction of these fractures. After the soft tissues have healed without infection, delayed cancellous bone grafting or delayed open reduction and internal fixation with plate and screws and cancellous bone grafting can be performed, if needed.

Complications

The complications of injuries of the forearm include malunion, nonunion, synostosis (associated with heterotopic ossification), infection, refracture, and subluxation or posttraumatic arthrosis of the distal or proximal radioulnar joints.

Nonunion of these fractures occurs most frequently when an inadequate internal fixation has been performed. It may also be associated with failure to do primary cancellous bone grafting when indicated and infection. To avoid failure of internal fixation, 3.5-mm dynamic compression plates should be used, with an adequate number of cortices fixed proximal and distal to the fracture. Semitubular plates do not provide adequate fixation. Symptomatic nonunions are reduced, stabilized with an adequate dynamic compression plate, and grafted with autogenous cancellous bone. Malunion should be prevented by performing open reduction and internal fixation for most diaphyseal forearm fractures. The major cause for malunion following a fracture of the shaft of the radius or ulna is failure to obtain adequate radiographic follow-up and perform open reduction and internal fixation as soon as an undisplaced fracture begins to displace (Fig. 11-10). Corrective osteotomy is most efficacious when performed as soon as possible after the injury. Satisfactory osseous contact for stable internal fixation can be difficult to obtain. Complications increase, and gains in range of forearm rotation decrease in patients undergoing operative treatment more than 1 year after the initial fracture. The usual indications for correc-

FIG. 11-10   This malunion of a fracture of both bones of the forearm was initially undisplaced. It has resulted in a severe cosmetic deformity, with the forearm fixed in neutral rotation.

tive osteotomy are loss of forearm rotation, cosmetic deformity, and instability of the distal radioulnar joint.

Wound infection is managed by returning the patient to the operating room, where the wound can be adequately opened and cleaned. Cultures are obtained. If a plate and screws are still providing adequate fixation, they are left in place. The wound is left open and supported with a splint. Delayed wound closure is performed after 5 days if the infection is under control. In some instances, the wound will be left open and allowed to heal secondarily with skin grafting as required. The fracture should unite if infection is controlled; however, cancellous bone grafting may be required.

Nerve injuries are uncommon except for penetrating wounds (i.e., gunshot fractures). The prognosis for these injuries is frequently poor without surgical exploration and repair. This is usually done as a secondary procedure because the extent of nerve damage at the time of primary exploration is difficult to determine.

Compartment syndrome after forearm fractures is not uncommon. It is very important when performing open reduction and internal fixation to deflate the tourniquet and provide adequate hemostasis prior to wound closure. The forearm fascia must not be closed.

Synostosis can be treated by resection after the synostosis has had a chance to mature, if the functional impairment is significant. Indications of maturity are a well-ossified mass with corticalized margins, a cold bone scan, a normal serum alkaline phosphatase, and the passage of approximately 12 months since the time of the injury. Heterotopic ossification with synostosis is more frequently encountered following injuries resulting from high-energy trauma or in patients with concommitant head injury. The synostosis is more likely to recur after excision when located in the proximal or distal paraarticular part of the forearm.

Painful subluxation and posttraumatic osteoarthritis of the radioulnar articulations are managed with antiinflammatory medication or local steroid injection. If these measures fail, distal radioulnar arthrosis can be managed by arthrodesing the distal radius and ulna and resecting a 1-cm section of distal ulnar metaphysis to produce a nonunion, thus preserving forearm rotation (Sauve–Kapandji procedure).

Routine removal of a diaphyseal plate after fracture fixation is not usually necessary or desirable because bone mineral density and grip strength are not affected. Plate removal can be complicated by neurovascular injury and refracture.

SELECTED READINGS

Elstrom JA, Pankovich AM, Egwele R: Extraarticular low velocity gunshot fractures of the radius and ulna. *J Bone Joint Surg* 60A:335–341, 1978.

Grace TG, Eversman WW Jr: Forearm fractures: Treatment by rigid fixation with early motion. *J Bone Joint Surg* 62A:433–438, 1980.

Henry AK: Extensile exposure applied to limb surgery, 1st ed. (3rd reprint). Edinburgh: E and S Livingstone Ltd. 53–64, 1950.

Lamey DM, Fernandez DL: Results of the modified Sauve–Kapandji procedure in the treatment of chronic posttraumatic derangement of the distal radioulnar joint. *J Bone Joint Surg* 80A:1758–1769, 1998.

Pollack FH, Pankovich AM, Prieto JJ, Lorenz M: The isolated fracture of the ulnar shaft. Treatment without immobilization. *J Bone Joint Surg* 65A:339–342, 1983.

Reckling FW: Unstable fracture–dislocations of the forearm (Monteggia and Galeazzi lesions). *J Bone Joint Surg* 64A:857–863, 1982.

Ring D, Jupiter JB, Simpson NS: Monteggia fracture in adults. *J Bone Joint Surg* 80A:1733–1744, 1998.

Thompson, JE: Anatomical methods of approach in operations on the long bones of the extremities. *Ann Surg* 68:309, 1918.

Trousdale RT, Amadio PC, Cooney WP, Morrey BF: Radio-ulnar dissociation. A review of twenty cases. *J Bone Joint Surg* 74A:1486–1497, 1992.

Trousdale RT, Linscheid RL: Operative treatment of malunited fractures of the forearm. *J Bone Joint Surg* 77A:894–902, 1995.

12 | Fractures of the Distal Radius and Distal Radioulnar Joint Injuries

Donald L. Pruitt

This chapter covers fractures of the distal radius (within 5 cm of the articular surface) and dislocations of the distal radioulnar joint.

ANATOMY

Important anatomic considerations are the bones, the joints, their x-ray appearance, and the surrounding soft tissue structures.

The **distal radius** is fan shaped when viewed from the anterior. The styloid projects past the ulna. On the dorsal surface of the radius is Lister's tubercle, which is grooved along the medial side for the extensor pollicis longus tendon. The pronator quadratus muscle inserts along the volar surface of the radius. Elevation of this muscle provides access to the volar surface of the radius for fracture fixation. The sigmoid notch articulates with the ulna.

The **distal ulna** is made up of the head and styloid. It is grooved dorsally for the extensor carpi ulnaris tendon. The distal portion of the head is separated from the lunate and triquetrium by the triangular fibrocartilage complex. This consists of a central articular disc and dorsal and volar marginal ligaments on the respective sides. Three-fourths of the ulna head is covered with articular cartilage (270°), which articulates with the sigmoid notch of the radius. On the volar surface of the distal ulna is the origin of the pronator quadratus.

The **wrist joint** is biaxial (i.e., it moves along two axes). The distal radius has two lesser articulations: the radioscaphoid and radiolunate joints. The radial portion of the radioscaphoid joint is part of the radial styloid, which is fractured in a Chauffeur fracture. The lunate fossa is separated from the scaphoid fossa by a small ridge. When fractured and depressed, the central portion of the lunate fossa is known as a *die punch fragment*. Normal range of motion at the wrist is 80° palmar flexion, 70° dorsiflexion, 20° radial deviation, and 40° ulnar deviation.

The **distal radioulnar joint** is a uniaxial pivot joint. The radius rotates around a fixed axis, the ulnar styloid. The triangular fibrocartilage complex attaches to the base of the ulnar styloid and helps hold the radius and ulna together. Normal range of motion for the distal radioulnar joint is 70° for pronation and for supination.

Important features of the **radiographic appearance** of the distal radius are radial length, radial angle, and volar tilt. **Radial length** is measured from a line perpendicular to the radial shaft drawn through the lunate fossa to the tip of the radial styloid (normally 12 to 15 mm; Fig. 12-1). **Radial angle** is the angle between a line drawn through the dis-

FIG. 12-1   Radial length and radial angle.

tal radioulnar joint and the radial styloid and a line perpendicular to the radial shaft through the lunate fossa (normally 23°; Fig. 12-1). **Volar tilt** is measured on the lateral film and is the angle between a line drawn through the dorsal and volar rims and a line drawn perpendicular to the radial shaft (normally 10° volarly; Fig. 12-2). These measurements should be kept in mind when assessing post reduction films.

Surrounding **soft tissue** structures are an important consideration in distal radius fractures. Strong ligaments surround the volar aspect of the radiocarpal joint; the dorsal ligaments are not as stout. Extensor tendons travel through six retinacular compartments on the dorsal aspect of the wrist. Although rarely injured acutely, attritional rupture (especially the extensor pollicis longus tendon) may occur in the presence or absence of malunion. Volar to the distal radius is the carpal tunnel, containing nine tendons and the median nerve. Symptoms of median nerve dysfunction should be checked in all distal radius fractures. The ulnar artery, ulnar nerve, and flexor carpi ulnaris tendon lie volar and ulnar to the distal radius. The ulnar artery and nerve enter Guyon's canal more distally between the pisiform bone and the hook of the hamate, the roof of which is formed by the volar carpal ligament blended with the tendinous distal extension of the flexor carpi ulnaris insertion, the pisohamate ligament. The radial artery and the flexor carpi radialis tendon are found outside the carpal tunnel on the volar radial side of the distal radius.

FIG. 12-2   Volar tilt of the distal radius.

FRACTURES OF THE DISTAL RADIUS

Classification

The AO and Frykman classification systems are the most widely used. We classify distal radius fractures into three major groups: nondisplaced; displaced extraarticular; and displaced intraarticular.

Nondisplaced fractures may be extra- or intraarticular.

Displaced extraarticular fractures do not involve the radiocarpal or radioulnar articulation. They are further classified according to the direction of displacement: dorsally (e.g., Colles fracture) or volarly (Smith's type I or II; Fig. 12-3). Displaced comminuted extraarticular fractures are high-energy injuries and often have a nondisplaced component entering one of the joints.

Displaced intraarticular fractures involve the radiocarpal joint, the distal radioulnar joint, or both. Uncorrected articular step-off larger than 2 mm has a poorer prognosis, especially in younger patients. Most often, the articular incongruity involves the lunate fossa (die punch fragment). Displaced intraarticular fractures are further classified according to whether they are simple (few fracture lines) or comminuted. Other eponyms for these fractures are dorsal Barton, volar Barton, and Chauffeur fractures (Fig. 12-4).

Diagnosis and Initial Management

History and Physical Examination

There are two patient populations that sustain distal radius fractures. The first is older, has osteopenic bone, and has sustained the fracture

FIG. 12-3 The three types of extraarticular fractures of the distal radius: (*A*) a dorsally displaced, or Colles, fracture; (*B*) a volarly displaced, metaphyseal fracture, or Smith type I fracture; and (*C*) a volarly displaced fracture that starts at the dorsal rim, or a Smith type II fracture.

FIG. 12-4   Types of intraarticular fractures of the distal radius: (*A*) dorsal Barton fracture; (*B*) volar Barton fracture; (*C*) fracture of the radial styloid, also known as a Chauffeur fracture; and (*D*) a die punch fracture of the lunate fossa.

FIG. 12-4 *Continued.*

during relatively minor trauma. The fracture is usually metaphyseal and extraarticular. The second group of patients is younger and has sustained the fracture as a result of a high-energy injury (e.g., fall from a height). Most of these patients have dense bone, and the fracture is often intraarticular and comminuted and has associated injuries.

There is pain, swelling, and deformity of the wrist. A neurovascular examination is performed, and the wrist is examined for the presence of open wounds.

Radiographic Examination

Anteroposterior, lateral, and oblique radiographs are obtained, with anything that might hinder assessment of the fracture, such as splints, removed. The amount of displacement seen on prereduction films provides a clue to the stability of the fracture. Radiographs taken with traction applied to the fracture, such as when the patient is suspended in finger traps with a counter force above the elbow, are useful in determining the extent of the fracture (whether there is intraarticular extension in an apparent extraarticular fracture) and the likelihood of obtaining and maintaining satisfactory reduction without opening the fracture site. Postreduction films, with traction removed, are important in assessing the stability of the reduction. Computed tomography is often useful to determine the extent of the injury and to assess alignment of articular fracture fragments.

Initial Management

Displaced fractures are reduced. This maneuver can be the definitive management, but even in fractures that will require surgery, early reduction often achieves reasonable alignment that may decrease the incidence of neurovascular compromise.

Patients with severely displaced or comminuted fractures are often admitted overnight, with the arm elevated and iced. The neurovascular status is frequently checked. Compartment syndrome or acute carpal tunnel syndrome may occur and need to be managed aggressively. Open fractures will need a tetanus toxoid booster, debridement and irrigation in the operating room, and intravenous antibiotics. Cultures obtained from these wounds are probably of no value in predicting infection or directing antibiotic therapy.

Associated Injuries

Injuries to the neurovascular structures about the wrist and bony or ligamentous injuries of the elbow are associated with fractures of the distal radius. The neurovascular status of the hand must be carefully examined. Median nerve compression, the most common nerve injury, is indicated by decreased sensation on the palmar aspect of the thumb and index and long fingers. Loss of palmar abduction of the thumb can also occur but is a later sign of median nerve compromise. Injury to the ulnar nerve is indicated by loss of sensation on the ulnar border of the hand and inability to abduct the fingers. Compartment syndrome of the forearm or hand may be associated with penetrating injuries and high-energy fractures of the distal radius. It may be delayed in onset and is most commonly manifested by tense swelling in the forearm and/or hand. Paresthesias and increasing pain are usually present if the patient is not obtunded. Fasciotomy must be performed in the presence of clinical signs and an elevated intracompartmental pressure. Good response to capillary refill in the nailbeds indicates vascular perfusion of the hand and digits.

High-energy fractures of the distal radius can be associated with injuries in the elbow joint, including fractures of the radial head and elbow dislocations. The elbow is examined for pain and swelling; radiographs are taken when indicated. Other associated injuries include scaphoid fracture, scapholunate dissociation, and other carpal, metacarpal, and phalangeal fractures. Displaced radial styloid fractures are frequently associated with scapholunate dissociation. Radiographs of the hand and wrist will show most of these injuries.

Definitive Management

The definitive management is based primarily on the type of fracture. Factors that enter into the treatment decision include the patient's age, occupation, degree of osteopenia, and associated medical conditions.

Nondisplaced fractures are managed with a short arm cast, unless considerable swelling is present, in which case a sugar tong splint is applied. The patient returns in 7 to 10 days for a follow-up radiograph. The cast is changed as the swelling decreases and is usually removed between 4 and 6 weeks. A wrist cock-up splint is worn between range-of-motion exercise sessions for an additional 2 weeks. Strengthening exercises are started once the splint is discontinued.

Displaced extraarticular fractures are displaced either dorsally (Colles) or volarly (Smith). The definitive management is based on the direction of displacement.

Indications for reduction of a **Colles fracture** are greater than 5-mm loss of radial length or 10° or more dorsal tilt. Parenteral analgesia, hematoma block, or regional or general anesthesia is administered. The thumb and index fingers are suspended in finger traps, with a roll of 3-inch webril placed between them to open up the first web space. Countertraction is provided with 10 to 20 lbs. of weight draped over the arm with a felt pad. A waiting period of 5 to 10 min helps disimpact the fragments. Reduction is performed by reproducing the injury first with hyperextension and then with flexion of the wrist. The distal radius is molded with the surgeon's thumbs on the dorsal and radial surfaces to push the distal fragment back onto the metaphysis. The distal fragment is pushed volarly to bring the volar cortices into opposition. Palpation to find step-offs along the dorsal and radial surfaces helps to confirm adequate reduction. While the wrist is being palmar flexed at 20° to 30° with traction maintained, a sugar tong splint or plaster cast is applied. Once the short arm portion of the cast has set, traction is released and the above-elbow portion is applied. Postreduction x-rays are obtained. If a cast has been applied, it is best to split the cast to allow for swelling. All patients are instructed in cast care, elevation of the arm, and warning signs of excessive swelling and are asked to return the next day for a cast check.

Postreduction films are evaluated for reestablishment of radial length, radial angle, volar tilt, and the presence of intraarticular step-off. Distal radius fractures are notoriously unstable and often redisplace in the cast despite an initial anatomic reduction. Factors associated with instability are excessive comminution, initial loss of more than 15 mm in radial length, initial dorsal tilt greater than 20°, or comminution of both the dorsal and volar cortices seen on the postreduction film. In general, any fracture that requires a manipulative reduction is carefully followed for potential loss of reduction. Radiographs are obtained weekly for at least the first 3 weeks after reduction. If the alignment is unchanged after 3 weeks, the patient is placed in a short arm cast and started on elbow range-of-motion exercises. At 6 weeks, the cast is removed, the wrist is placed into a removable splint, and range-of-motion exercises are begun. Emphasis is on regaining motion for the first 3 weeks; strengthening is started later. If the patient does not recover a reasonable range of motion within 3 weeks of cast removal, dynamic splinting is indicated.

Criteria indicating the need for remanipulation and possible fixation are loss of radial length or angle and dorsal tilt greater than 10°. It is difficult to obtain good anesthesia in the office more than 5 days postinjury, so it is best to treat patients with loss of reduction in the operating room. Fractures can often be remanipulated for up to 3 weeks postfracture; beyond this period, open reduction would be necessary.

Remanipulation is performed by using the same technique as for fresh fractures. An image intensifier can be used to assist in the reduction, but permanent radiographs should be obtained to assess the adequacy of the reduction. Kirschner wires can be inserted percutaneously into the fracture site, if necessary, to free the fracture. After alignment has been restored, the fracture is stabilized with percutaneous pins. A 0.062-inch Kirschner wire is inserted into the radial styloid and driven across the fracture site and out the proximal metaphysis. A second wire is inserted from the dorsal ulnar corner of the distal fragment to the volar radial metaphysis. Two wires are often enough, but additional wires are added as necessary. Percutaneous pins do not provide firm fixation and a cast is still necessary to maintain reduction. The pins are cut off beneath the skin and can be removed in the office with local anesthesia. Alternatively, an external fixator or pins and plaster can be used to stabilize the fracture if adequate reduction is obtained.

Smith fractures are unstable. The pull of the flexor muscles across the wrist exerts shear forces across the fracture site, resulting in redisplacement after closed reduction. If the fracture is displaced on the initial film, fixation is indicated. In younger patients with good bone stock, these fractures can be reduced closed and pinned percutaneously. In older patients or those with osteopenic bone, the fracture is managed with a volar buttress plate. A short arm cast is applied, and the postoperative management is as described for Colles fractures.

Open or severely comminuted Colles and Smith fractures present a different set of management priorities. Open distal radius fractures are managed with emergent irrigation and debridement of the fracture site. After debridement, grade I and grade II fractures are treated like the corresponding closed fracture. Grade III fractures are managed with external fixation.

Comminution causes instability, and frequently reduction is impossible to maintain with casting alone. In general, if the metaphyseal comminution is not extensive and the patient has good bone stock, the fracture can be stabilized with percutaneous pins (Figs. 12-5 to 12-7); otherwise, the fracture is managed with external fixation or open reduction and plate fixation.

Prior to application of the **external fixator**, the fracture is reduced in the operating room with sterile finger traps and brachial countertraction. An image intensifier is used to confirm reduction. Metacarpal pins are placed through incisions just large enough to retract the soft tissues out of the way. Radial pins are placed through an incision large enough to visualize the radial nerve and retract it out of harm's way. Fixators are kept on for approximately 8 weeks. Autologous bone grafting or use of new bone graft substitutes including allograft chips allows for earlier fixator removal.

FIG. 12-5   Anteroposterior view of a dorsally displaced extraarticular distal radius fracture. There is loss of radial angle (5°) and radial length (4 mm).

FIG. 12-6   Lateral view of case shown in Fig. 12-5. The tilt is 30° dorsal.

FIG. 12-7   Anteroposterior radiograph after closed reduction and percutaneous pin fixation of the same patient (Figs. 12-5 and 12-6). Note the restoration of radial length and radial angle.

Displaced intraarticular fractures have a poorer prognosis than an equivalent extraarticular fracture and demand more aggressive management. The two types of displaced intraarticular fractures are simple fractures and comminuted fractures.

Simple intraarticular fractures involve the radial styloid (Chauffeur fracture), the dorsal rim (dorsal Barton fracture), and the volar rim (volar Barton fracture).

Chauffeur fractures usually run from the radial metaphysis into the radiocarpal joint between the scaphoid and lunate fossa. Nondisplaced fractures are managed with cast immobilization. Displaced fractures are reduced and pinned by one of three techniques: closed by using image intensification, arthroscopically, or open.

Volar Barton fractures are unstable because of the pull of the flexor muscles, resulting in volar subluxation of the carpus. They are best managed with a volar buttress plate. The radius is approached through an incision paralleling the flexor carpi radialis tendon. Dissection proceeds between the flexor carpi radialis tendon and the radial artery to the pronator quadratus muscle, which is detached sharply from its insertion on the radius. The exposed fracture is reduced, and a buttress plate is applied. The distal screw holes in the plate may be left unfilled, especially in osteopenic patients. Postoperatively, a short arm cast is maintained for 4 weeks.

Management of **dorsal Barton fractures** differs depending on the size of the fragment. Small dorsal fragments are treated with closed reduction and cast immobilization with the wrist in extension. Careful follow-up is important to ensure that dorsal subluxation does not occur. For larger fragments or those with comminution, either percutaneous pin fixation or a dorsal buttress plate is used. Postoperatively, a short arm cast is applied for 4 weeks.

Comminuted displaced intraarticular fractures are the most difficult distal radius fractures to manage. If the fracture can be reduced closed, management is done with an external fixator. An external fixator is needed because the reduction of a comminuted fracture will be unstable and lost in a cast. If the fracture cannot be reduced closed, an open reduction is performed.

First the fracture is reduced, and then the external fixator is applied, as described above. Final adjustments in fracture position are made, and the frame is tightened. Percutaneous Kirschner wires or plates and screws are added to secure major fragments. Intraarticular step-off can be corrected either by using an arthroscope to visualize the fragments or through a dorsal incision. Major volar fragments may require a separate volar approach (usually the volar–ulnar corner). There are several plates available that allow for strong fixation and make the external fixator unnecessary.

Practically, the best that the dorsal tilt can be corrected is to neutral with external fixation. Factors that make external fixation alone unreliable include extensive dorsal comminution, interposition of soft tissues between fracture fragments, depression of the lunate fossa (die punch fragment), and rotation of fragments.

The primary indication for **open reduction** of comminuted intraarticular distal radial fractures is displacement that cannot be reduced by closed manipulation. The articular incongruity most commonly involves the lunate fossa. External fixation and limited operative exposure or arthroscopy has been a useful technique for these fractures. The lunate fossa can be elevated through a limited dorsal incision, supported with Kirschner wires and autogenous bone graft, and may be used in conjunction with an osteoinductive material such as Graft-on. Alternate bone graft materials such as Interpore® are also useful. Open reduction is necessary when there is soft tissue interposition or malrotation. Application of an external fixator initially helps in maintaining alignment and holding the fragments apart. After exposure, fragments are stabilized by using a combination of Kirschner wires, plates, and screws. Kirschner wires placed just beneath the subchondral surface help support the restored articular surface (Fig. 12-8). The fixator may be removed if good stability is obtained with a plate.

Postoperatively, the arm is placed in a long arm splint and elevated, and early finger and shoulder motion is encouraged. Most fractures involve the distal radioulnar joint, so a long arm splint is maintained for the first 3 weeks. The fixator is removed once callus formation is visible. Bone grafting allows for earlier fixator removal. Aggressive physical therapy is necessary, including the use of dynamic splints once the fixator is removed. Even with optimal surgical treatment, some degree of residual pain and loss of motion and grip strength are inevitable.

Complications

Acute complications include carpal tunnel syndrome, compartment syndrome, reflex sympathetic dystrophy, loss of reduction, and insta-

FIG. 12-8   Use of external fixator and pin fixation for treatment of a comminuted intraarticular distal radius fracture.

bility of the distal radioulnar joint. Transient neuropathy may occur because of the initial trauma and displacement of the fracture. If neuropathy does not improve after reduction, all circumferential dressings are loosened and the wrist is placed into a neutral position. If the sensory changes persist, operative decompression of the carpal canal and the distal forearm fascia is performed. Tense, painful swelling of the forearm and/or hand with paresthesias following high-energy fractures of the distal radius are signs of compartment syndrome and may occur as late as 3 days after injury. Compartment pressures need to be obtained and decompression performed if pressures are elevated. Failure to diagnose and treat compartment syndrome, especially in obtunded patients who cannot complain of pain, usually results in a catastrophic loss of function.

Reflex sympathetic dystrophy is also associated with increasing pain, swelling, progressive stiffness of the fingers, and dysesthesias. Early diagnosis with bone scintigraphy, aggressive physical therapy, and stellate ganglion blocks are the usual methods of management. Loss of reduction is common after distal radius fractures. Frequent x-ray follow-up is necessary to diagnose a loss of reduction early, when it can be more easily corrected.

Late complications are malunion, posttraumatic arthritis, and residual stiffness of the fingers and wrist.

DISLOCATIONS OF THE DISTAL RADIOULNAR JOINT

Isolated dislocations of the distal radioulnar joint are rare injuries. Dislocations associated with a distal radial fracture (i.e., Galeazzi fracture) are covered in "Fractures of the Forearm" (Chap. 11).

Classification

Dislocations of the distal radioulnar joint are classified according to the direction of displacement of the ulna in relation to the radius as either dorsal or volar.

Initial Diagnosis and Management

History and Physical Examination

There is pain on the ulnar side of the wrist, accompanied by snapping and crepitation with forearm rotation, or there is inability to rotate the forearm. The history of the injury frequently includes forced pronation or supination. Physical findings of a dorsal dislocation include a prominent ulnar head, increased mobility of the ulnar head, and limited supination. Physical signs of a volar dislocation include an apparently absent ulnar head, narrowing of the wrist, and limited pronation.

Radiographic Examination

Radiographically, the anteroposterior and lateral projections may not be diagnostic unless compared with identical views of the opposite, uninjured wrist. CT is used to confirm the diagnosis.

Initial Management

Once the diagnosis has been made, a closed reduction is attempted. A hematoma block and sedation are used. Dorsal dislocations are reduced with supination and immobilized in a long arm splint or cast. Volar dislocations are reduced with pronation. If closed reduction is not possible, then open reduction is indicated.

Definitive Management

Factors indicating surgical management include a dislocation that cannot be reduced with closed methods, reductions that are unstable after reduction, and a sizable fracture of the ulnar styloid base, indicating a repairable avulsion of the triangular fibrocartilage. Volar dislocations are approached from the volar side, and the head of the ulna is levered from under the volar surface of the radius. Dorsal dislocations are approached from the dorsal side; usually an osteochondral fragment or tendon is in the sigmoid notch, blocking reduction. If the ulnar styloid is to be repaired, it is reduced and held in place with a small screw or Kirschner wires. This is done through a separate ulnar incision if a volar approach has been used. Once the forearm has been reduced, it is held in neutral rotation, and the ulna is pinned to the radius. Use at least a 0.062-inch Kirschner wire to prevent pin breakage. A long arm cast is maintained for 6 weeks, at which time the cast and pin are removed and gentle rotation exercises are begun.

If closed management is chosen, a long arm cast in supination (dorsal dislocation) or pronation (volar dislocation) is maintained for 6 weeks.

Complications

Complications unique to this injury include chronic radioulnar instability or arthritis. Management consists of either excision of part or all of the ulnar head or arthrodesis of the ulnar head to the sigmoid notch and extraperiosteal resection of 2 cm of the distal ulnar diaphysis to produce a nonunion (Sauve-Kapandji procedure).

SELECTED READINGS

Bass RL, Blair WF, Hubbard PP: Results of combined internal and external fixation for the treatment of severe AO–C3 fractures of the distal radius. *J Hand Surg* 20A:373–381, 1995.

Clancey GJ: Percutaneous Kirschner wire fixation of Colles fractures. A prospective study of thirty cases. *J Bone Joint Surg* 66A:1008–1014, 1984.

Fernandez DL: Correction of posttraumatic wrist deformity in adults by osteotomy, bone grafting, and internal fixation. *J Bone Joint Surg* 64A:1164–1178, 1982.

Knirk JL, Jupiter JB: Intra-articular fractures of the distal end of the radius in young adults. *J Bone Joint Surg* 68A: 647–659, 1986.

Leung KS, Shen WY, Tsang KH, Chiu KH, Leung PC, Hung LK: An effective treatment of comminuted fractures of the distal radius. *J Hand Surg* 15A:11–17, 1990.

Louis, DS: Barton's and Smith's fractures. *Hand Clin* 4:399–402, 1988.

Ouellette EA, Kelly R: Compartment syndromes of the hand. *J Bone Joint Surg* 78A:1515–1522, 1996.

Seitz WH Jr: External fixation of distal radius fractures. Indications and technical principles. *Orthop Clin North Am* 24:255–264, 1993.

Simpson NS, Jupiter JB: Delayed onset of forearm compartment syndrome: a complication of distal radius fracture in young adults. *J Orthop Trauma* 9:411–418, 1995.

Trumble TE, Culp R, Hanel DP, Geissler WB, Berger RA: Intraarticular fractures of the distal aspect of the radius. *J Bone Joint Surg* 80A:582–600, 1998.

Fractures and Dislocations of the Wrist

Donald L. Pruitt

This chapter covers fractures and dislocations of the carpus.

ANATOMY

The eight carpal bones are divided into a proximal row (scaphoid, lunate, triquetrum, and pisiform) and a distal row (trapezium, trapezoid, capitate, and hamate). The proximal row has no tendon insertions and functions as an intercalated segment between the forearm and the hand. The shape of the carpal bones and their ligamentous connections maintain stability, however, they are predisposed to collapse.

Articular cartilage covers 80% of the surface of the **scaphoid.** The proximal pole is intraarticular, with no external blood suply. Two vessels supply the scaphoid, and both enter at the distal end. Thus, fractures of the middle third interfere with the blood supply of the proximal pole, leading to a high incidence of avascular necrosis and nonunion.

The two types of **ligaments** in the wrist are intrinsic and extrinsic. Intrinsic ligaments, also known as interosseous ligaments, connect two or more carpal bones and lie within the synovial cavity. The **scapholunate** and the **lunotriquetral** ligaments are the most important interosseous ligaments. Extrinsic ligaments are specialized thickenings of the wrist capsule and lie outside the synovial cavity. The major extrinsic ligaments are the **radioscaphoid, radiocapitate, and radiotriquetral** ligaments, all located on the volar surface. The neck of the capitate gives origin to the **intercarpal deltoid** ligament, which fans out toward the scaphoid and triquetrum in an inverted "V" configuration. This leaves a space between the head of the capitate and the lunate, known as the **space of Poirier,** through which lunate dislocations occur.

Biomechanically, the carpus is a link joint, with the lunate acting as a potentially unstable segment between the distal row and the radius. The scaphoid functions as a bridge by providing stability to an otherwise unstable intercalated segment (Fig. 13-1).

DISLOCATIONS OF THE WRIST

Classification

Dislocations of the wrist are classified as perilunate, lunate, transscaphoid perilunate, radiocarpal, and radioulnar translocation. Less severe stages of perilunate dislocation present as scapholunate dissociation.

Perilunate, lunate, and transscaphoid perilunate dislocations are variations of the same injury caused by hyperextension of the wrist. There are five stages in this type of injury: I, tearing of the scapholunate

FIG. 13-1 Link joint concept of carpal stability: *(A)* the lunate acts as an intercalated segment between the capitate and radius; *(B)* the segment is unstable, tending to collapse; and *(C)* the scaphoid acts as the stabilizing link to prevent collapse.

and volar radioscaphoid ligaments, resulting in **scapholunate dissociation,** or rotary subluxation of the scaphoid; II, dislocation of the capitate head through the space of Poirier; III, tearing of the lunotriquetral ligament, resulting in separation of the lunate and triquetrum; IV, disruption of the dorsal ligaments and dislocation of the carpus dorsally (the lunate remains in the lunate fossa of the radius), resulting in a **perilunate dislocation;** and V, the carpus drives the lunate volarly and articulates with the radius, resulting in a **lunate dislocation.**

Variations in the path of force transmission result in a variety of related injuries. For example, if the path goes through the body of the scaphoid, causing a fracture, **a transscaphoid perilunate fracture dislocation** results.

Radiocarpal dislocation, or dislocation of the entire carpus from the radius, is often associated with a radial styloid fracture (Fig. 13-2).

Ulnar translocation is another form of a radiocarpal dislocation in which the ligaments between the radius and proximal row are disrupted, allowing the carpus to slide ulnarly on the radius (Fig. 13-3).

Diagnosis and Initial Management

History and Physical Examination

There is pain localized to the wrist, usually after falling onto an outstretched hand. Swelling varies from barely perceptible to significant in the case of a major dislocation. Begin the clinical examination by noting areas of ecchymosis, active range of motion, and neurovascular status. Try to localize tender points over specific bones or ligaments. When dislocated, the wrist appears shortened, with a fullness over the dorsum

FIG. 13-2 Radiocarpal dislocation and fracture of the radial styloid.

FIG. 13-3 Ulnar translocation. The carpus has shifted ulnarly.

or in the carpal tunnel. Any movement will produce pain. Determine if there are signs of median nerve compression.

Scapholunate dissociation is difficult to diagnose clinically. In many cases, no specific traumatic incident can be recalled. There is an area of point tenderness dorsally over the scapholunate joint. Motion may not be restricted much by the pain. In Watson's **clunk test,** the examiner's thumb is placed against the volar aspect of the scaphoid (distal pole), and the other hand is used to move the wrist from ulnar to radial deviation. If there is a scapholunate dissociation, this maneuver forces the scaphoid dorsally out of the scaphoid fossa of the radius, thereby eliciting a painful clunk the examiner can feel.

Radiographic Examination

A minimum of four views of the wrist are obtained: anteroposterior (AP) in neutral, AP in ulnar deviation, oblique, and true lateral.

A series of arcs that are helpful in detecting carpal abnormalities are seen on the AP projection (Fig. 13-4). Arc I is formed by the proximal borders of the scaphoid, lunate, and triquetrum. Arc II is formed by the distal borders of these same three bones. Arc III consists of the proximal borders of the capitate and hamate. Normally, the three arcs form smooth lines; a break in the arc is a sign of fracture, dislocation, or instability.

If carpal instability is suspected, the scapholunate and capitolunate angles are measured. These are determined on the lateral radiograph (Fig. 13-5). To determine the **scapholunate angle,** one line is drawn along the longitudinal axis of the scaphoid and another line is drawn at

FIG. 13-4 Carpal arcs. A break in an arc indicates intercarpal ligament injury, fracture, or dislocation.

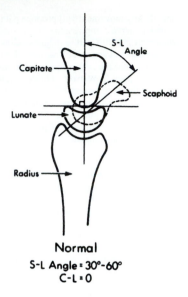

FIG. 13-5   The scapholunate (S-L) and the capitolunate (C-L) angles.

a right angle to a line connecting the dorsal and volar poles of the lunate (essentially bisecting the lunate). The angle between the two lines normally ranges from 30° to 60°. Angles greater than 60° indicate a dorsal intercalated segmental instability (DISI), and angles less than 30° indicate a volar intercalated segmental instability (VISI; Fig. 13-6). The capitolunate angle is formed by a line along the capitate axis and the line bisecting the lunate. This angle should normally be less than 15°; if greater and pointing dorsally, DISI is present, and if pointing volarly, VISI is present.

Radiographic findings of a perilunate dislocation are a triangular lunate on the AP view, loss of parallelism between adjacent articular surfaces of the radius and proximal carpal row, and the head of the capitate dorsal to the lunate on the lateral view. A lunate dislocation is characterized by the absence of the lunate from its fossa on the AP radiograph and displacement of the lunate volarly on the lateral radiograph. A transscaphoid perilunate dislocation is characterized by the signs of a lunate or perilunate dislocation and a fracture of the scaphoid. Distraction films separate the fragments, making the diagnosis more obvious.

VISI

S-L = <30°
C-L = >15°

FIG. 13-6   VISI deformity of the carpus.

The key finding of scapholunate dissociation is a widened space between the scaphoid and lunate seen on the AP view (Fig. 13-7). On the lateral view, there is a more horizontal orientation to the scaphoid and the scapholunate angle is greater than 70°. Comparison views of the uninjured side help in making the diagnosis. When the clinical examination points to a scapholunate dissociation but radiographic signs are equivocal, cineradiographs, or arthrograms, are obtained.

The diagnosis of radiocarpal dislocation is obvious on the lateral view. The lunate and entire carpus are displaced off the radius. On the AP radiograph, there is often a fracture of the radial styloid, and the carpus overrides the distal radius (Fig. 13-2).

The diagnosis of ulnar translocation is made on the AP radiograph (Fig. 13-3). There are two types: (1) the entire carpus is displaced ulnarly off the radius, or (2) the scaphoid remains in place and the rest of the carpus is shifted ulnarly.

Initial Management

Perilunate, lunate, and transscaphoid perilunate dislocations are reduced as soon as possible to minimize the incidence of median nerve in-

FIG. 13-7 Scapholunate dissociation.

jury. Axillary block or intravenous (IV) regional anesthesia provides adequate muscular relaxation, whereas IV sedation or local injection will not. A preliminary period of traction (10 to 15 lbs.) relaxes the muscles. This is an excellent time to take radiographs because the carpal bones are distracted and additional injuries are easier to detect. After 5 to 10 min of traction, the finger traps are removed and the surgeon maintains traction. One thumb is placed over the carpal tunnel to push the lunate back into the lunate fossa. Extension of the wrist followed by gradual palmar flexion allows the head of the capitate to slip back into the concavity of the lunate. A thumb spica plaster splint is applied, with the wrist in neutral with slight plamar flexion. Postreduction films are obtained, the patient is admitted overnight with hourly neurovascular checks, and the arm is elevated and iced.

Radiocarpal dislocation is reduced by using the same technique used for fractures of the distal radius. Plaster splints are applied, and the patient is observed for signs of median nerve compromise. Postreduction films are examined for signs of concomittant injuries, especially carpal instability.

Closed reduction of a **scapholunate dissociation and radioulnar translocation** is usually not possible. The wrist is splinted for comfort until asymptomatic or surgery is performed.

Associated Injuries

The most frequently associated injury is median nerve compromise. This is indicated by the loss of sensation on the palmar surface of the thumb, index and long fingers, and occasionally the inability to oppose the thumb. Loss of median nerve function is an indication for immediate reduction of dislocations or fractures and possible emergent carpal tunnel release.

Other less commonly associated injuries include disruption of the radial or ulnar arteries and injury to the ulnar nerve. These are ruled out by a focused neurovascular examination.

Definitive Management

We percutaneously pin most perilunate and lunate dislocations using fluoroscopy because of the high likelihood of late collapse, even with an adequate initial reduction. A short arm thumb spica cast is applied and split on both sides to allow for swelling. The pins are removed at 8 weeks, and an orthoplast splint is worn for an additional 4 weeks. Range-of-motion exercises are started after pin removal, and strengthening is delayed until the orthoplast splint is removed.

When anatomic reduction is not achieved by closed means, open reduction and internal fixation is performed from an extended carpal tunnel approach. The lunate is located in the carpal canal and reduced through the rent in the volar capsule. Percutaneous pin fixation of the scaphoid and lunate is performed by using fluoroscopy. If an anatomic reduction is not achieved, a dorsal exposure is employed to better visualize the scaphoid and lunate relationship while pins are placed. Pins are placed between the scaphoid and lunate, between the scaphoid and capitate, and usually between the radius and lunate. The tear in the volar capsule is repaired.

Postoperatively, the wrist is immobilized in a thumb spica sugar tong plaster splint. The plaster splint is changed to a short arm thumb spica cast at the time of suture removal in 7 to 10 days. The Kirschner wires are kept in place for 8 to 10 weeks. Range-of-motion exercises are begun after pin removal.

Transscaphoid perilunate dislocation is reduced as described in the section "Initial Management." The adequacy of the scaphoid reduction is carefully assessed on the postreduction radiographs. If there is any doubt, magnetic resonance imaging (MRI) or a computed tomographic (CT) scan is obtained. Pay special attention to DISI instability or a dorsal "hump back" deformity of the scaphoid (apex dorsal angulation at the fracture site). If the reduction is acceptable, a thumb spica cast is applied. Follow-up radiographs are taken weekly for the first 3 weeks. Cast immobilization is maintained until healing of the scaphoid fracture occurs (often several months).

If the scaphoid fracture is displaced more than 1 mm or is angulated, open reduction is performed through a modified Russe approach that can be extended to allow access to the volar wrist capsule. The fracture is stabilized with either Kirschner wires or a screw designed for use in the scaphoid. Radiographs are obtained, and the relationship between the scaphoid and lunate is evaluated. If there is residual malalignment, the Russe approach is extended into a carpal tunnel approach or a separate dorsal approach is added. Kirschner wires are used to stabilize the lunate, capitate, and scaphoid into their normal relationship. When open reduction is performed late, bone grafting of the scaphoid fracture is necessary.

A sugar tong thumb spica splint is applied after wound closure. The postoperative splint is changed to a short arm thumb spica cast at 1 week. Patients are followed at 4-week intervals when the cast is changed and radiographs obtained. If there is no progression toward fracture healing 4 to 6 months after injury, bone grafting is indicated. Kirschner wires are removed after scaphoid fracture healing. Physical therapy, including the use of dynamic splints, is usually necessary.

Closed reduction and pin fixation of **scapholunate dissociations** is performed under image intensification or arthroscopic guidance. Permanent films are obtained, and if the relationship between the scaphoid and lunate is normal, the pins are kept in place for 10 weeks. Range-of-motion exercises are started after pin removal. Ligament healing after closed reduction and pinning of scapholunate dissociation is not always reliable, and carpal malalignment may later recur. For this reason, we usually prefer open scapholunate ligament repair and a dorsal capsulodesis procedure.

The scapholunate ligament is repaired through a dorsal approach. The ligament is usually found to be torn off the scaphoid. Mini-suture anchors containing nonabsorbable sutures are attached to the scaphoid. The suture is passed through the ligament ends by using a mattress suture technique. The scaphoid and lunate are placed into anatomic alignment and held with Kirschner wires. The sutures are tied down. A strip of dorsal capsule 1 cm wide based over Lister's tubercle is attached to the scaphoid along the dorsal surface distal to the midpoint of rotation (Blatt capsulodesis). Postoperative treatment is the same as that for a perilunate dislocation.

Radiocarpal dislocation is managed with closed reduction unless there is an associated carpal instability, in which case open reduction, Kirschner wire fixation, and primary ligament repair of both palmar and dorsal ligaments are performed. Isolated palmar radiocarpal dislocation is almost invariably associated with postreduction instability.

Treatment options for **ulnar translocation** are reduction and ligament repair or radiocarpal arthrodesis.

Complications

The complication unique to dislocations of the carpal bones is late instability. After the lunate is reduced, DISI may occur because of the loss of the stabilization provided by the scaphoid and/or the scapholunate ligament. Left uncorrected, the DISI pattern leads to progressive intercarpal arthritis. A similar instability pattern, VISI, is seen on the volar side of the wrist. In this case, forces first destabilize the lunotriquetral articulation. This less common form of wrist instability also results in arthritis but not as rapidly as with the DISI deformity.

FRACTURES

Fractures of the wrist occur in isolation or in combination with other fractures and dislocations. The scaphoid is the most commonly fractured carpal bone, followed in order of frequency by the triquetrum, lunate, capitate, pisiform, and the other carpal bones.

Classification

Scaphoid fractures are classified according to whether they are displaced and the location of the fracture. The mechanism of injury is that, during wrist hyperextension, the dorsal rim of the radius is driven into the scaphoid waist, simultaneously tensile stresses are developed on the volar surface of the scaphoid, and a fracture results. The scaphoid tends to open up dorsally and compress the volar surfaces together, gradually assuming the "humpback" deformity, which is associated with an increased likelihood of nonunion. There are displaced and undisplaced fractures of the proximal pole, waist, and distal pole. Displaced fractures include any fracture with larger than 1 mm step-off on the AP view, an intrascaphoid angle greater than 45° seen on lateral tomograms or CT (normal is 30° or less), or the presence of an associated carpal instability pattern.

Triquetral Fractures

The most common triquetral fracture is an avulsion off the dorsal surface. These are best seen on the lateral view. Fractures of the triquetral body also occur.

Lunate Fractures

Fractures of the lunate are uncommon unless associated with Kienbock's disease. There are two types of acute lunate fractures: lunate body fractures and rim fractures.

Lunate body fractures are the result of either a compression force applied to the wrist or the normal compressive forces from the capitate head pressing on an avascular lunate in Kienbock's disease. It is often difficult to assess displacement on plain radiographs, and CT is recommended.

Dorsal and volar rim fractures of the lunate occur in association with other wrist injuries, especially perilunate dislocations. Most of these injuries are small and best left alone unless they become symptomatic. If the fracture involves a significant portion of the lunate articular surface, open reduction and internal fixation is indicated.

Capitate Fractures

Fractures of the neck of the capitate occur either in isolation or in association with other injuries. They are displaced or undisplaced. Capitate neck fractures may occur in association with a transscaphoid perilunate dislocation (scaphocapitate syndrome).

Pisiform Fractures

The pisiform is a sesamoid bone located within the flexor carpi ilnaris tendon and has an articulation with the hamate. Fractures of the pisiform occur due to direct trauma, usually from a fall. These fractures are best visualized radiographically on the oblique view. Displaced fractures of the articular surface may lead to painful arthritis of the pisohamate joint.

Other Carpal Fractures

Fractures have been described for all of the carpal bones. In general, fractures that involve significant portions of the body of a bone or articular surface should be carefully evaluated for displacement. Fractures of the hook of the hamate require a high index of suspicion to find, especially in patients with repetitive trauma (e.g., using a jackhammer) or a sudden blow to the palm of the hand (e.g., a baseball bat or errant golf swing).

Associated Injuries

Intercarpal dislocations and ligamentous injuries are frequently associated with displaced fractures of the carpus. These injuries are ruled out with the appropriate radiographic studies. Neurovascular injuries are rare but are ruled out with a focused examination.

Diagnosis and Initial Management

History and Physical Examination

There is wrist pain with point tenderness directly over the involved bone. The scaphoid is the most commonly fractured carpal bone. Scaphoid fractures are frequently seen in young men. The physical findings unique to scaphoid fractures are pain: with thumb pinch, on palpation of the proximal pole in the snuffbox, and on palpation of the distal pole on the volar surface of the wrist.

Radiographic Examination

A minimum of four views are obtained: AP with the wrist in neutral, AP with the wrist in ulnar deviation, oblique, and true lateral. Special scaphoid views are obtained by angulating the wrist 20° to bring the long axis of the scaphoid parallel to the x-ray cassette and perpendicular to the x-ray beam as described by Stecher. Other tests that are useful in establishing the diagnosis of a fracture of a carpal bone are bone scans, CT, and the MRI.

Fractures of a hook of the hamate may occasionally be seen on a carpal tunnel view. However, if these views are negative and the patient has localizing tenderness, an MRI should be obtained.

Nonunions are distinguished from acute fractures on plain films by resorption or cyst formation, sclerosis at the fracture site, displacement of the fracture, and dorsal angulation.

Initial Management

The key initial decision is whether the fracture will be managed with closed methods or surgery. If closed methods are to be used, the initial management is the definitive management. If the fracture is to be managed with surgery, a thumb spica splint is applied, with the wrist elevated and iced. If the physical examination is suspicious for a fracture but the x-rays are negative, a thumb spica splint is applied and repeat radiographs are obtained in 2 weeks. If the radiographs are still negative and the clinical examination remains suspicious for a fracture, a bone scan or MRI is obtained.

Definitive Management

Scaphoid Fractures

Nondisplaced scaphoid fractures are managed with a long arm thumb spica cast, with the wrist in neutral for the first 4 weeks, followed by a short arm thumb spica cast until healing occurs. The only exception is a tuberosity fracture, which will heal in a short arm cast. The cast is changed every 4 weeks, and radiographs are obtained out of plaster. Immobilization is continued until there is bony bridging across the fracture. CT scans are helpful when there is any question about union.

Open reduction through a Russe approach and fixation with Kirschner wires or a Herbert screw is indicated for displaced fractures. Arthroscopic reduction and pinning is only recommended for those surgeons with extensive arthroscopic experience. Bone grafting is not necessary in acute fractures unless there is comminution, in which case graft is usually obtained from the distal radius. The wrist is immobilized in a short arm thumb spica cast until union occurs. Wires are removed in the office, and screws are removed only if they become symptomatic. The use of a Herbert screw is technically challenging even for those with extensive experience and has little to recommend it over Kirschner wires.

Triquetral fractures are managed in a short arm cast until asymptomatic, usually 2 to 4 weeks. Fractures of the triquetral body occur with more extreme trauma. If significantly displaced, body fractures are managed with open reduction and fixation.

Displaced **lunate body fractures** are managed with open reduction and fixation. Fractures of the dorsal or volar rim, if small and not associated with other injuries such as perilunate dislocation, are managed for 4 to 6 weeks with a short arm cast extending to the metacarpalphalangeal joints. Rim fractures involving a significant portion of the articular surface are managed with open reduction and fixation.

Nondisplaced **capitate neck fractures** are managed with cast immobilization but are followed with frequent radiographs to ensure that displacement does not occur. Displaced neck fractures are managed with anatomic reduction and fixation, usually through a dorsal approach.

Pisiform fractures are managed with splinting initially. If symptomatic due to nonunion or pisohamate arthritis, the pisiform is excised.

Other **carpal fractures** with significant displacement of the articular surface are managed with open reduction and internal fixation. Avulsion fractures usually indicate a ligament injury and are managed with immobilization until healed. When diagnosed and treated within the first week after injury, fractures of the hook of the hamate can heal with a short arm cast. Symptomatic, ununited fractures of the hook of the hamate are excised.

Complications

The complications most frequently encountered following fracture of one of the bones of the carpus are arthritis, nonunion, and avascular necrosis.

Arthritis is initially managed conservatively with activity restriction, splinting, and nonsteroidal antiinflammatory medications. If arthritis is sufficiently symptomatic, management with arthrodesis of the joint involved (i.e., a limited intercarpal arthrodesis) or full wrist arthrodesis may salvage the situation.

Nonunion and avascular necrosis are not uncommon problems following a fracture of the scaphoid (Fig. 13-8). Ten percent of all acute scaphoid fractures will go on to a nonunion. Factors associated with increased likelihood of nonunion include delayed initial diagnosis, initial displacement or angulation, and proximal pole fractures. Important considerations in the treatment of scaphoid nonunion include preservation of blood supply, bone grafting of the nonunion site, internal fixation for stability, correction of humpback deformity, and associated carpal instability.

Symptomatic scaphoid nonunion associated with advanced arthritis has no management options that will restore normal function and is best

FIG. 13-8   Nonunion of the scaphoid.

treated with a salvage procedure. Options include a fascial interposition arthroplasty, four-corner fusion with scaphoid excision, proximal row carpectomy, and wrist fusion.

SELECTED READINGS

Adkison JW, Chapman MW: Treatment of acute lunate and perilunate dislocations. *Clin Orthop* 164:199–207, 1982.

Gilula LA, Destouet JM, Weeks PM, Young LV, Wray RC: Roentgenographic diagnosis of the painful wrist. *Clin Orthop* 187:52–64, 1984.

Herbert TJ, Fisher WE: Management of the fractured scaphoid using a new bone screw. *J Bone Joint Surg* 66B:114–123, 1984.

Howard RF, Slawski BP, Gilula LA: Isolated palmar radiocarpal dislocation and ulnar translocation. *J Hand Surg* 22A:78–82, 1997.

Lavernia CJ, Cohen MS, Taleisnik J: Treatment of scapholunate dissociation by ligamentous repair and capsulodesis. *J Hand Surg* 17A:354–359, 1992.

Mayfield JK, Johnson RP, Kilcoyne RK: Carpal dislocations: Pathomechanics and progressive perilunar instability. *J Hand Surg* 5:226–241, 1980.

Stecher WR: Roentgenography of the carpal navicular bone. *AJR* 37:704–705, 1937.

14 | Fractures and Dislocations of the Metacarpals and Phalanges

Mark Gonzalez

This chapter covers fractures and fracture dislocations of the metacarpals and phalanges.

ANATOMY

The **metacarpals 2 through 5** have an expanded cuboidal base, with facets for articulation with the carpus and neighboring metacarpals. Dorsal and palmar intermetacarpal ligaments and interosseous ligaments stabilize these articulations. The first **carpometacarpal joint** (CMC) is a biconcave saddle joint stabilized primarily by the anterior oblique ligament and the intermetacarpal ligament.

The **metacarpal phalangeal joints** (MCP) are complex hinge joints that allow medial and lateral movement when they are fully extended. The volar aspect of these joints is supported by a volar plate. The collateral ligaments are medial and lateral to the joints and are the primary medial and lateral stabilizers. The metacarpal head is cam shaped, and the collaterals are under maximal stretch in flexion. The MCP joint is safely splinted in 70° to 90° of flexion. The cam effect of the metacarpal head maintains collateral ligament length and prevents an extension contracture (Figs. 14-1 and 14-2). The MCP joint of the thumb is structurally similar to the other MCP joints, but its intrinsic muscles (adductor pollicis, abductor pollicis brevis, and flexor pollicis brevis) and three extrinsic tendons (flexor pollicis longus, extensor pollicis brevis, and extensor pollicis longus) are dynamic stabilizers. The thumb is splinted to avoid contracture of these intrinsic muscles (i.e., the first web space).

Proximal and middle phalanges have a slight apex dorsal curve. The **proximal and distal interphalangeal joints** (PIP and DIP) are true hinge joints. Stabilizing ligaments are similar to those of the MCP joint, but unlike the MCP joints there is no side to side motion. The PIP joints are splinted in 0° to 10° flexion, thereby preventing the development of checkrein ligaments about the volar plate and a flexion contracture.

The **extensor hood** is dorsal to the PIP joint; its central slip inserts on the middle phalanx and the lateral bands form the DIP joint extensor. The flexor digitorum sublimis (FDS) inserts on the middle phalanx, and the flexor digitorum profundus (FDP) inserts on the distal phalanx.

FRACTURES OF THE METACARPALS

Classification

Fractures of the metacarpals are classified as involving: the base, the diaphysis, the neck, or the head. Additional factors that influence man-

FIGS. 14-1 and 14-2   The cam shape of the metacarpal head results in the collateral ligaments being stretched maximally when the MCP joint is flexed.

agement are whether the fracture is open, closed, or the result of a high energy injury, and whether more than one metacarpal is fractured.

Fractures of the **metacarpal bases** are frequently associated with dorsal subluxation of the CMC joint (Fig. 14-3). This is particularly true of fractures of the base of the fifth metacarpal, which are displaced proximally by the extensor carpi ulnaris (Fig. 14-4).

Metacarpal neck fractures, also known as **boxer's fractures,** are due to a volarly directed force to the metacarpal head. The intrinsics maintain the fracture in a flexed position.

FIG. 14-3 Dorsal dislocation of the fifth MCP joint and a fracture of the base of the fourth metacarpal.

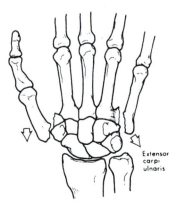

Extensor carpi ulnaris

FIG. 14-4 Fracture with subluxation of the base of the fifth metacarpal and Bennet fracture of the first metacarpal.

Fractures of the **metacarpal head** are due to avulsion of a collateral ligament or to impaction from a longitudinal blow. Fracture of the metacarpal head due to impaction of a tooth during a fist fight is also known as a **fight bite** and is particularly likely to become infected.

Diagnosis and Initial Management

History and Physical Examination

There is pain localized to the area of injury and a history of trauma. Deformity and swelling may be present. In particular, correct rotational alignment must be confirmed or malalignment detected. Digital scissoring may occur in spiral fractures of the metacarpal diaphysis, and it is essential to flex the injured MCP joint and observe rotational alignment of the nail bed to check for this deformity. It will not be evident on x-ray.

Radiographic Examination

Anteroposterior, lateral, and oblique views of the hand are obtained. A 30° pronation anteroposterior view of the fifth CMC joints allows visualization of subluxation of this joint. Computed tomography (CT) may help in the evaluation of the CMC joints.

Initial Management

Initial management of a metacarpal fracture is reduction if the fracture is displaced and immobilization in a splint. The splint extends from the DIP joints to the elbow. The position of immobilization is: the MCP joints flexed to 90°, the PIP joints extended, and the wrist dorsiflexed to 20°. In cases in which reduction is required, a hematoma block is administered.

Fracture dislocations of the **base of the metacarpals** are reduced by longitudinal traction and pressing the metacarpals volarly. Fractures of the metacarpal diaphysis and neck are angulated with the apex dorsal. **Diaphyseal fractures** are reduced with longitudinal traction and application of pressure to the apex of the deformity. **Spiral fractures** of the diaphysis are often underestimated. They require immobilization with the MCP joints flexed so that rotational deformity does not occur. **Boxer's fractures** are reduced by flexing the MCP and PIP joints and by pushing the proximal phalanx dorsally while maintaining volar pressure on the metacarpal. Fractures of the **metacarpal head** usually do not require closed reduction and are splinted.

Associated Injuries

A wound over the metacarpal head should raise suspicions of a fight bite. Because of the likelihood of infection, these injuries should be surgically explored for impaction fractures of the metacarpal head and then thoroughly irrigated. There are no other injuries specifically associated with metacarpal fractures and dislocations.

Definitive Management

Most metacarpal fractures are managed with splinting for 3 to 6 weeks. Immobilization is discontinued when there are clinical (i.e., absence of pain at the fracture site) and radiographic signs of healing. There are specific indications for surgery for each type of metacarpal fracture.

An unstable or less than anatomic reduction of fractures of the **metacarpal bases** are indications for operative reduction and pinning. The fracture is either reduced under direct vision through a dorsal incision or reduced with the aid of fluoroscopy. Kirschner wires are driven across the fracture, into an adjacent metacarpal, or into the carpus. Postoperatively, the hand is splinted for 3 to 6 weeks, when the wires are removed. During this time, the splint is removed daily for range-of-motion exercises of the PIP and MCP joints.

Indications for internal fixation of fractures of the **metacarpal diaphysis** are shortening of more than 3 mm, rotation resulting in digital scissoring when the MCP joints are flexed, dorsal angulation of the fourth and fifth metacarpals greater than 40°, dorsal angulation of the second and third greater than 10°, multiple metacarpal fractures (because of instability), and gunshot wounds or crush injuries with comminution and loss of bone. The fracture is reduced closed under fluoroscopy or exposed through a dorsal incision. Fractures reduced closed are stabilized with percutaneous Kirschner wires. Screws, plates, cerclage wires, interosseous wires, and intramedullary wires are used to stabilize fractures that have been opened and reduced. Fractures with a deficient or contaminated soft tissue envelope are managed with external fixation, wires, or polymethylmethacrylate spacers prior to the definitive reconstruction. Postoperatively, simple fractures are immobilized 6 weeks, the splint is removed daily for range-of-motion exercises, and the pins are removed at 6 to 8 weeks. Postoperative management of fractures with loss of bone and severe soft tissue injury is individualized.

Indications for internal fixation of fractures of the **metacarpal neck** are rotational deformity resulting in digital scissoring and excessive apex dorsal angulation. Up to 40° of angulation in the fourth and fifth and up to 10° in the second and third metacarpals are acceptable. More angulation is acceptable in the fourth and fifth metacarpals because the second and third CMC joints are more rigid, and significant angulation results in a prominent metacarpal head and painful grasp. The fracture is reduced closed under fluoroscopy and stabilized with percutaneous Kirschner wires driven into an adjacent metacarpal or used as intramedullary rods and inserted through the MCP joint. When inserted through the MCP joint, they are left long, and the MCP joint is maintained in flexion until the fracture heals (usually 4 to 6 weeks), when the pins are removed.

Undisplaced fractures of the **metacarpal head** are splinted, as described in the section "Initial Management," for 3 weeks. Fractures with large displaced intraarticular fragments are exposed through a dorsal incision, reduced, and stabilized with Kirschner wires, a Herbert screw, or intraosseous wires. Comminuted fractures that cannot be reduced are managed with distraction in an external fixator.

Ligamentous avulsions of the collaterals are managed with buddy taping. Collateral avulsion with bony displacement of more than 5 mm is managed with open reduction and pinning. **Fight bites** are always opened through a dorsal incision, debrided, and irrigated. Postoperatively, systemic antibiotics are administered a minimum of 2 weeks.

Complications

Complications include malunion, nonunion, and tendon adhesions. **Malunion** is managed with osteotomy and internal fixation. **Nonunion** is managed with stable fixation and bone grafting. **Adhesions** are managed initially with intensive physical therapy and surgical release, if necessary. Silicone arthroplasty and MCP fusion are salvage procedures and are only considered if there are no alternatives.

FRACTURES AND DISLOCATIONS OF THE PHALANGES

Fractures of the phalanges are classified as involving the base of the proximal phalanx, the diaphysis of the proximal or middle phalanx, PIP joint, DIP joint, or distal phalanx. Dislocations are of the MCP, PIP, or DIP joints.

Fracture of the **base of the proximal phalanx** is due to avulsion of the collateral ligament or impaction by the metacarpal head.

Fracture of the **diaphysis of the proximal or middle phalanx** is caused by a direct blow or torsion.

Fractures of the proximal phalanx have apex volar angulation secondary to the pull of the interossei. Deforming forces on the middle phalanx are the FDS tendon and the long extensor tendon. Distal fractures of the middle phalanx tend to have apex volar angulation; proximal fractures tend to have apex dorsal angulation.

Fractures of the **PIP joint** involve the proximal or middle phalanx. Fractures of the proximal phalanx are undisplaced, unicondylar, or bicondylar and comminuted.

Fractures of the base of the middle phalanx are undisplaced fractures, volar or dorsal lip fractures, lateral avulsions, and comminuted.

Fractures of the **DIP joint** involve either the head of the middle phalanx or the base of the distal phalanx. Fractures of the dorsal lip of the distal phalanx, or *mallet finger,* are caused by avulsion of the extensor tendon. Fractures of the volar lip of the distal phalanx are caused by avulsion of the FDP tendon or volar plate during hyperextension. FDP avulsions occur in contact sports such as rugby or football and most often involve the fourth finger.

Distal phalangeal fractures are caused by a direct blow and are longitudinal, transverse, or comminuted.

Dislocations of the **MCP and DIP joints** are usually dorsal and caused by hyperextension. Dislocations of the PIP joint are most commonly dorsal but can also be volar and can be associated with a rotatory component.

Diagnosis and Initial Management

History and Physical Examination

There is a history of trauma, and there is pain localized to the area of injury. There may be swelling and deformity. Malrotation, which can result in digital scissoring, will be evident by flexing the MCP joints while keeping the PIP joint extended or by checking the rotation of the nail bed. Dimpling of the skin associated with a dislocation indicates that reduction may not be possible by closed means.

Radiographic Examination

Anteroposterior, lateral, and oblique radiographs define the injury. Other studies are not necessary.

Initial Management

The majority of fractures of the phalanx are managed with closed methods. Buddy taping is used for fractures of the proximal and middle phalanges, which do not require reduction. In cases in which reduction is performed, a hematoma block or digital block is administered. Immobilization of reduced fractures of the proximal phalanx is done with a splint extending from the metacarpal heads to the elbow and an alumafoam extension for the involved digit. The wrist is immobilized in 20° of dorsiflexion, the MCP joint in 90° of flexion, and the PIP and IP joints in extension. Fractures of the PIP joint and distal phalanx are immobilized in an alumafoam splint.

Definitive Management

Small avulsion fractures of the **base of the proximal phalanx** are managed with buddy taping and early protected motion. Fragments comprising more than 30% of the articular surface are exposed through volar or dorsal incisions, depending on location, and fixed with small Kirschner wires, interosseous wires, or screws. **Impaction** fractures are managed with reduction of the joint surface, bone grafting to elevate depressed articular segments, and fixation of the joint surface to the diaphysis. The MCP joint is immobilized at 90° to "mold" the fracture to the shape of the metacarpal head. Motion is started at 3 to 5 weeks. When a comminuted impaction fracture cannot be reduced and stabilized, traction through the proximal phalanx maintains reduction and allows motion.

Undisplaced fractures of the **diaphysis of the proximal and middle phalanges** are managed with buddy taping.

Displaced fractures are managed with closed reduction and splinting. Up to 15° of angulation in the plane of motion is well tolerated. Rotational deformity results in digital scissoring, and angulation in the coronal plane results in spaces between the fingers when cupping the hand. "Bayoneting" of the fragments results in a prominent spike, causing soft tissue impingement and limiting motion.

Failure to maintain reduction, open fractures, and injuries with multiple fractures are indications for operative reduction and stabilization. Reduction is open through a dorsal incision or closed with fluoroscopy. Fixation is done with Kirschner wires, interosseous wires, screws, plates, or external fixators. Postoperatively, immobilization is maintained for 3 to 5 weeks, when vigorous range-of-motion exercises are initiated.

Undisplaced fractures of the **PIP joint** (proximal or middle phalanx) are managed with buddy taping. Displaced unicondylar or bicondylar fractures of the proximal phalanx are reduced open and stabilized. The surgical exposure splits the extensor tendon, thereby preserving the attachment of the central tendon on the middle phalanx. Stabilization is done with Kirschner wires, interosseous wires, or screws. Barton (1984) described an excellent extraarticular method of reduction and fixation of oblique unicondylar fractures. Comminuted fractures are managed with an external fixator or with dynamic traction.

Displaced **volar lip** fractures involving more than 30% of the joint surface are often associated with joint instability. They are exposed through a volar incision, the A-3 pulley is opened, flexor tendons are retracted, and the fragment is reduced and stabilized with Kirschner wires. Alternatively, comminuted fragments are excised, and the volar plate is advanced into the defect. The joint is pinned for 3 weeks, when protected motion is begun. Agee (1978) described a force coupling device for maintaining joint reduction while allowing motion. Fractures of the dorsal lip are rare and represent avulsion of the central slip of the extensor tendon. Displacement of more than 2 mm results in an extensor lag or Boutonniere deformity. If more than 30% of the articular surface is involved, the joint may be unstable. Exposure is through a dorsal approach, and stabilization is done with Kirschner wires or a pullout stitch tied over a volar button. Displaced lateral avulsion fractures are the result of collateral ligament avulsion. They are opened, reduced, and stabilized with Kirschner wires.

The **comminuted** fracture of the middle phalangeal base is similar to a pilon fracture. Up to four fragments can be reduced and stabilized with Kirschner wires or screws. Collapse of the joint surface requires elevation and bone graft. Severely comminuted fractures are managed with an external fixator or dynamic skeletal traction.

Fractures of the **DIP joint** involve the head of the middle phalanx or the base of the distal phalanx. Intraarticular fractures of the head of the middle phalanx are similar to condylar fractures of the proximal phalanx. Undisplaced fractures of the head of the middle phalanx are managed with splinting or buddy taping. Displaced fractures are pinned percutaneously or reduced open and pinned. The DIP joint is immobilized for 6 weeks, but the PIP joint is left unsplinted. A fracture of the **dorsal lip of the distal phalanx,** or **mallet finger,** is an avulsion of the extensor tendon. Most are managed with immobilization of the DIP joint in hyperextension for 6 weeks. Fractures comprising more than 30% of the articular surface may be reduced open and pinned through a dorsal incision, but there is a high rate of complication including stiffness. Most authors have recommended open reduction only for those fractures associated with subluxation of the joint. The joint is pinned for 6 weeks. Volar lip fractures that are FDP avulsions are explored, and the tendon is repaired or the fragment of bone is reduced and stabilized with a pullout wire or small-diameter Kirschner wires.

Undisplaced transverse tuft fractures of the **distal phalanx** are splinted. Displaced fractures are often associated with a soft tissue laceration and are pinned if unstable.

Longitudinal fractures may be intraarticular and, when displaced, are pinned percutaneously with the aid of fluoroscopy or under direct vision.

Dislocation of the MCP joint is most commonly dorsal and can be recognized with hyperextension of the digit. This can be reduced by distal- and volar-based pressure on the base of the proximal phalanx. Irreducible dislocation is caused by detachment of the proximal volar plate and interposition of the volar plate between the metacarpal head and base of the proximal phalanx. The digit is in slight hyperextension, and often the volar skin is puckered by the pull of the entrapped volar plate. Operative reduction can be through a volar or dorsal incision. The volar plate is divided longitudinally through the dorsal incision, allowing the metacarpal head to reduce. To affect reduction through the volar approach, the A-1 pulley is divided, allowing the tendon to be retracted and permitting the volar plate and proximal phalanx to fall into their reduced position.

Dislocation of the PIP joint is most commonly dorsal but can also occur volarly. Dorsal dislocation is associated with avulsion of the volar plate and is usually stable. This can be treated with immobilization or extension block splinting for 1 to 2 weeks. Unstable dorsal dislocations with volar fractures can be treated with extension block splinting for 3 to 4 weeks, extension block pinning, or open reduction of a large fragment. In extension block pinning, a Kirschner wire is placed through the head of the proximal phalanx, temporarily blocking extension.

Volar dislocation of the **PIP** joint can be straight volar or with a rotatory component. Straight volar dislocations usually involve avulsion of the central slip. Reduction is performed with gentle traction, and the **PIP joint** is splinted in hyperextension for 6 weeks to avoid a Boutonniere deformity. Rotatory dislocation of the **PIP joint** most frequently involves buttonholing of the condyle of the proximal phalanx between the central slip and lateral band. This can be irreducible, and open reduction is necessary to extricate the lateral band from the joint and reduce the entrapped condyle.

Dislocations of the **DIP** joint are generally dorsal and are reduced with gentle traction. Irreducible dislocations are rare and are associated with interposition of the volar plate or flexor tendon. Surgery is necessary to extricate the interposed structure.

Complications

Complications of phalangeal fractures and dislocations include malunion, nonunion, and stiffness. These are managed with osteotomy, stabilization with bone grafting, and aggressive physical therapy. Occasionally, symptomatic loss of motion will require a soft tissue release.

FRACTURES OF THE THUMB

There are two injuries unique to the first ray, or thumb: fractures of the base of the metacarpal and gamekeeper's thumb. Other fractures of the first ray are managed as their counterparts in the second through fifth rays.

Fractures of the base of the first metacarpal are classified as a Bennet fracture, Rolando fracture, or an extraarticular fracture. **Bennet fracture** is a fracture dislocation. The volar lip fragment is held by the anterior oblique ligament and varies in size. The metacarpal is subluxed radially, proximally, and dorsally by the pull of the adductor pollicus brevis and the abductor pollicus longus (Fig. 14-4). **Rolando fracture** is a comminuted fracture of the base of the first metacarpal. Extraarticular fractures of the base of the first metacarpal are usually transverse fractures within 1 cm of the articular surface.

Gamekeeper's thumb is an avulsion of the ulnar collateral of the first MCP joint. The collateral ligament often is torn in midsubstance, allowing the adductor to become interposed between the ends. This produces the Stener lesion (Figs. 14-5 and 14-6). Less commonly, the collateral ligament is avulsed from the proximal phalanx with an osteocartilaginous fragment of articular surface.

Diagnosis and Initial Management

History and Physical Examination

There is a history of injury to the thumb and pain localized to the area of injury. An x-ray of the injured MCP joint should be obtained prior to stressing the joint to avoid displacing a nondisplaced fracture. Stressing of the MCP joint with an ulnar opening of 10° to 15° greater than the unaffected side is indicative of an ulnar collateral avulsion.

FIGS. 14-5 and 14-6   Gamekeeper's thumb and the Stener lesion.

Radiographic Examination

Anteroposterior and lateral radiographs are obtained. Stress views of the first MCP joint can be diagnostic of gamekeeper's thumb.

Initial Management

Initial management is splinting.

Definitive Management

Bennet fracture is reduced closed under fluoroscopy with longitudinal traction, abduction, and pronation. Reduction is stabilized with percutaneous pinning. The first metacarpal is pinned to the carpus or to the second metacarpal. It is not necessary to transfix the small volar fragment as long as reduction is maintained. Fragments comprising more than 30% of the articular surface are reduced and pinned to ensure maintenance of reduction of the articular surface. Postoperatively, the hand is splinted from the first IP joint to the elbow for 4 weeks, when the pins are removed.

Rolando fracture is reduced open through a hockey-stick incision of the volar side of the MCP joint. The fracture is reduced, and Kirschner wires or small screws are used to stabilize the fragments. Comminuted Rolando fractures are not amenable to open reduction. A well-molded cast or percutaneous pinning of the metacarpal shaft to the second metacarpal can maintain length and an approximate reduction. Postoperatively, the hand is splinted from the first IP joint to the elbow for 4 weeks.

Extraarticular fractures are managed with closed reduction and casting for 4 to 5 weeks. Reduction is obtained by longitudinal traction and pronation of the distal fragment. Fifteen degrees of angulation is acceptable.

Gamekeeper's thumb is managed with open repair of the ulnar collateral ligament through an ulnar incision. The ligament is repaired, and bony avulsions are reduced and stabilized with Kirschner wires, a pullout wire, or screws. Postoperatively, the hand is splinted from the IP joint to the elbow for 4 weeks for bony avulsions and 6 weeks for ligament repairs.

Complications

The most common complication of Bennet and Rolando fractures is MCC joint arthritis. **MCC** arthritis is managed conservatively with nonsteroidal antiinflammatory drugs and local steroid injections. If these measures fail, the joint is arthrodesed. The most common complication of gamekeeper's thumb is instability of the MCP joint due to failure of repair. It is managed with ligamentous reconstruction with a tendon graft or **MCP joint** arthrodesis.

SELECTED READINGS

Agee JM: Unstable dislocation of the proximal interphalangeal joint of the fingers: A preliminary report of a new treatment technique. *J Hand Surg* 3:386–389, 1978.

Barton MJ: Fractures of the hand. *J Bone Joint Surg* 66B:159–167, 1984.

Becton JL, Christian JD Jr, Goodwin HN, Jackson JG: Simplified technique for treating the complex dislocation of the index metacarpal–phalangeal joint. *J Bone Joint Surg* 57A:698–700, 1975.

Burkhalter WE: Closed treatment of hand fractures. *J Hand Surg* 14A:390–393, 1989.

Dinowitz M, Trumble T, Hanel D, Vedder N, Gilbert M: Failure of cast immobilization for thumb ulnar collateral ligament avulsion fractures. *J Hand Surg* 22A:1057–1063, 1997.

Eaton RG, Malerich MM: Volar plate arthroplasty for the proximal interphalangeal joint. A ten year review. *J Hand Surg* 5:260–268, 1980.

Gonzalez MH, McKay W, Hall RF Jr: Low velocity gunshot wounds of the metacarpal: treatment by early stable fixation and bone grafting. *J Hand Surg* 18A:267, 1993.

Hastings H II, Carroll C IV: Treatment of closed articular fractures of the metacarpophalangeal and proximal interphalangeal joints. *Hand Clin* 4:503–527, 1988.

Lubahn JD: Mallet finger fractures: a comparison of open and closed technique. *J Hand Surg* 14A:394, 1989.

Mueller JJ: Carpometacarpal dislocations: report of five cases and review of the literature. *J Hand Surg* 11A:184–188, 1986.

Parsons SW, Fitzgerald JAW, Shearer JR: External fixation of unstable metacarpal and phalangeal fractures. *J Hand Surg* 17B:151–155, 1992.

Pellegrini VD Jr: Fractures at the base of the thumb. *Hand Clin* 4:87–102, 1988.

Schneider LH: Fractures of the distal phalanx. *Hand Clin* 4:537–547, 1988.

Stern PJ, Roman RJ, Kiefhaber TR, McDonough JJ: Pilon fractures of the proximal interphalangeal joint. *J Hand Surg* 16A:844–850, 1991.

Weiss AP, Hastings H II: Distal unicondylar fractures of the proximal phalanx. *J Hand Surg* 18A:594–599, 1993.

15 | Fractures and Dislocations of the Spine

Lawrence G. Lenke   *Michael F. O'Brien*
Keith H. Bridwell

Spinal trauma includes injuries occurring in the axial skeleton from the occipital-cervical junction to the coccyx. The anatomic classification of spinal trauma is organized into upper cervical, subaxial cervical, thoracic and lumbar, and sacral injuries. The pathophysiology of spinal trauma and the initial assessment of a patient with a suspected spinal injury are similar for all patients.

When presented with a spinal injury, the key questions are: What is the mechanism of injury? Are there other injuries, including life-threatening injuries? What are the injured anatomic structures of the spine? Is there actual or impending neurologic damage? Can the spine function as a weight-bearing column? What is the best treatment method (operative or nonoperative) for the particular fracture? The most important decision initially is whether definitive management should be operative or nonoperative.

ANATOMY

The function of the spine as a support column is broken down into the four anatomical segments: cervical, thoracic, lumbar, and sacrococcygeal. Normally, these segments align in a linear fashion in the coronal or frontal plane. However, in the sagittal plane, there are approximately 25° of cervical lordosis, 35° of thoracic kyphosis, and approximately 50° of lumbar lordosis, thereby allowing the skull to align directly over the midportion of the top of the sacrum.

The cross-sectional anatomy of the spine is organized into **three columns** (Fig. 15-1). The **anterior column** consists of the anterior longitudinal ligament, anterior half of the vertebral body, annulus fibrosis, and disc. The **middle column** consists of the posterior one-half of the vertebral body, annulus, disc, and posterior longitudinal ligament. The **posterior column** includes the facet joints, ligamentum flavum, posterior elements, and interconnecting ligaments.

The three-column theory of the spine produces a basic classification system of spinal injuries. Thus, spinal injuries are classified into four different categories dependent on the specific column(s) injured: compression fractures, burst fractures, seat-belt-type flexion–distraction injuries, and fracture–dislocations (Table 15-1). **Compression fractures** are characterized by failure of the anterior column under compression, with an intact middle and posterior columns. When the anterior and middle columns fail under axial-loading forces, a **burst fracture** is produced. Distraction of the middle and posterior column produces a seat-belt type of **flexion–distraction** injury. **Fracture–dislocations** are

187

POSTERIOR

MIDDLE

ANTERIOR

FIG. 15-1   The three columns of the spine.

TABLE 15-1 Classification of Spinal Injuries

| | Columns injured | | |
Type of injury	Anterior	Middle	Posterior
I Compression fractures	yes	no	no
II Burst fractures	yes	yes	no
III Flexion–distraction injuries	yes/no	yes	yes
IV Fracture–dislocations	yes	yes	yes

characterized by involvement of all three columns in compression, distraction, rotation, and/or shear.

Although the three-column theory of the spine provides an excellent model to describe the individual spinal segments injured, it is essential to determine the overall structural stability of the spine. For example, compression injuries to the anterior and/or middle column may cause kyphosis. Because spinal injuries result from a combination of various forces acting on the spinal column, including compression, distraction, axial load, rotation, torsion, or shear, careful attention is paid to alignment in the coronal and sagittal planes to identify potential subluxation or dislocations of the spine.

Osseous Anatomy

The **cervical spine** comprises the first seven vertebrae and connects the skull to the thoracic spine. The cervical spine functions to protect the spinal cord and nerve roots while supporting the skull and allowing flexibility to position the head. Approximately one-half of the neck flexion–extension occurs between the base of the skull and C1. Similarly, half of the rotation of the head on the neck occurs at the C1-to-C2 articulation. The remaining motions of flexion, extension, rotation, and side-bending occur between the C2-to-T1 articulations.

The atlas (C1) and the axis (C2) differ markedly in structure from the lower five cervical vertebrae (C3 through C7). The atlas is unique among vertebrae in that it has no vertebral body but a thick anterior arch that has two bulky lateral masses and a thin posterior arch. The axis has the odontoid process or dens, which is the fused remnant of the body of the first cervical vertebra. The odontoid process sits cephalad on the body of C2 and rests just posterior to the anterior arch of the atlas, where it is held tightly by ligaments. The remaining lower cervical vertebrae (C3 through C7) have small vertebral bodies that are convex on the superior surface and concave on the inferior surface. Arising anterolaterally from the bodies are transverse processes that have both anterior and posterior tubercles. The foramen transversarium is located between the posterior tubercle and the lateral part of the vertebral body. The vertebral artery passes through this foramen, entering at C6 and exiting at C2. The exiting nerve roots pass just posterior to the vertebral arteries at the level of the disc space.

Posterior to the vertebral foramina are the lateral masses that comprise that portion of bone between the superior and inferior facets. The lateral masses are important anatomic structures for the placement of screws in posterior plating procedures of the cervical spine. The cervical facet joints are oriented more in a horizontal than in a vertical plane, with the superior facet sitting anterior to the inferior facet of the level above. This allows for a great amount of flexion and extension of the neck but limits side-bending. The remainder of the posterior elements of the cervical spine include the lamina and spinous processes, which are posterior and medial to the facet joints and lateral masses.

There are 12 vertebrae of the **thoracic spine.** The differential features of thoracic vertebrae are thin pedicles that connect the vertebral body to the posterior elements, the transverse processes that project superolaterally from the posterior part of the pedicle and are larger in size than the cervical transverse processes, and the ventral surface of the transverse process that has a costal articulation. The thoracic spine is a more rigid column than the cervical or lumbar spine because of the rib cage. As in the cervical spine, the facets of the thoracic spine are oriented in the coronal plane, with the superior facet anterior to the inferior facet. At the thoracolumbar junction, the facet joints change gradually from a coronal to a more sagittal orientation.

The vertebrae of the **lumbar spine** are larger than the cervical or thoracic vertebrae. The pedicles are wider and broader, and they are usually able to accept bone screws. The facet joints are oriented sagittally, with the inferior facet of the segment above medial to the superior facet of the segment below. The transverse processes project straight lateral from the superior facets and are quite large. The posterior elements (lamina and spinous processes) are also larger in the lumbar spine.

The **sacrum and coccyx** are normally fused and attach the axial skeleton to the pelvis by sacroiliac articulation, the sacrotuberous ligaments, and sacrospinous ligaments.

Ligamentous Anatomy

The ligaments of the spinal column support the osseous structures. We distinguish between those supporting the anterior and middle columns and those stabilizing the posterior column. The stabilizers of the anterior and middle columns are the **anterior longitudinal ligament** and the **posterior longitudinal ligament.** These ligaments extend the entire length of the spine and insert on the vertebral bodies. They are the major stabilizers of the vertebral bodies and discs during flexion and extension. The anterior longitudinal ligament is closely attached to the intervertebral disc and has a ribbon-like structure. The posterior longitudinal ligament is widest in the upper cervical spine and narrows as it proceeds caudally. It thins over the vertebral bodies and thickens over the intervertebral discs.

The ligamentous structures stabilizing the posterior column include the **supraspinous ligament, the interspinous ligament, the facet joint capsule,** and **the ligamentum flavum.** The ligamentum flavum runs from the superior margin of the caudad lamina to the ventral surface of the cephalad lamina. There are right and left ligaments separated by a small fissure that merges with the interspinous ligaments posteriorly and medially and with the fibrous facet capsules laterally. The posterior ligamentous structures are stabilizers during flexion.

The ligamentous structures of the upper cervical spine are unique. The odontoid process is held snugly against the posterior wall of the anterior arch of the atlas by the **transverse ligament.** Additional stability is afforded by the **apical ligament** and the paired **alar ligaments** that run superiorly from the odontoid process to the anterior rim of the foramen magnum. This allows rotation of C1 on C2 but prevents posterior translation of the dens within the ring of the atlas, which would place the spinal cord at risk.

The **intervertebral discs** are complex structures made up of an outer annulus fibrosis and an inner nucleus pulposus. The **annulus fibrosis** is a laminated structure consisting of collagen fibers that are oriented 30° from horizontal. The inner layers are attached to the cartilaginous endplates, whereas the outer fibers are firmly secured to the osseous vertebral bodies. The annulus surrounds and contains the **nucleus pulposus,** a matrix of protein, glycosaminoglycans, and water. Injury to the intervertebral disc may not be obvious on conventional radiography, but it must be considered when evaluating overall spinal stability and potential neurologic compromise. Magnetic resonance imaging (MRI) allows direct visualization of the intervertebral disc.

BIOMECHANICS

In the sagittal projection, the spine is made up of three smooth curves: cervical lordosis, thoracic kyphosis, and lumbar lordosis, with a smooth transition between these curves. The center of gravity passes anterior to the midthoracic spine and just posterior to the midlumbar spine before intersecting the top portion of the sacrum. This implies that most of the spinal column experiences compressive forces anteriorly through the vertebral bodies and tensile forces through the posterior elements and ligaments.

The distribution of materials and their properties match the function of the spine. The vertebral bodies are well equipped for handling compressive loads. The majority of the vertebral bodies are made of trabecular bone. Trabecular bone is the primary weight-bearing component of the vertebral bodies in compression. Removing the cortex of the vertebral body reduces its strength by only 10%. The marrow contents of the vertebral body act as a hydraulic system when compressed. This visco-elastic property allows the vertebral body to absorb more energy.

Posteriorly, the major stabilizers of the spine are the ligamentous structures of the posterior column. These structures are predominantly made of collagen and are very strong when loaded in tension.

The intervertebral discs are important to the structural stability of the spine. The inner layers of the annulus and the nucleus transmit loads from vertebra to vertebra. With significant force application, the annular fibers fail, allowing the potential for segmental instability and traumatic disc herniations.

The rib cage stabilizes the thoracic spine. This increased thoracic spine stability creates stress risers at the junction of the more mobile cervical spine above and lumbar spine below.

The criteria for determining traumatic **spinal instability** are controversial. The three-column concept of spinal anatomy provides a framework in which to consider specific anatomical areas of injury. Thus, when only one column is injured, the spine is usually stable. When two or three columns are injured, it is usually unstable (i.e., unable to function adequately as a support column and to protect the neural elements). This definition is applicable both acutely and chronically. Thus, in many situations, the question of spinal stability is unclear and rests on the interpretation of pertinent radiographs, the neurologic examination, and sound clinical judgment.

Neurologic Injuries

Based on the anatomic location of the spinal injury, there are three categories of neurologic injury: spinal cord, conus medullaris, and cauda equina lesions. Injuries to the cervical and thoracic spine may directly affect the spinal cord or nerve roots (Table 15-2). The distal spinal cord

TABLE 15-2 Upper Extremity Neurologic Examination

Root	Motor	Sensory	Reflex
C4	Diaphragm	Top of shoulder	
C5	Elbow flexion (biceps)	Lateral arm	Biceps
C6	Wrist extensors (ECRL/ECRB)	Lateral forearm, thumb/index finger	Briachioradialis
C7	Elbow extension (triceps)	Middle finger	Triceps
C8	Finger flexors (FDP)	Medial forearm, ring/little finger	
T1	Finger abduction (interossei)	Posterior shoulder	

is termed the *conus medullaris* and usually lies at the thoracolumbar junction at the pedicle level of L1. The sacral nuclei, which control bowel and bladder function, are located in the conus. The cauda equina consists of all lumbar and sacral roots below the conus (usually L2 and below). Injuries to the cauda equina are peripheral nerve root injuries; they have a better prognosis for return of function than do spinal cord or conus injuries.

Spinal cord injuries in the cervical or thoracic spine are designated as complete or incomplete. **Complete** lesions are characterized by total loss of motor, sensory, and reflex function below the level of injury. These injuries result in quadriplegia in the upper cervical spine and paraplegia in the thoracic spine. Complete spinal cord injuries of the cervical spine are described by the lowest level of cervical root function. This has implications for functional independence of the patient. A C3 quadriplegic is ventilator dependent without any upper or lower extremity function. Patients with C6 or below quadriplegia function independently.

Complete spinal cord injuries in the thoracic spine produce paraplegia. The location of the lesion is irrelevant to the functional outcome for the patient because the segmental thoracic nerve roots only supply sensation to the thorax and innervation to the intercostal muscles. However, a proximal thoracic paraplegic versus a distal thoracic paraplegic has an increased risk of respiratory problems because of increased intercostal paralysis.

Incomplete spinal cord injuries are categorized into four types based on the cross-section location of the injury within the spinal cord: anterior cord, posterior cord, central cord, and Brown–Séquard syndrome. In the **anterior cord syndrome,** the injury is to the anterior spinal cord, which contains the corticospinal motor tracts. This results in motor paralysis with preservation of deep pressure sensation and proprioception due to the intact posterior columns. The **posterior cord syndrome** is rare and results from damage to the posterior columns. This results in loss of proprioception and deep pressure sensation but in the maintenance of motor function due to the intact anterior motor columns. **Central cord syndrome** results from damage to the central gray matter and centrally oriented white matter tracts. In the cervical spine, the centrally oriented white matter tracts provide motor innervation to the upper extremities. As a result, the upper extremities will be more involved than the lower. In the thoracic region, a central cord injury affects the proximal musculature of the lower extremities more than the distal. In **Brown–Séquard syndrome,** half the cord is damaged in the coronal projection. Thus, there is ipsilateral motor paralysis, loss of position sense, and contralateral loss of pain and temperature sensation because the motor tracts and posterior columns decussate in the brainstem, whereas the sensory tracts decussate one to two levels above where they enter the spinal cord. Frequently, there is overlap between these syndromes.

The second group of neurologic injuries involves the **conus medullaris.** These injuries occur with trauma to the thoracolumbar junction and frequently involve elements of the lower spinal cord and cauda equina. Injuries at this level are very difficult to diagnose accurately in the acute setting, especially in the face of spinal shock. Because the conus medullaris usually ends at the level of the L1 pedicle, spinal injuries at this level may damage the upper motor neurons of the sacral cord or the lower motor neurons to the sacral or lumbar roots, which have already exited the spinal cord. Thus, it is not unusual to regain motor strength in the lower extremities, which are innervated by lumbar nerves, but continue to have absent bowel and bladder function because of a conus injury damaging sacral nerve root innervation to the bowel and bladder.

Cauda equina injuries occur with fractures or dislocations of the L2 level and below. The neurologic deficit may range from a single nerve root injury to a **cauda equina syndrome** in which there is marked weakness of the lower extremities and involvement of the nerve roots supplying the bowel and bladder.

The decrease in spinal canal cross-sectional area following fracture or dislocation does not always correlate with the severity of neurologic injury or the prognosis for recovery because the size of the canal and the presence of bone or disc material within it only reflect the final resting place of these fragments, not the magnitude of energy absorbed, the maximum displacement, or the trajectory of the displaced fragments. However, residual spinal canal compromise of greater than 50% or absolute spinal canal dimensions less than 10 to 13 mm indicate acute or impending neurologic dysfunction.

Decompression of the spinal canal in complete spinal cord injuries does little or nothing to improve neurologic outcome. Surgical decompression is recommended for incomplete spinal cord, conus, or cauda equina lesion. Significant improvement in neurologic outcome is possible, especially with cauda equina (lower motor neuron) lesions.

The incidence of penetrating spinal trauma from **gunshot wounds** is increasing. Rarely is the spinal column rendered unstable from a gunshot wound; however, neurologic injury is frequent. Cervical and thoracic level injuries often produce quadriplegia or paraplegia, respectively. Similarly, injury to the cauda equina occurs with lumbar gunshot wounds. Most of the neural damage is secondary to the kinetic energy transference to the neural tissues. Surgical removal of bullet is rarely indicated except in incomplete spinal cord or cauda equina lesion with a space-occupying fragment of bone or bullet identified. Because of the heat generated, these bullet wounds have a low infection rate, except when they have traversed the colon prior to entering the spinal column. This is one indication for elective removal of the bullet if lodged in the spinal column or canal.

Diagnosis and Initial Management

The diagnosis and initial management of patients with spinal fractures and dislocations depend to a great degree on the area of the spine involved. Nevertheless, there are commonalities.

Patients with spinal injuries may have additional life-threatening injuries; therefore, initial priorities are to secure an airway, ventilation, and hemodynamic stabilization.

Precautions for the stabilization of the entire spinal column begin at the accident site. Patients with a history of trauma to the head, neck, or back, or conscious patients who report any neurologic symptoms are immobilized in a cervical collar with complete head and neck immobilization on a spine board until an appropriate evaluation is performed. A history of the mechanism of injury and a detailed report of any neck or back pain and motor or sensory changes in the extremities are essential. Unconscious patients with major trauma are a more difficult challenge, and suspicion must remain high until a thorough examination for potential spinal injury is performed.

A thorough neurologic examination is performed as soon as possible. Neurologic examinations include complete assessment of motor, sensory, and reflex function for both upper and lower extremities. Perianal sensation and a rectal examination are critical to determine the function of the sacral roots and sacral cord. Sacral sensory sparring or any trace of distal motor function implies possible return of function. Also, spinal shock for the first 24 to 48 h may have the appearance of a complete spinal cord injury in patients who will later be found to have sensory and motor function. The resolution of spinal shock is indicated by the return of the **bulbocavernosus reflex.** This is tested while performing a digital rectal examination. Pulling on the Foley catheter will result in contraction of the anal sphincter when the bulbocavernosus reflex is present. When the bulbocavernosus reflex returns in the face of a complete spinal cord injury, the chances are that the neurologic deficit is permanent.

Radiographic Examination

Screening radiographs include anteroposterior and lateral views. On the lateral radiograph, one should examine the height of all the vertebral bodies and the intervening disc spaces. These heights should be fairly uniform and symmetric. When the vertebral body height is decreased, an angulatory deformity (i.e., kyphosis) is produced on the lateral radiograph. The anterior and posterior vertebral body lines should align throughout the whole spine. With injury to the middle column (posterior vertebral body), retropulsion of bone into the spinal canal may be evident on the lateral view. The lateral radiograph also will show the posterior elements, including the facets, lamina, and spinous processes. Widened interspinous process distance is indicative of distraction injury to the posterior column.

The anteroposterior radiograph of the spine is examined. Each vertebral body should sit directly on top of the one below, with symmetric and evenly placed disc spaces between the bodies. The right and left borders of the vertebral bodies should be well aligned. The two round pedicle shadows of each vertebral body should be present and symmetric. Widening of the interpedicular distance at one level may be indicative of a middle column burst-type injury. Careful examination delineates the posterior elements of the spine. The posterior elements of a segment are somewhat distal to the corresponding vertebral body. The spinous process shadow is usually visible, allowing for comparison of the interspinous process distance at each level. The transverse processes at each level are examined for fracture, as are the ribs in the thoracic spine, the sacrum, sacroiliac articulations, and iliac wings of the pelvis.

It is very important in patients with spinal trauma to not miss additional spinal injuries. Up to 10% of patients with spinal trauma at one site will have another injury to the spinal column at an adjoining or distant site. This is especially important in cervical or thoracic spine-injured patients who may have spinal cord injuries resulting in sensory loss to more distal areas of their thoracic and lumbar spine, adding to the difficulty of diagnosis of injuries in these areas.

Initial Management

All patients are kept supine on a well-cushioned mattress and are log-rolled every 2 h to decrease pressure on sensitive areas. Antiembolism stockings are used for deep vein thrombosis prophylaxis. Cardiac status and oxygen saturation are monitored continuously. A nasogastric tube is placed for the accompanying gastrointestinal ileus. A Foley catheter allows accurate determination of urine output and simplifies nursing care. Intravenous fluids maintain an adequate fluid volume. Complete blood counts are obtained at presentation and then several times in the early postinjury period. Intravenous pain medications are dictated by the age, medical status, and amount of pain. Physical therapy for range-of-motion exercises of uninjured extremities is begun early in the hospital course.

The initial care for a patient with cervical spine injury is somewhat different. Patients with a cervical spine injury causing spinal malalignment, regardless of the neurologic status, are placed in **skeletal tong traction.** We use graphite Gardner–Wells tongs that are MRI compatible. They are placed one finger breadth above the earlobe in line with the external auditory canal. The skull bolts are finger tightened until the pressure valve is released in the center of the bolt, indicating adequate force. Tongs are applied in the emergency room when spinal malalignment is identified. Approximately 5 lbs. per level of injury is slowly added to the traction apparatus under close neurologic and radiographic surveillance. Thus, a patient with a C4-to-C5 facet dislocation may require 25 lbs. or more for reduction of the malalignment. It is not uncommon to require anywhere from 50 to 100 lbs. of traction weight for lower cervical spine dislocations to accomplish reduction in large adults. Once reduction is achieved, a load of 10 to 15 lbs. is sufficient to maintain reduction. A lateral cervical spine radiograph ensures maintenance of proper cervical spine alignment and should be checked frequently, especially after returning from tests that require mobilization of the patient.

The pharmacologic treatment of acute spinal cord injury is administration of steroids in an attempt to diminish edema around the neural elements following injury. Indications for steroids are all cervical spine-injured patients with any neurologic deficit, thoracic spine injuries with incomplete paraplegia, incomplete cauda equina lesions with neurologic deterioration, and the inability to take the patient promptly to surgery. Steroids are administered to complete cervical spine-injured patients. They are not administered to complete thoracic spine-injured patients because of the significant benefit of saving or gaining a functional root level in a complete cervical spine-injured patient. Thirty milligrams per kilogram of methylprednisolone is administered as a loading dose intravenously over 30 min. A continuous intravenous drip of methylprednisolone at a dose of 5.4 mg/kg per hour is continued for 24 h and then discontinued. Any neurologic deterioration while on methylprednisolone merits reconsideration of its use. The risk of this high-dose steroid regimen is gastrointestinal hemorrhage; therefore, all patients are protected with H2 antagonists such as Cimetidine or Ranitidine for a minimum of 72 h.

Spine injuries are divided into four groups based on the involved segment: upper cervical, subaxial cervical, thoracic and lumbar, and sacral.

UPPER CERVICAL SPINE INJURIES (OCCIPUT TO C2)

Classification

There are eight types of upper cervical spine injuries encountered. The four most frequently encountered are atlas fractures, atlantoaxial subluxations, odontoid fractures, and traumatic spondylolisthesis of the axis (C2 hangman's fractures). The four less common injuries are occipital condyle fractures, atlantooccipital dislocation, atlantoaxial rotary subluxation, and C2 lateral mass fractures.

Atlas fractures result from impaction of the occipital condyles on the arch of C1. This causes single or multiple fractures of the ring of C1, which usually splay apart and thus increase the space for the spinal cord; therefore, neurologic injury is rare. There are four types of atlas fractures. The first two are stable injuries: isolated anterior or posterior arch fractures. Anterior arch fractures are usually avulsion injuries from the anterior portion of the ring. Posterior arch fractures result from hyperextension, with compression of the posterior arch of C1 between the occiput and C2. The third type of atlas fracture is a lateral mass fracture. The fracture lines run anterior and posterior to the articular surface of the C1 lateral mass, with asymmetric displacement of the lateral mass from the remainder of the vertebrae. This is best seen on an open-mouth odontoid view of the C1-to-C2 complex. The fourth type, burst fractures of the atlas (or Jefferson fracture), classically has four fractures in the ring of C1: two in the anterior portion and two in the posterior ring. Potential instability of these fractures is best identified by examining the overhang of the C1 lateral masses on the C2 articular facets, as noted on the open-mouth odontoid view. Total lateral displacement on both sides of more than 6.9 mm indicates rupture of the transverse ligament with resultant atlantoaxial instability.

Atlantoaxial subluxation is secondary to rupture of the primary stabilizer of the atlantoaxial articulation, the transverse ligament. This produces atlantoaxial instability that may place the spinal cord at risk. Thus, potential complications from this injury include neurologic injury resulting from the odontoid compressing the upper cervical cord against the posterior arch of C1.

Identification of **odontoid process fractures** requires a high index of suspicion. Odontoid process fractures must be ruled out in all patients with neck pain following a motor-vehicle accident and elderly patients involved in trivial trauma to the head and neck region. If there is significant anterior or, more commonly, posterior displacement of the odontoid process, spinal cord injury may result. The incidence of neurologic injury is approximately 10%. Odontoid fractures are further classified into three types based on the anatomic level at which they occur (Fig. 15-2).

Type I fractures represent an avulsion fracture from the tip of the odontoid process, where the alar ligament inserts.

Type II fractures are the most common type of odontoid fracture and occur in the midportion of the dens proximal to the body of the axis. The limited blood supply and small cross-sectional cancellous surface area lead to a high incidence of nonunion. Other risk factors for nonunion are angulation, anterior or posterior displacement of more than 4 mm, and patient age older than 40 years.

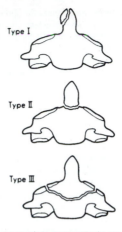

ODONTOID PROCESS FRACTURES

FIG. 15-2   The three types of odontoid fractures.

Type III injuries are those in which the fracture line extends into the vertebral body of C2. Because of the larger cross-sectional area and the presence of cancellous bone with a rich blood supply, these type III fractures consistently unite, providing they are adequately aligned (Fig. 15-3).

FIG. 15-3   An open-mouth view indicating a type III odontoid fracture.

Traumatic spondylolisthesis of the axis, or hangman's fracture, is a bipedicle fracture with disruption of the disc and ligaments between C2 and C3, resulting most commonly from hyperextension and distraction. This fracture is named for the injury resulting from judicial hanging with a rope in the submental position.

Hangman's fractures are further classified based on the amount of displacement and angulation of the C2 body in relation to the posterior elements (Figs. 15-4 through 15-7).

FIG. 15-4   Type I hangman's fracture.

FIG. 15-5   Type II hangman's fracture.

FIG. 15-6   Type IIA hangman's fracture.

FIG. 15-7   Type III hangman's fracture.

Type I injury is a fracture of the neural arch without angulation and with as much as 3 mm of anterior displacement of C2 on C3.

Type II fractures have anterior displacement greater than 3 mm or angulation of C2 on C3. These fractures usually result from hyperextension and axial load followed by severe flexion that stretches the posterior annulus and disc and produces the anterior translation and angulation. **Type IIA** injuries are a flexion–distraction variant of type II fractures. They demonstrate severe angulation of C2 on C3, with minimal displacement, apparently hinging on the anterior longitudinal ligament. It is important to recognize this type of hangman's fracture because the application of traction may distract the C2-to-C3 disc space and further displace the fracture.

Type III injuries are bipedicle fractures associated with unilateral or bilateral facet dislocations. These are serious, unstable injuries and have a high incidence of neurologic sequelae.

Fractures of the **occipital condyles** result from combined axial loading and lateral bending. There are two types: avulsion fractures or comminuted compression fractures.

Atlantooccipital dislocations are rare injuries resulting from total disruption of all ligamentous structures between the occiput and the atlas. The mechanism of injury is usually extension or flexion. Death is usually immediate due to severe brainstem involvement with complete respiratory arrest.

Atlantoaxial rotary subluxation occurs most often secondary to vehicular accidents. The main difficulty is lack of early recognition.

Lateral mass fractures of the axis are the result of combined axial-loading and lateral-bending forces.

Associated Injuries

Associated injuries include spinal cord or cervical nerve root compression, head injuries, and other spine fractures, particularly of the cervical spine. Fractures of the occipital condyles are associated with severe head trauma and are accompanied by cranial nerve palsies. Fifty percent of patients with a fracture of the posterior arch of the atlas have another cervical spine injury, the most common being a traumatic spondylolisthesis of the axis or a displaced odontoid fracture. A high index of suspicion and careful physical and radiographic examinations are the best method of finding associated injuries.

Diagnosis and Initial Management

Physical Examination

The patient has pain localized to the neck, and there may be a feeling of instability or fixed deformity. The initial assessment is performed as described.

Radiographic Examination

Initially, a cross-table lateral radiograph is obtained in all patients with suspected cervical spine injuries. This radiograph includes all seven cervical vertebrae and the C7-to-T1 junction. When this is not possible due to interposition of the shoulders in patients with short necks, the patient's arms are pulled down to lower the shoulders, or one arm is extended above the head while keeping the other arm at the side while shooting (swimmer's view; Fig. 15-8).

FIG. 15-8   Swimmer's view of cervical spine.

Additional required views include an anteroposterior view and an odontoid, or open-mouth, view, which details the C1-to-C2 articulation in the coronal plane (Fig. 15-3). Right or left oblique and voluntary flexion–extension views are obtained as indicated.

Four lines are essential to examine on the lateral radiograph: the anterior vertebral body line, the posterior vertebral body line, the spinal laminar line, and the line connecting the tips of the spinous processes. All of these landmarks should align in a smooth arc from C1 to T1 (Fig. 15-9). Any malalignment indicates potential vertebral subluxation or dislocation occurring with a spinal injury.

The soft tissue shadows on the lateral cervical spine radiographs represent the retropharyngeal and retrotracheal shadows. These soft tissue shadows are expanded by the accompanying hematoma produced following cervical spine injury and may be the only indication of subtle injuries. The soft tissue shadow should be no more than 6 mm from the anterior aspect of C2 and no more than 2 cm at the anterior edge of C6 (i.e., **6 at 2 and 2 at 6**).

Fractures of the occipital condyles are difficult to visualize on plain radiographs and require axial computed tomography (CT) for delineation.

Atlantooccipital dissociation is identified on the lateral radiograph of the cervical spine or lateral view of the skull, which profiles the at-

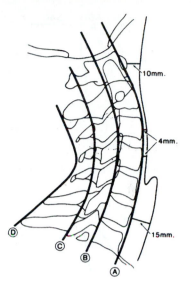

FIG. 15-9   Normal bony arcs and soft tissue shadows seen on the lateral view of the cervicle spine: (A) anterior vertebral body line, (B) posterior vertebral body line, (C) laminar line, and (D) spinous process line.

lantooccipital junction quite well. There is dissociation between the base of the occiput and the C1 arch and severe soft tissue swelling.

Fractures of the atlas are diagnosed on a lateral cervical spine radiograph and/or an open-mouth odontoid view. The lateral cervical spine radiograph demonstrates fracture lines within the posterior arch of C1. The open-mouth view indicates splaying of the lateral masses of C1 on the articular surfaces of the axis. Axial CT is helpful in the evaluation.

Atlantoaxial subluxation due to disruption of the transverse ligament is best demonstrated on lateral flexion–extension views and is indicated by an increase in the atlantodental interval, which is normally less than 3.5 mm. This is measured from the posterior aspect of the anterior arch of C1 to the anterior aspect of the odontoid process (Figs. 15-10 and 15-11). However, spinal extensor muscle spasm accompanying an acute injury may prevent adequate voluntary flexion–extension radiographs. Once recognized, an axial CT scan is obtained to ascertain whether instability is purely ligamentous or due to a bony avulsion.

Radiographs following atlantoaxial rotary subluxation are often reported as normal because it is difficult to obtain radiographs parallel to

FIG. 15-10   Normal relation of the atlas and dens seen on the lateral view.

FIG. 15-11   Atlantoaxial subluxation as indicated by an increase in the atlantodental interval (ADI).

the plane of both C1 and C2 due to the accompanying torticollis. Open-mouth radiographs often help recognize this injury by demonstrating a "wink sign." This occurs because of the unilateral overlap of the lateral mass of C1 on C2. CT is helpful in describing the direction and rotation of C1 on C2.

Odontoid fractures are seen on lateral cervical spine radiographs or an open-mouth view. Occasionally, three-dimensional CT reconstruction or conventional tomography may be necessary to identify and fully evaluate these fractures. Axial CT may miss the fracture line as it is in the plane of the axial image.

Hangman's fractures are seen on the lateral radiograph. Lateral mass fractures with minimal comminution may require CT for identification.

Initial Management

Occipital condyle fractures are managed initially in a cervical orthosis. Fractures of the occipital condyles are generally stable injuries that can be treated with orthotic immobilization with a two-poster orthosis or a rigid Philadelphia collar. Most of these fractures heal uneventfully, although occasionally posttraumatic arthritis occurs, requiring posterior atlantooccipital fusion.

Traction is contraindicated following atlantooccipital dislocation. Even 5 lbs. may overdistract and stretch the brain stem, with catastrophic results. Initial treatment is application of a halo vest to maintain stability of the spine, while attention is placed on the patient's respiratory and neurologic status. Once the patient is stabilized, a posterior occiput to upper cervical spine fusion is performed, with continued immobilization in a halo vest for approximately 3 months.

Initial management of type I, II, and III fractures of the atlas is a cervical orthosis. Jefferson fractures are placed in traction.

Atlantoaxial subluxation and atlantoaxial rotary subluxation are managed initially with a cervical orthosis.

Type I odontoid fractures are managed with a cervical orthosis. Type II and III fractures are initially managed with cervical tong traction to reduce and/or maintain sagittal alignment.

Type I and II hangman's fractures are managed with a cervical orthosis. The initial management of type III fractures is application of traction to reduce the facet dislocation. Reduction by closed means may not be possible because of the dissociation between the vertebral body and the posterior elements.

Definitive Management

Definitive management of fractures of the atlas is based on the type of fracture. Type I and II fractures may be managed in a cervical orthosis in a compliant patient, whereas type III injuries are managed with a halo vest. Type IV, or Jefferson, fractures with a competent transverse ligament (less than 6.9 mm displacement of the lateral masses) are stable and are also managed with a halo vest. Jefferson fractures with an incompetent transverse ligament (more than 6.9 mm displacement) are unstable and are managed with extended cervical traction to reduce the splaying until the bony fragments are sticky. This is necessary because the halo vest is unable to provide the axial distraction necessary to maintain fracture reduction. After preliminary healing, application of a halo vest for the remainder of the 3- to 4-month period allows complete healing. When a C1 fracture is presumed healed, voluntary lateral flexion–extension radiographs of the cervical spine are obtained to ensure there is no significant atlantoaxial subluxation. If there is more than 5 mm of atlantoaxial subluxation in an adult, posterior C1-to-C2 fusion is performed with or without transarticular C1-to-C2 screw fixation.

Atlantoaxial subluxation due to bony avulsion of the transverse ligament is managed with a halo vest for 3 months. Purely ligamentous injuries are managed with a C1-to-C2 posterior fusion, possibly with C1-to-C2 transarticular screws.

Atlantoaxial rotary subluxation recognized within several weeks of injury is reduced with cervical traction. This may require up to 30 to 40 lbs. of traction to reduce the rotary dislocation. Often a "pop" is heard and felt at reduction. A halo vest is applied. Even with prolonged halo vest treatment, long-term stability may not be achieved because the C1-to-C2 facet joint is a saddle-type joint and depends on ligamentous restraint for stability. Atlantoaxial arthrodesis is the treatment of choice for chronic instability and pain or for patients with an associated neurologic deficit. For chronic injuries, closed reduction through cervical traction is not possible; they are managed with open reduction and C1-to-C2 arthrodesis.

Type I odontoid fractures are stable injuries that are managed with an orthosis for symptomatic comfort. However, the type I avulsion injury is often associated with atlantooccipital dislocations; therefore, this more serious injury must be ruled out. There are four types of definitive treatment for type II odontoid fractures: halo vest management of minimally displaced or angulated fractures followed by posterior C1-to-C2 arthrodesis if healing does not occur within 4 months; primary posterior C1-to-C2 arthrodesis as long as the posterior arch of C1 is intact; posterior C1-to-C2 transarticular facet screw fixation and fusion; and anterior screw fixation of the dens under biplanar fluoroscopy. The theoretical advantage of anterior screw fixation is that it does not require a C1-to-C2 fusion and thus preserves motion of the upper cervical spine. Provided type III odontoid fractures are adequately reduced, halo vest immobilization for 3 months is the treatment of choice. When reduction is lost after halo vest placement, cervical traction for 3 to 4 weeks to allow early fracture healing before continuing with the halo vest is required or reduction by traction and posterior C1-to-C2 fusion may be performed.

Type I hangman's fractures are stable injuries and are managed with a cervical orthosis for 3 months in compliant patients. Type II fractures displaced less than 5 mm and minimally angulated are managed with a halo vest if reduction can be maintained. Fractures displaced more than 5 mm are managed in cervical tong traction, with slight extension prior to application of the halo vest, which will also need to be applied with neck extension. Traction is contraindicated for type IIA fractures. These fractures are managed with early halo application under fluoroscopic guidance and with compression across the fracture site for maintenance of reduction. Type III fractures are reduced open when closed reduction is not possible, and posterior spinal fusion of C2-to-C3 is performed. Postoperatively, halo vest immobilization is maintained 3 months for these injuries.

Lateral mass fractures of the atlas are stable injuries that only require orthotic immobilization. Occasionally, with late symptomatic facet degeneration, some of these may require posterior fusion for pain relief.

Complications

The complication of high cervical fractures is bony or ligamentous instability. Management is posterior fusion of the unstable segments. Failure to identify an upper cervical spine injury is not too infrequent an occurrence, especially in multiply traumatized patients. Fortunately, neurologic injury is rare because of the large amount of space available for the spinal cord in the upper cervical spine.

SUBAXIAL CERVICAL SPINE INJURIES

Although bony injuries are often the obvious manifestation of cervical spine trauma, it is essential to accurately identify ligamentous components of injury to the subaxial cervical motion segments. It is often this ligamentous failure which allows cervical motion segment translation that may account for severe neurologic damage. It is also well accepted that ligaments heal with scar tissue that is weaker than the preinjured ligamentous structure and may result in chronic instability.

An important difference between upper and subaxial cervical spine injuries is the increased risk of cervical cord injuries in the lower cervical spine. This is a reflection of two factors: the overall diminished size of the spinal canal in the lower cervical spine and the increasing prevalence of injuries that narrow rather than expand the canal. Thus, the immediate and long-term goals for injuries in the lower cervical spine are to obtain and maintain spinal column alignment to optimize the environment for the spinal cord and existing nerve roots.

Classification

There are five types of **subaxial cervical spine** injuries: isolated posterior element fractures, minor avulsion and compression fractures, vertebral body-burst fractures, teardrop fractures, and facet injuries causing spinal malalignment.

Isolated posterior element fractures of the lamina, articular process, or spinous process may occur by a compression extension sequence with impaction of the posterior elements upon one another. Additional lesions include unilateral or bilateral laminar fractures and, often, contiguous posterior element fractures secondary to the impaction of the adjacent posterior elements.

Minor avulsion and compression fractures of the subaxial cervical spine include anterior compression or avulsion injuries of the vertebral body and combined anterior and posterior bony injuries with minimal displacement and angulation.

Vertebral body-burst fractures are usually the result of axial-loading injury with different amounts of flexion possible, as seen in diving accidents. They involve the anterior column and the middle column, with the potential for bony retropulsion into the spinal canal.

Teardrop fractures of the subaxial cervical spine are a particular group of fractures with a high association of severe spinal cord injury and spinal instability. These injuries occur when the neck is in a flexed position, with axial compression as the main loading force. The inferior tip of the proximal vertebral body is driven down into the caudad body by compression and flexion. This produces the typical teardrop fragment on the anteroinferior aspect of the affected body. The true significance of this injury lies in the three-column instability pattern produced. The typical fracture line proceeds from superior to inferior and exits through the disc space, which is severely damaged. Posterior element ligament and bony damage is characteristic of the teardrop injury. This produces a grossly unstable injury of all three spinal columns in which the entire vertebral body is retropulsed into the spinal canal, causing either partial or complete spinal cord injury.

Facet injuries are divided into fractures and ligamentous injuries. Both may allow segmental translation with subluxation or dislocation of the vertebral segments. The primary mechanism of injury is a posterior distraction force applied to the already flexed spine. This produces a spectrum of injury that ranges from an interspinous ligament sprain to complete posterior ligamentous and facet joint failure producing facet subluxation or facet dislocation. These injuries are further divided into unilateral and bilateral facet injuries. Thus, facet injuries are described as unilateral or bilateral facet fractures with or without subluxation, unilateral facet dislocations, perched facets, or bilateral facet fractures. Unilateral facet fractures or dislocations display a variety of neurologic injuries, ranging from a normal examination to single root deficits or spinal cord syndromes. The increasing spectrum of distraction and flexion injuries produces the perched facet injury. This occurs with bilateral facet injuries causing perching of the inferior facet on the superior facet, with segmental kyphosis between the two affected vertebral body segments. Neurologic deficits are variable but most commonly include isolated root deficits. The most severe facet injury is bilateral facet dislocation. This is a purely ligamentous injury, with disruption of the entire posterior ligamentous complex, including the interspinous ligament, ligamentum flavum, both facet capsules, and, in severe cases, disruption of the posterior longitudinal ligament and intervertebral disc. This injury produces the highest incidence of neurologic deficit of any facet injury because of the loss of space available for the spinal cord as a result of vertebral translation. The incidence of bilateral facet fractures associated with dislocations is extremely small. Both of these injuries predispose to rotational and translational instability.

Diagnosis and Initial Management

Physical Examination

The primary sign of a subaxial cervical spine injury may be the associated neurologic deficit. Other than neck pain and a sense of instability, there may be no symptoms indicating a cervical spine fracture without neurologic deficit. Patients with unilateral facet dislocation have a mild rotational deformity of the neck: the head is tilted and rotated to the contralateral side of the facet dislocation.

Radiographic Examination

A common, isolated posterior element fracture, the unilateral vertebral arch fracture, often is not evident on the initial lateral cervical spine radiograph. Oblique views or nonstandard views, such as a 20° oblique or pillar view, may be necessary to establish the diagnosis. When both an ipsilateral pedicle and laminar fracture occur, the articular process may rotate into the frontal plane and be viewed as a "transverse facet" on the anteroposterior radiographic view.

Vertebral body-burst fractures involve the anterior and middle columns of the cervical spine. The lateral radiograph indicates compression of the anterior and middle columns, with retropulsion of the middle column posteriorly into the spinal canal. Burst fractures always require an axial CT or MRI examination to document the amount of middle column retropulsion. As anterior compression approaches 50%, middle column injuries or concomitant posterior ligamentous injuries must be considered. It is difficult to identify posterior ligamentous injuries in a patient with a burst fracture because voluntary flexion–extension views are unobtainable. Warnings include a widened interspinous process distance, fractured posterior elements including facet fractures, or sagittal MRI evidence of ligamentous damage.

Teardrop fractures are first suspected on the lateral cervical spine radiograph, which will show retrodisplacement of the cephalad vertebral body on the caudad and, possibly, the anteroinferior teardrop fragment. Posterior element fractures may also be noted on the lateral or the anteroposterior radiograph. CT or MRI through the involved segment also demonstrates the fractures and the diminished spinal canal diameter due to the significant retrolisthesis.

Facet dislocations are identified on the lateral radiograph. Unilateral dislocations are characterized by approximately 25% anterior olisthesis of the cephalad vertebra on the caudad vertebra; bilateral dislocations have 50% anterior olisthesis (Fig. 15-12). Axial CT further defines the injury. Perched facets are diagnosed on the lateral radiograph by the increased distance between the spinous processes. There is also an obvious segmental kyphosis seen between the involved vertebral bodies and anterior translation of the cephalad vertebral body on the caudad body.

Initial Management

Initial management of isolated fractures of the posterior elements and minor avulsion and compression fractures is a cervical orthosis.

Initial management of burst fractures with greater than 25% loss in height, retropulsion, or neurologic deficit is cervical tong traction to

FIG. 15-12   Bilateral facet dislocation of C4 on C5.

stabilize the spinal segment and attempt an indirect reduction of retropulsed fragments via ligamentotaxis, thereby decompressing the neural canal.

Initial management of teardrop fractures is application of cervical tong traction to increase the spinal canal diameter by indirect reduction via ligamentotaxis.

Initial management of unilateral or bilateral facet injuries causing any spinal subluxation or dislocations, perched facets, and bilateral facet dislocations is cervical tong traction for reduction (Fig. 15-13). The one caveat is that there is a small but significant incidence of disc herniations accompanying bilateral facet dislocations. In these patients, there is the potential that a closed reduction maneuver will retropulse the injured disc into the spinal canal and cause further neurologic compromise. The disc herniation is best identified by MRI but is suspected when the disc space at the dislocated level is markedly decreased in height on the lateral radiograph. Therefore, in patients with a normal neurologic examination, reduction is performed in an incremental fashion, with careful attention paid to the neurologic examination and ra-

FIG. 15-13   Same patient as in Fig. 15-12 following closed reduction.

diographic reduction sequence. The threshold must be low for obtaining a cervical MRI prior to or during closed reduction in these patients to rule out a herniated disc.

In an awake patient with a complete neurologic injury, reduction is attempted prior to obtaining an MRI examination. In an awake patient with an incomplete neurologic deficit, reduction is attempted as long as the neurologic examination does not deteriorate. If at any time the neurologic examination deteriorates, the reduction maneuver is halted and the patient is immediately taken for an MRI examination or cervical myelography if MRI is not available. Treatment of a traumatic disc herniation associated with a facet dislocation is anterior discectomy and fusion preceding a single-level posterior instrumentation and fusion. Unilateral facet dislocation is often difficult, if not impossible, to reduce with pure longitudinal cervical traction. These require a manual reduction maneuver after application of the appropriate amount of cervical traction weight. Manually turning the rotated head and chin toward the ipsilateral side of injury often produces a palpable clunk and feeling of reduction for the patient. This obviously must be done with careful neurologic monitoring and radiographic control. This reduction maneuver unlocks the dislocated facet and places it back into the normal position, that is, the superior facet sits anterior to the inferior facet. A prereduction MRI should be performed to determine whether a concomitant cervical disc herniation is present.

Associated Injuries

Associated injuries are identical to those of the upper cervicle spine.

Definitive Management

Definitive treatment options for subaxial cervical spine injuries include (1) orthotic immobilization with sternal–occipital–mandibular immobilizer (SOMI; Fig. 15-14); (2) halo vest immobilization (Fig. 15-15); (3) posterior fusion and stabilization using wires, cables, clamps and/or screws, and plates; (4) anterior approaches for decompression and strut graft fusion with or without plate and screw stabilization; and (5) a com-

FIG. 15-14 SOMI orthosis.

FIG. 15-15   Halo vest.

bination of these four treatment modalities. The two primary considerations for choosing a particular treatment plan include the presence of neural compression and actual or anticipated spinal instability.

Traditionally, posterior stainless steel wire constructs have provided adequate stabilization for fusion in the subaxial cervical spine by using spinous processes and/or facet wiring techniques. Sublaminar wire techniques are not recommended in the subaxial cervical spine following trauma because of the risk of iatrogenic neurologic injury. In addition, with the presence of posterior bony element injury, these wiring techniques may be impossible or must be extended to normal levels above and/or below the injury. Recently, lateral mass-plating techniques have been developed in an attempt to provide stabilization to areas with spinous process and lamina injuries but intact lateral masses. This technique requires screw placement into the lateral masses, which has some risk of neurologic and vascular complications associated with it; long-term results are not yet available for this technique (Fig. 15-16).

The halo vest is often a useful modality in the management of subaxial cervical spine bony injuries. As a general rule, the more osseous the

FIG. 15-16 Same patient as in Fig. 15-12 following posterior plating and fusion.

injury (i.e., the less ligamentous), the more useful the halo vest. Ligamentous injuries will heal with scar tissue in a halo, and this scar tissue will not maintain long-term spinal stability. For single-level or multilevel bony injuries, the halo vest is often the optimal treatment device. However, there are many potential complications of halo vest management. The most commonly encountered complication is pin tract infection causing pin loosening. Thus, these patients must be followed closely when being treated as an outpatient.

The majority of isolated posterior element fractures are stable and are not associated with a major neurologic deficit (except for isolated cervical root deficits). These injuries are managed in a SOMI. Occasionally, with multiple injuries spanning several segments, a halo vest provides better control of alignment.

Minor avulsion and compression fractures are managed in a cervical orthosis or halo vest.

The definitive management of cervical burst fractures is dependent on the loss of height of the vertebral body, retropulsion, neurologic status, kyphosis, and the presence of posterior element injury. Fractures with less than 25% loss of height, minimal retropulsion, and kyphosis in a neurologically intact patient are managed in a halo vest for approximately 3 months. With increasing middle column retropulsion, there is an increased likelihood of spinal cord injury. These patients are candidates for anterior decompression via corpectomy and strut graft stabilization. If the posterior ligaments are intact, stability is maintained with an anterior strut graft and halo vest for approximately 3 months. An alternative to provide additional stability is an anterior cervical plate attached to the segments above and below the fractured vertebral body, thereby internally stabilizing the strut graft and possibly obviating the halo vest. In patients with vertebral body-burst fractures and posterior ligamentous disruption, anterior strut grafting with anterior plate fixation cannot resist flexion forces, and thus posterior stabilization is also necessary.

Definitive management of teardrop fractures is based on the extent of bony, ligamentous and neurologic damage. When there is significant spinal canal compression, anterior corpectomy of the retropulsed vertebral body is performed with autogenous iliac crest strut grafting. Application of an anterior cervical plate is an option to further stabilize these segments. Because of the posterior column instability, either halo vest placement (for posterior bony injuries) or posterior instrumentation and fusion is performed.

Unilateral facet fractures without subluxation are managed in a SOMI orthosis or halo vest for 3 months or until bony healing is noted. The residual rotatory instability of a facet fracture with subluxation may be uncontrolled in a halo vest; therefore, these may heal in a malunited rotated position, which may exacerbate a nerve root deficit. For those injuries in which reduction cannot be maintained with a halo vest, management is anterior cervical discectomy and fusion with anterior cervical plating in addition to a halo vest to provide reduction and stability for posterior column healing.

When closed reduction of a facet dislocation is successful, the patient's neurologic status and overall medical condition are monitored. When the patient is considered neurologically and medically stable, single-level posterior instrumentation with fusion is performed. Posterior wiring techniques are the traditional method of internal stabilization. Posterolateral mass plating techniques are also being used for internal stabilization of these injuries (Fig. 15-16). With both of these techniques, patients are kept out of a halo, which aids in both pulmonary and psychologic recovery. As an alternative, these patients may also be treated with an anterior discectomy, fusion, and plating technique followed by a cervical orthosis from 3 months. Bilateral facet fractures are approached anteriorly because the posterior column involvement precludes posterior instrumentation. Anterior cervical discectomy and fusion with or without anterior cervical plating is performed at the involved level. Postoperative treatment with a halo vest may be necessary to immobilize the posterior element fractures.

Complications

Complications of burst fractures include progressive kyphosis with potential neurologic sequelae due to failure to diagnose a posterior ligamentous injury. In cases in which there is greater than 50% loss of height of a vertebrae in the neurologically intact patient, voluntary flexion–extension radiographs after healing of the compression fracture are necessary to rule out posterior ligamentous injury, which will result in chronic instability. Complications associated with the use of anterior strut grafts include anterior dislodgment with esophageal compression, posterior dislodgment with potential spinal cord compression, and breakage or nonunion of the strut graft.

Complications of teardrop fractures revolve around the difficulty in stabilizing unrecognized posterior ligamentous injuries. Management with anterior corpectomy and strut graft in the face of posterior column injury has resulted in graft dislodgment, late kyphotic deformities, and the need for reoperation even with postoperative halo vest treatment. Anterior and posterior surgical approaches with internal stabilization via plates anteriorly and posteriorly appear to stabilize these injuries maximally.

Complications of cervical facet injuries are the development of acute or chronic instability. This is frequently due to inadequately treating ligamentous injuries in a halo, which will not produce long-term stability, failure to recognize a concomitant disc herniation in the presence of a facet subluxation or dislocation during the closed reduction maneuver, and failure to anticipate rotational instability and using interspinous wiring techniques that do not control rotational instabilities. Acute and chronic cervical instability has been quantified to be present when more than 3.5 mm of segmental translation or greater than 11° of segmental angulation are present. Patients who have this degree of instability, even if asymptomatic, should be considered for posterior instrumentation and fusion.

THORACIC AND LUMBAR SPINAL INJURIES

Fractures of the thoracic, thoracolumbar, and lumbar spine are classified into four general categories: compression fractures, burst fractures, flexion–distraction injuries (Chance fractures), and fracture–dislocations.

The most common and benign of thoracic and lumbar fractures are simple **compression fractures.** These typically are wedge-shaped fractures of the vertebral body involving only the anterior column. They occur after trivial trauma in elderly patients with osteoporosis or following more significant trauma in younger patients. They are located in any part of the thoracic or lumbar spine, most frequently in the midthoracic to the midlumbar spine (Fig. 15-17).

Burst fractures involve the anterior and middle columns with or without injury to the posterior column. The mechanism of injury is high-energy axial loading with slight flexion. The vertebral body liter-

FIG. 15-17   Compression fracture of the lumbar spine.

ally explodes or "bursts," often resulting in posterior vertebral body wall retropulsion into the spinal canal (Fig. 15-18).

Flexion–distraction injuries (Chance fractures) are three-column injuries with the fracture propagating through the posterior elements, pedicle, and exiting through the vertebral body. These can also be completely ligamentous injuries entering through the posterior ligaments and exiting through the disc space or combined bony and ligamentous injuries. Chance fractures often occur during a head-on automobile collision in which the patient is wearing a lap belt. The mechanism of injury is acute flexion of the torso on the lap belt. During impact, the upper part of the body is accelerated anteriorly over the seat belt, producing a distraction force posteriorly around a fixed fulcrum just anterior to the abdomen (Fig. 15-19).

FIG. 15-18   Burst fracture of the lumbar spine.

FIG. 15-19   Flexion–distraction, or Chance, fracture of the lumbar spine.

Fracture–dislocations are the result of significant energy applied to the spine with a variety of forces including flexion, distraction, extension, rotation, shear, and axial-loading components producing spinal malalignment. These injuries always involve all three columns of the spine and are extremely unstable. They have a high propensity for profound neurologic injury (Fig. 15-20).

Diagnosis and Initial Management

History and Physical Examination

The neurologic examination is critical in patients with thoracic and lumbar spinal injuries and particularly so in burst fractures. Clinically, patients may have tenderness to palpation over the affected posterior elements if these are injured also.

The diagnosis of flexion–distraction spinal injuries includes a high index of suspicion from the mechanism of injury, as noted previously. Often, these patients present to the emergency room with a seat-belt type of abrasion over the anterior abdominal wall. A tender, palpable gap may be present when examining the back, indicative of the distracted spinous processes. The incidence of neurologic complications in flexion–distraction injuries is low in patients without an associated dislocation. Patients with fracture–dislocations often have multisystem injuries due to the violent nature of the trauma. Gross spinal malalignment may be obvious when examining the back, which may have a palpable step-off in the posterior spinal contour.

FIG. 15-20   Dislocation of the lumbar spine.

Radiographic Examination

The diagnosis of a compression fracture is normally made on routine lateral radiographs of the affected region of the spine. Typically, loss of anterior body height versus posterior height is noted, depending on the amount of compression seen. For more subtle injuries, technetium bone scanning with or without CT may be necessary to identify the injury. Axial CT can reliably document an intact posterior vertebral body wall, thereby confirming an intact middle column and thus verifying an anterior compression injury.

The diagnosis of burst fracture is made on either plane radiographs or CT. Radiographic signs of a burst fracture include a widened interpedicular distance at the fractured level on the anteroposterior projection, vertebral body compression with segmental kyphosis, and retropulsion of the posterior cortex of the vertebral body on the lateral projection. The plane radiographs are also examined for subluxation or dislocation in the coronal or sagittal planes and for evidence of posterior column injury. Axial CT demonstrates a break in the posterior cortical wall with different degrees of spinal canal compression from retropulsed bone (Fig. 15-21).

Plain radiographs are essential in the diagnosis of flexion–distraction injuries. The lateral radiograph indicates widening of the posterior column either within or between the bony elements and localized kyphosis. There are also different degrees of distraction of the middle column and thus either a fracture propagating through the pedicles or a widening of the posterior disc space. The anteroposterior radiograph indicates a widened interspinous distance indicative of ligamentous posterior column injury, fracture through the spinous process lamina, or splayed posterior

FIG. 15-21   Fracture–dislocation of T11 on T12.

elements. If translational forces are present and sustained, ligamentous flexion–distraction injuries may progress to unilateral or bilateral facet subluxation or dislocation. Unilateral dislocation is characterized by anterior displacement of the superior vertebra on the inferior by 25% on the lateral radiograph. When displacement is 50% or greater, a bilateral facet dislocation is likely.

Plain radiographs indicate fracture–dislocations of the thoracic and lumbar spine in either the coronal or sagittal planes, or both (Fig. 15-22). Occasionally, thoracic subluxations are quite subtle and may involve only a slight lateral or anterior translation of one vertebral body on another. When subluxation proceeds to frank dislocation, the spinal malalignment is obvious on the lateral radiograph. CT is mandatory for these fractures to assess unrecognized posterior element fractures that may affect operative management. Axial CT often demonstrates two vertebral bodies in the same transaxial slice, indicating dislocation of a vertebral segment. The empty facet sign is present when there is complete facet dislocation. Unlike burst fractures, the middle column is often intact when the primary mechanism of injury is a shearing force. In this instance, the vertebral canal compromise is

FIG. 15-22   CT scan indicating compromise of the spinal canal following a burst fracture.

secondary to the extreme vertebral malalignment rather than retropulsed bone.

Initial Management

The initial treatment of a patient with a spinal thoracic or lumbar fracture includes supine bed rest with log-rolling to minimize pressure-dependent areas. A thorough system review for associated injuries is performed. It is essential to perform serial neurologic examinations on patients who are awaiting definitive treatment of fractures. Deterioration in the neurologic examination is an indication for emergent surgery.

Associated Injuries

There is a high incidence of multisystem trauma, such as liver or spleen lacerations, aortic arch tears, and intraabdominal trauma associated with high-energy thoracolumbar fractures. Twenty-five percent of patients with flexion–distraction injuries have associated intraabdominal injuries. Conversely, 25% of patients with intraabdominal injuries from wearing a lap belt have a flexion–distraction spine injury. Patients with thoracic spinal injuries also may have concomitant rib fractures with hemothorax or pneumothorax.

Definitive Management

Definitive management of thoracic and lumbar compression fractures depends on the age of the patient, location of the injury, amount of compression deformity, and any evidence of posterior column distraction injury. Elderly patients with multiple osteoporotic compression fractures of the spine often are treated symptomatically without any immobilization. Concern for possible pathologic involvement with tumor or infection must be maintained in the elderly patient population. Compression fractures with less than 50% loss of height are usually stable injuries that can be treated with a spinal orthosis for pain control during healing in younger patients. For lesions in the thoracolumbar junction and lumbar spine, a hyperextension orthosis attempts to limit the kyphosis that occurs after these injuries. However, even with a well-molded hyperextension cast or orthosis, some settling does occur during the healing process in the majority of these patients, but usually it is of little significance as long as the middle and posterior columns are intact.

For patients with greater than 50% compression deformity, it is essential to rule out middle column involvement and posterior column distraction. Radiographs demonstrate a widened intraspinous process distance or posterior element fracture, and the sagittal MRI also may document a posterior ligamentous injury. These injuries may require surgery with posterior compression instrumentation and fusion with or without an anterior corpectomy and anterior fusion to prevent a progressive kyphosis and neurologic sequelae.

Definitive management of thoracic and lumbar burst fractures depends on neurologic status, patient age, fracture location, spinal canal compromise, posterior element involvement, coronal or sagittal subluxation, amount of segmental sagittal kyphosis present, concomitant multisystem injuries, and body habitus. Methods of management are nonoperative bracing or casting or operative stabilization via anterior, posterior, or combined surgical approaches.

Burst fractures are managed **non-operatively** when the patient is neurologically intact, there is minimal segmental kyphosis and bony retropulsion (less than 50% canal compromise), no coronal or sagittal subluxation, and no posterior column involvement. A molded two-piece hyperextension spinal orthosis is applied. Younger patients with kyphosis and a thin body habitus are managed with a hyperextension risser cast to limit the post-injury settling of the fracture. When L4 or L5 is fractured, a single thigh is incorporated into the cast or brace to increase control of the lower lumbar spine sagittal alignment. The nonoperative treatment of lumbar burst fractures in neurologically intact patients with greater than 50% canal compromise is controversial. The majority of patients with this clinical scenario heal their burst fractures uneventfully without neurologic sequelae. The spinal canal remodels over time to increase the space available for the neural elements. However, settling of the burst fracture usually results in an increase in segmental kyphosis.

Indications for **operative** management of a burst fracture in a **neurologically intact** or minimally involved patient are three-column injuries, subluxation in the coronal or sagittal plane, significant segmental sagittal kyphosis at the fracture site, spinal canal compromise greater than 50%, and concomitant injuries or body habitus that will not allow orthotic or cast treatment. Fractures of the thoracolumbar junction or upper lumbar spine are approached posteriorly, reduced, bone grafted, and stabilized. The preservation of sagittal alignment and maintenance of motion segments are important and accomplished by using posterior pedicle screw fixation systems when the pedicles are of sufficient size. In cases in which there is inadequate anterior and middle column support, anterior corpectomy and strut grafting are performed as a second-stage procedure. Significant burst fractures of the thoracic spine in the neurologically intact patient are usually managed with combined anterior corpectomy and fusion, followed by posterior compression instrumentation and fusion to minimize the risk of further bony retropulsion and neurologic injury.

Operative management of burst fractures associated with **significant neurologic deficit** is individualized. The primary concern is spinal canal decompression. The anterior approach to the spine is the most thorough method of clearing the spinal canal of retropulsed bone and disc material, and it is the treatment of choice for this group of patients. The surgical approach is dictated by the level of pathology: a thoracotomy for T1 to T10 fractures; a thoracoabdominal approach usually through the tenth rib for T11, T12, and L1 fractures; and a retroperitoneal flank approach below the diaphram for L2 to L5 fractures. The intervertebral discs above and below the fracture are excised, and a subtotal corpectomy of the injured vertebra is performed, leaving the anterior and deep cortex intact. As an alternative, a reach-around posterior approach can provide anterior decompression and strut grafting via a costotransversectomy or far lateral lumbar approach.

Following spinal canal decompression, a strut graft or titanium mesh cage is placed from the inferior end plate of the cephalad vertebra to the superior end plate of the caudad vertebra. Success or failure of the surgery rests mainly on the stability and healing of the graft more than on any instrumentation placed. Anterior instrumentation devices secure the strut graft and at times may act as a stand-alone device along with postoperative bracing. However, the spine may also be instrumented and fused posteriorly in a second stage with rods and hooks over the same levels as the anterior construct for further stabilization.

The spine is approached posteriorly first for burst fractures with significant posterior column disruption or subluxation. The posterior instrumentation is used for reduction and restoration of sagittal plane alignment. At the same sitting, anterior corpectomy and strut graft fusion are performed.

Definitive management of flexion–distraction injuries depends on the anatomic structures involved and the amount of displacement. Lesions occurring entirely through bone are managed in a hyperextension cast. This is particularly successful when the fracture line has propagated through the pedicles bilaterally. Injuries in which the fracture involves the pars interarticularis and pure soft tissue are managed operatively because the pars has very little cancellous bone, which means fracture healing is less reliable, and ligamentous healing does not result in adequate stability. It is important to identify traumatic disc disruptions and herniations prior to the surgical reduction of displaced posterior elements because posterior compression forces may displace herniated disc material into the spinal canal, causing neurologic injury. A short segment fixation with pedicle screw instrumentation and fusion is performed via a posterior approach. A thoracolumbar orthosis is worn 4 months postoperatively. Definitive management of fracture–dislocations is posterior operative reduction, stabilization, and fusion. Thoracic injuries are instrumented three to four segments above and below the fracture dislocation by using hook and/or screw and rod constructs. Thoracolumbar and lumbar injuries are instrumented with pedicle screw and rod constructs, limiting the number of distally instrumented and fused motion segments, if possible. Postoperative bracing increases the fusion rate by protecting the instrumentation until fusion occurs.

The timing of operative reduction and stabilization is determined by the neurologic status and overall medical condition. The primary indication for emergent operative reduction is a neurologically incomplete patient with a progressing neurologic deficit. Patients with complete spinal cord injuries are stabilized as soon as possible to decrease the duration of enforced bedrest. A patient with an incomplete neurologic injury that is improving is observed until improvement plateaus. The spine is then reduced and stabilized.

Complications

The most significant complication of compression fractures is progressive kyphosis resulting from: settling of the vertebral body, unrecognized posterior column ligamentous injuries, multiple contiguous compression fractures, and pathologic fractures. Neurologic abnormalities are not seen with typical compression fractures, which involve only the anterior column.

Complications of nonoperative management of burst fractures are residual segmental kyphosis, progressive kyphosis secondary to unrecognized posterior column injury, and vertebral collapse due to settling. All these have a potential for increasing neurologic deficits. Complications of operative management of burst fractures are failure of instrumentation due to inadequate anterior column reconstruction, vascular or neurologic injury during the surgical approach, and dislodgment of strut grafts. Pseudarthrosis is rare with either operative or nonoperative treatment.

Complications of flexion–distraction injuries are inadequate posterior column reduction with casting for bony injuries, unrecognized ligamentous components of the injury, and rare traumatic disc herniations. The latter may retropulse into the spinal canal during operative reduction by posterior compression forces.

Complications of fracture–dislocations of the spine are an increase in spinal deformity due to inadequate treatment in a spinal orthosis or a charcot spinal arthropathy below a complete spinal cord injury.

SACRAL FRACTURES

Classification

Sacral fractures are classified anatomically into zones I, II, and III. **Zone I fractures** are lateral to the neural foramen. Neurologic deficits result from superiorly displaced sacral fracture fragments compressing the L5 nerve root against the undersurface of the L5 transverse process. Zone I injuries also include various ligamentous avulsion injuries around the periphery of the sacrum.

Zone II fractures are longitudinal fractures through the sacral foramen. These are associated with a 28% incidence of neurologic deficits. The neurologic injury is usually characterized by S1 compression associated with sciatica. L5 is involved when fracture fragments are displaced superiorly, and other sacral nerve roots can be involved if the fracture extends through these levels, causing displacement. Because these fractures are unilateral, incontinence is rare, but sensory changes over the involved dermatomes are common.

Zone III fractures involve the central canal and have a high (57%) incidence of neurologic deficits, with loss of sphincter control, saddle anesthesia, and acute cauda equina symptoms. Transverse fractures occur as isolated injuries as the result of a flexion force imparted to the lower part of the sacrum and the coccyx. Below S4, there is little chance of a significant neurologic deficit because the sacral nerve roots have exited proximal to this area.

Diagnosis and Initial Management

History and Physical Examination

Sacral fractures occur most frequently in high-energy trauma. Physical findings are back and buttock pain, ecchymosis over the sacrum, and sacral pain on rectal examination. Specific low lumbar and sacral root neurologic deficits should prompt consideration of sacral fractures. The fifth lumbar root is often involved when it is trapped between the transverse process of L5 and the superiorly migrating fragment of the sacral ala. Evaluation of the Achilles and bulbocavernosus reflex is mandatory when assessing sacral root function. Sacral fractures may result in anesthesia over the sacral dermatomes, impotence, and a flaccid bowel and bladder. Incontinence rarely occurs with unilateral root injury between

S2 and S5. Decreased sensation is a more usual consequence. When in doubt about the integrity of the structures innervated by the sacral segments, urodynamics is helpful in the assessment of motor function of the bladder.

Radiographic Examination

Radiographic documentation of sacral fractures is difficult because of the complex shape of the sacrum and pelvis. Fifty percent of sacral fractures without neurologic deficit is missed on initial examination. The initial radiographic examination includes lateral and anteroposterior, or Fergusson, projections. The Fergusson projection centers the proximally directed beam on the sacrum. Radiographic findings associated with sacral fractures are low lumbar transverse process fractures, asymmetrical sacral foramen, and irregular trabeculation of the lateral masses of the proximal sacral segments. CT is the most accurate method of evaluating sacral fractures. Suspected fractures are identified on bone scan when the sacral segments are too osteopenic to produce reliable radiographic images.

Initial Management

The focus of initial management of sacral fractures is pain relief. The patient is kept at bed rest and log-rolled from side to side until the pain subsides to the point where mobilization can be initiated, usually 7 to 10 days.

Associated Injuries

Multisystem injuries and neurologic injuries are associated with fractures of the sacrum.

Definitive Management

Isolated sacral fractures without anterior pelvic ring fractures or neurologic deficits are stable and do not require treatment beyond relief of symptoms. After the initial period of bed rest, the patient is mobilized with nonweight-bearing on the affected side for 4 to 8 weeks and then with weight-bearing as tolerated. Sacral fractures that present as elements of a pelvic injury are managed to reestablish the pelvic ring.

Complications

Complications of sacral fractures are chronic pain secondary to sacroiliac arthritis or change of alignment of the sacrum and loss of voluntary control of bowel and bladder. Sacroiliac arthritis is managed with arthrodesis.

Neurologic deficits associated with zone II injuries are managed with observation because many of these injuries are neuropraxias that will resolve spontaneously. Symptoms that persist beyond 6 to 8 weeks may benefit from foraminal decompression. Deficits associated with zone III injuries should undergo aggressive radiologic examination to identify the cause of the neurologic injury because early posterior decompression may result in return of bowel and bladder control and reversal of foot drop. Late decompression is often complicated by epidural fibrosis and minimal return of function.

SELECTED READINGS

Allen GL, Ferguson RL, Lehmann TR, O'Brien RP: A mechanistic classification of closed, indirect fractures and dislocations of the lower cervical spine. *Spine* 7:1–27, 1982.

Bohlmann HH: Acute fractures and dislocations of the cervical spine, an analysis of 300 hospitalized patients and review of the literature. *J Bone Joint Surg* 61A:1141, 1979.

Bohlmann HH: Treatment of fractures and dislocations of the thoracic and lumbar spine-current concepts review. *J Bone Joint Surg* 67A:165–169, 1985.

Clark CR, White AA III: Fractures of the dens. A multi center study. *J Bone Joint Surg* 67A:1340, 1985.

Denis F: The 3-column spine and its significance in the classification of acute thoracolumbar spinal injuries. *Spine* 8:817–831, 1983.

Haher TR, Selnly WF, O'Brien MO: Diagnosis and management of thoracic and lumbar spinal fractures. *In* Bridwell KH and Dewald RL (eds). *Textbook of spinal surgery*, 1st ed. Philadelphia, Lippincott, 1991.

McAfee PC, Bohlman HH, Yuan HA: Anterior decompression of traumatic thoracolumbar fractures with incomplete neurological deficit using a retroperitoneal approach. *J Bone Joint Surg* 47A:89–103, 1985.

Sabiston CP, Wing PC: Sacral fractures: Classification and neurologic implications. *J Trauma* 26:1113–1115, 1986.

Vaccaro AR, An HS, Lin S, Sun S, Balderston RA, Cotler JM: Noncontiguous injuries of the spine. *J Spinal Disord* 5:320–329, 1992.

White AA, Southwick WO, Panjabi MM: Clinical instability in the lower cervical spine, a review of past and current concepts. *Spine* 1:15–27, 1976.

Fractures and Dislocations of the
Pelvic Ring and Acetabulum

D. Kevin Scheid

This chapter reviews fractures and dislocations of the pelvic ring and
acetabulum and dislocations of the hip.

ANATOMY OF THE PELVIC RING

The bony pelvic ring consists of two innominate bones (hemipelvis) and
the sacrum, which are held together by an intricate ligamentous network.
Each innominate bone consists of three parts: ilium, ischium, and pubis,
which fuse at the acetabulum upon skeletal maturity. The **anterior column,** or iliopubic column, includes the anterior wall of the acetabulum,
the anterior ilium, and the superior pubic ramus. The **posterior column,**
or ilioischial column, includes the posterior wall of the acetabulum and
extends from the posterior-inferior ilium at the greater sciatic notch to
the ischial tuberosity (Fig. 16-1). Specific landmarks on the anterior column helpful during surgery include the anterosuperior iliac spine, anteroinferior iliac spine, iliopubic line, iliopubic eminence, and pubic
tubercle. Landmarks on the posterior column include the greater sciatic
notch, lesser sciatic notch, ischial spine, and ischial tuberosity.

Each innominate bone articulates with the sacrum posteriorly at the
sacroiliac joints. The joints are covered with hyaline cartilage on the
sacral side and fibrocartilage on the iliac side. All sacroiliac joint stability is derived from **interosseous, posterior sacroiliac, and anterior
sacroiliac ligament complexes** (Fig. 16-2). The anterior pelvic ring is
joined at the cartilage-covered pubic symphysis and is held by an en-
veloping fibroligamentous complex. Two additional (sacroischial) ligaments, the sacrospinous and sacrotuberous, confer stability to the pelvic
ring. Together, these ligament complexes resist vertical and rotational
forces on each hemipelvis. The pelvic brim divides the upper (false
pelvis) and lower (true pelvis).

Vascular, neurologic, and genitourinary structures lie within and
along the inner pelvis, making them susceptible to injury during pelvic
disruption. The **common iliac artery** gives rise to the **internal iliac and
external iliac arteries.** The **superior and inferior gluteal, vesical, and
lumbosacral arteries** all arise from the internal iliac artery. The **sacral
venous plexus** is particularly susceptible to injury and is difficult to
control or embolize.

The **lumbosacral plexus,** which includes the fourth and fifth lumbar
and sacral nerve roots, lies along the anterior sacrum. The sciatic, gluteal,
and splanchnic nerves arise from this plexus. The obturator nerve runs
along and below the pelvic brim to exit the obturator foramen.

FIG. 16-1   *(A)* Anterior and *(B)* posterior columns of the pelvis.

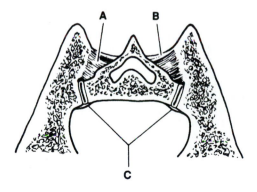

FIG. 16-2   Transverse section through sacroiliac joints: *(A)* in-terosseous ligaments, *(B)* posterior sacroiliac ligaments, and *(C)* anterior sacroiliac ligaments.

The bladder, urethra, vagina, and rectum are all susceptible to puncture or tear by bony spicules, shear forces, and compression.

FRACTURES AND DISLOCATIONS OF THE PELVIS

Classification

Pelvic fractures have previously been classified according to the presumed mechanism of injury as lateral compression, anteroposterior compression, vertical shear, and complex. The more useful AO classification of Tile is based solely on pelvic stability and therefore better dictates treatment.

Type A fractures are both vertically stable and rotationally stable. They do not truly disrupt the pelvic *ring* as do **type B** and **type C** fractures. An iliac wing fracture involving the crest that does not disrupt the integrity of the pelvic ring or an isolated transverse sacrum fracture are examples of type A fractures. Avulsions of the ischeal tuberosity or iliac spines are also type A injuries.

Type B fractures are vertically stable but rotationally unstable. They include the lateral compression and anteroposterior compression injuries. The hemipelvis is disrupted rotationally, causing both anterior and posterior ring injuries. Although these injuries can be quite severe and cause gross *rotational* instability to the hemipelvis, the hemipelvis is not vertically unstable and will not displace vertically because of intact ligamentous structures. The two common subgroups of type B injuries include the "open book" (B1) injury, with anterior pelvic ring disruption and disruption of the *anterior* sacroiliac ligaments. The hemipelvis is unstable to *external* rotation but vertically stable because of intact posterior sacroiliac ligaments (Fig.16-3). The second most common subgroup of B injuries are those unstable to *internal* rotation and include the "lateral compression" (B2) injuries. The internally rotated hemipelvis disrupts the *posterior* sacroiliac ligaments and crushes the anterior ring (pubic rami). The anterior sacroiliac ligaments and sacrospinous and sacrotuberous ligaments remain intact. The rotating hemipelvis frequently crushes the anterior sacrum or sacral ala. The intact ligaments keep the hemipelvis vertically stable. The disrupted anterior ring and posterior sacroiliac ligaments cause internal rotational instability (Figs. 16-4 and 16-5).

Type C fractures are *vertically* and thus *rotationally* unstable. Like type B injuries, the anterior and posterior pelvic ring is disrupted. Unlike type B injuries, sufficient bony or ligamentous disruption has occurred, allowing the hemipelvis to displace vertically. The posterior injury can involve the sacrum, sacroiliac joint, posterior ilium, or any combination thereof. The anterior injury can involve the symphysis or ischial and pubic rami (Figs. 16-6 and 16-7). Because of the combined

FIG. 16-3   B1 injury with anterior ring and anterior sacroiliac ligament disruption. The posterior sacroiliac ligaments remain intact, providing vertical stability.

Fig. 16-4   B2 injury with anterior ring and posterior sacroiliac ligament disruption. The anterior sacroiliac, sacrospinous, and sacrotuberous ligaments remain intact, providing vertical stability.

bony and ligamentous injuries, these fracture-dislocations can migrate vertically because of the pull of the torso muscles.

Diagnosis and Initial Management

History and Physical Examination

There is always a history of significant trauma. A rapid initial physical examination includes inspection for pelvic, abdominal, and perineal

Fig. 16-5 B2 injury with fracture of the ilium posteriorly. Like the fracture pictured in Fig. 16-4, this fracture is unstable to internal rotation but not vertically unstable.

FIGS. 16-6 and 16-7 C-type injuries showing vertical instability of the hemipelvis. The posterior injury can involve the posterior ilium, sacroiliac joint, or sacrum. The anterior injury can involve the symphysis (Fig 16-6) or the ischial and pubic rami (Fig 16-7).

bruising; rectal or vaginal tears, indicating an open fracture; blood at the urethral meatus, indicating possible urethral tear; pelvic asymmetry; iliac crest mobility; lower extremity malrotation; leg length discrepancy; and a focused neurologic and vascular examination of the lower extremities.

Radiographic Examination

An anteroposterior pelvis film usually raises suspicion of a pelvic ring disruption. Inlet and outlet views and CAT scans define the posterior injury and, thus, probable pelvic ring stability. If equivocal, suspected instability is documented fluoroscopically by examination under anesthesia.

Initial Management

Hemodynamically stable patients are closely monitored. Hemodynamic instability is a life-threatening emergency. Hemodynamically unstable patients are put in a MAST suit (antishock trousers) to increase peripheral vascular resistance and decrease motion of the fracture by direct pressure. Use of the MAST suit for other than initial transport and stabilization is not indicated because of complications secondary to prolonged inflation. Immediate intervention for the bleeding pelvis after removal of the MAST suit is rapid reduction and external fixation to tamponade bleeding vessels. Anterior ring stabilization alone will usually suffice to tamponade retroperitoneal hemorrhage, even if there is vertical instability; however, skeletal traction is added to prevent vertical migration of the hemipelvis. If bleeding persists, as indicated by continued hemodynamic instability, selective arterial embolization is attempted. Indications for emergent open control of hemorrhage or packing are rare: open fracture and inability to control hemorrhage, major vessel disruption uncontrollable by embolization, and life-saving hemipelvectomy.

Associated Injuries

Pelvic fractures frequently are associated with vascular and genitourinary system injuries. B1 injuries, unstable in external rotation, have a greater incidence of associated vascular injuries than do B2 injuries, unstable to internal rotation. **Vascular injuries** are life-threatening and must be aggressively managed. Rapid evaluation is required to rule out thoracic, intraperitoneal, or external bleeding and to direct management of the patient in extremis toward the retroperitoneum and the pelvic fracture. The hypovolemic patient with an unstable pelvic ring fracture is assumed to have significant retroperitoneal hemorrhage due to injury of the sacral venous plexus, bleeding fractured bone, and major or minor arterial injuries.

Genitourinary injury is suspected with any pelvic fracture and is more common in B2 injuries. Blood at the urethral meatus, fractures of the ischial and pubic rami, and a floating prostate on rectal examination indicate urethral injury. A retrograde urethrogram determines the presence of a urethral tear prior to catheterization of the bladder. A cystogram determines whether the bladder is intact.

Definitive Management

The goal of early management is stabilization of the unstable pelvis. This is most frequently accomplished by application of an anterior external fixator.

In **rotationally unstable (B)** fractures, only anterior ring stability is required to convert an unstable pelvic ring to a stable structure. Displaced or grossly unstable lateral compression (B2) fractures require anterior ring stabilization only. Often, an external fixator is used to externally rotate and reduce the internally rotated hemipelvis. Open book (B1) injuries with instability on stress views greater than 2.5 cm of symphysis dissociation or gross radiographic and clinical instability also warrant stabilization of the anterior pelvic ring. In equivocal cases, examination with imaging under general anesthesia will assess the degree of rotational instability. An external fixator or pubic symphysis plate is sufficient to internally rotate and stabilize the externally rotated hemipelvis.

In **vertically unstable** fractures, anterior and posterior stabilization is required.

Anterior stabilization is accomplished in many cases with an external fixator. Relative indications for internal fixation of the disrupted symphysis pubis or pubic rami fractures include exposure of the area for laparotomy or bladder repair, an acetabular fracture stabilized with an anterior column plate that can be continued across the pubic symphysis, and when external fixator pins would violate an acetabular surgical incision, thereby increasing the chance of postoperative infection. The **technique of external fixation** follows many of the guidelines set forth for external fixator use in long bones. Two to three pins at least 5 mm in diameter are placed in each hemipelvis. Increased pin spacing improves stability. External fixator systems that do not require parallel pin placement allow individual angling of pins for optimum positioning. The shape of the iliac wing makes it a challenge to insert the pins between the two cortical tables. Pins are placed through small horizontal incisions over the iliac crest. The starting point for the first pin is 2 cm posterior to the anterosuperior iliac spine. The second pin is inserted in the broad iliac tubercle 6–10 cm posterior to the first pin. A drill hole is made in the cortex of the crest only, and pins are inserted by hand with a T-handled chuck. Imaging can be used with tangential views to ensure that the pins remain between the cortical tables. Directing each pin toward the rectum offers an initial three-dimensional mental landmark for pin placement within the cortical tables. Maximum pin depth, with the tip of the pins ending in the ilium just above the acetabulum, affords the greatest stability and longevity of the pin. Rotating the fluoroscope in different directions allows tangential views of each pin, verifying placement between the cortical tables. A simple quadrilateral frame is attached to the pins, the pelvis is reduced by manipulation under fluoroscopy, and the frame is tightened to hold the reduction.

The **technique of open reduction and internal fixation** of the anterior pelvic ring is with a horizontal Pfannenstiel or vertical laparotomy incision. Two anterior plates oriented 90° to each other are much more stable than a single plate. A Foley catheter in the bladder not only decompresses the bladder but also serves as an easily palpable landmark for bladder location.

There are no external fixator constructs or anterior internal fixation alone that provide enough stability to maintain reduction of a vertically unstable fracture. Therefore, when vertical instability is present, the posterior ring must be stabilized. This can be done acutely in a stable patient or delayed until the patient has stabilized. Traction must be employed if posterior fixation is delayed. Various **techniques of posterior fixation** have evolved and their use depends on the location of the posterior injury and the surgeon's experience. **Posterior iliac fractures** are stabilized by using standard plating techniques. Lag screws compress the fracture, and a neutralization plate is applied. The approach is anterior through an iliac crest incision, exposing the inner table, or posterior, with the patient in a lateral decubitus or prone position. Exposure of the more lateral iliac fracture is easier through an inner pelvic approach. Posterior iliac fractures are more easily exposed through a posterior approach, especially in the obese patient.

Sacroiliac joint stabilization is most commonly accomplished by image-guided, percutaneously placed iliosacral screws. In experienced hands, one and usually two screws placed into S1 or S1 and S2 are sufficient. Anterior iliosacral plating can also be done if it offers certain advantages in a given case. Sacral bars are rarely used.

The majority of patients presenting for delayed posterior fixation have had an external fixator placed on admission or during the resuscitation. The external fixator may need to be detached to allow mobility of the hemipelvis for anatomic reduction. After anatomic posterior reduction is obtained, the fixator is resecured.

Anterior fixation with two- or three-hole plates has been used successfully for many years. Stability of fixation is increased by the use of two plates. This is important when there is room for only one screw on the sacral side due to the proximity of the L5 nerve root. Occasionally, the sacroiliac joint is approached posteriorly. A **posterior approach** is most commonly employed when a large iliac fragment is present and is attached to the sacrum by the iliolumbar and iliosacral ligaments. Direct exposure of this fragment facilitates its reduction and fixation.

The advantage of **percutaneous iliosacral lag screws** is the direct fixation of the ilium to the sacrum. The disadvantages are potential iatrogenic neurologic injury from screw penetration into the sacral foramina or spinal canal and violation of the sacroiliac joint itself with the screws. Two large-diameter cannulated screws are inserted from the posterolateral ilium into the Sl body or sacral ala. Washers or small plates are used to prevent migration of the screw head through the ilium as the screw is tightened. The technique requires clear visualization by using image intensification. Patient position must allow enough undertable clearance to obtain appropriate inlet, outlet, and lateral views with the fluoroscope. When there is inadequate visualization of the sacral foramina on the outlet view because of obesity or bowel gas, alternative methods of fixation are used, or the procedure is delayed until the bowel is well prepped. On the inlet view, the pin is angled slightly anteriorly to pass through the vestibule of the sacral ala at a perpendicular angle. The tip of the guidepin is placed in the anterior one-third of the S1 body to maintain the maximum distance between it and the sacral spinal canal. On the outlet view, the guidepin should be angled slightly cephalad, ending in the upper one-half of the Sl body. A final check with a true lateral view ensures accurate guidepin placement.

Sacral fractures are stabilized in situ by using the percutaneous iliosacral screw technique described for sacroiliac joints. Problems unique to sacral fractures are loss of foraminal landmarks secondary to the fracture pattern and crushing of interposed nerves between bone fragments while the screws are being tightened. When anatomic reduction of the sacral fracture is not achieved by closed methods, a combination posterior open and percutaneous approach is used. The patient is positioned prone, and the sacrum is exposed through a posterior longitudinal incision. The fracture is reduced, and nerves are decompressed. With the help of fluoroscopy, percutaneous iliosacral screws are placed. Even with a direct approach to the sacrum or sacroiliac joint posteriorly, exposure of the outer posterior ilium is not required to place percutaneous screws. This will help prevent posterior wound breakdown.

Complications

Complications include posttraumatic arthritis of the sacroiliac joint, symptomatic malunion resulting in leg length discrepancy, malrotation, and neurologic symptoms due to inflammation and entrapment of lumbar and sacral nerve roots. **Arthritis** of the sacroiliac joint is managed conservatively initially, and with arthrodesis if necessary. Symptomatic **malunion** is managed with a shoe lift and gait modification. Occasionally, a correctional osteotomy is indicated. **Neuritis** is managed with nonsteroidal antiinflammatory drugs, neuroleptics and occasionally nerve decompression.

ACETABULAR FRACTURES

Classification

The anatomic classification of acetabular fractures was published by Judet et al. in 1964 and refined by Letournel in 1981. Acetabular fractures are classified into five **simple** and five **associated** fractures.

Simple Fractures

Posterior wall fractures represent posterior dislocations of the femoral head. They involve different amounts of the posterior rim of the acetabulum. Sciatic nerve injury and marginal impaction of the remaining intact posterior wall are common (Fig. 16-8). A frequent mistake is classifying a large posterior wall fracture as a posterior column fracture.

Posterior column fractures by definition require disruption of the ilioischial line on the anteroposterior pelvis view. They include the ischial portion of the bone and often involve a disruption of the obturator foramen (Fig. 16-9).

Anterior wall fractures are rare. They involve different portions of the anterior rim or half of the acetabulum. The fracture does not involve the inferior pubic ramus (Fig. 16-10).

Anterior column fractures are characterized by disruption of the iliopectineal line. Low-column fractures involve the inferior acetabulum and have disruption of the inferior pubic ramus. Superior fractures involve different parts of the anterior one-half of the ilium (Fig. 16-11).

Transverse fractures divide the hemipelvis into superior and inferior halves. The line can traverse the articular surface at any level, and the obturator foramen is intact (Figs. 16-12 and 16-13).

Associated Fractures

Posterior column–posterior wall fractures represent a dislocation of the hip with an associated posterior column fracture. There is a break in the obturator foramen (Fig. 16-14).

FIG. 16-8   Posterior wall fracture.

FIG. 16-9   Posterior column fracture.

FIG. 16-10   Anterior wall fracture.

FIG. 16-11   Anterior column fracture.

FIG. 16-12   Transverse fracture.

T-shape fractures are transverse with an associated vertical fracture into the obturator foramen and out through the inferior ramus (Fig. 16-15).

Anterior wall or column fracture with posterior hemitransverse, as the name implies, combines an anterior wall or column fracture with the posterior one-half of a transverse fracture (Fig. 16-16).

FIG. 16-13   Transverse fracture.

FIG. 16-14   Posterior column–posterior wall fracture.

Both-column fractures are diagnosed more often than they occur. A true both-column fracture has no articular surface attached to the *intact* portion of the ilium, which remains attached to the sacrum (Fig. 16-17).

Transverse with posterior wall fractures usually do not have a break in the obturator foramen (Fig. 16-18).

FIG. 16-15   T-shaped fracture.

FIG. 16-16   Anterior wall or column fracture with a posterior hemitransverse fracture.

Diagnosis and Initial Management

History and Physical Examination

There is always a history of significant injury. The patient has pain localized to the hip. The leg may be rotated and shortened. Motion of the hip elicits severe pain. A partial or complete sciatic nerve injury may exist.

Radiographic Examination

Radiographic evaluation is important for preoperative planning. Virtually all fractures can be classified with an anteroposterior pelvis film and two oblique views. Although both-column outlines can be seen on the anteroposterior view (Fig. 16-19), the two oblique, or Judet, views at 45° best display the individual columns. The **iliac oblique** view is taken with the fractured side tilted down, or away, from the x-ray tube. This view profiles the ilium and best displays the posterior column of the affected side (Fig. 16-20). The **obturator oblique** view, taken with the fractured side tilted up toward the tube, best displays the outline of the anterior column (Fig. 16-21). Computed tomography provides additional information not easily found on plain films including undisplaced ilium fragments or impacted segmental fragments of the acetabulum. Downfalls of axial CT include the inability to determine dome step-off and difficulty in classification without comparison to plain films. Three-dimensional CT scans are accurate representations of the fracture but usually add little additional information.

FIG. 16-17   Both-column fracture.

FIG. 16-18 Transverse with posterior wall fracture.

AP

A **Iliopectineal line**
B **Ilioischial line**
C **Anterior rim**
D **Posterior rim**

FIG. 16-19 Anteroposterior view of the hemipelvis.

ILIAC-OBLIQUE

P   Outline post column
GS   Greater sciatic notch
IS   Ischial spine

FIG. 16-20   Iliac oblique projection.

OBTURATOR-OBLIQUE

A   Pelvic brim of anterior
column

FIG. 16-21   Obturator oblique projection.

Associated Injuries

Associated injuries of the femoral head, pelvis, genitourinary system, and sciatic nerve occur frequently. Unfortunately, the best acetabular reconstruction may have a poor result because of **damaged articular surface of the femoral head.** Some of this damage occurs postinjury as the subluxed head articulates with fractured bony edges. For this reason, the patient is placed in skeletal traction until it is determined that the fracture is undisplaced and that there are no intraarticular fragments. A concomitant **pelvic ring** injury complicates the preoperative planning. **Genitourinary** injuries are less frequent than with pelvic ring disruptions. **Sciatic nerve** contusion with selective injury to the peroneal section of the nerve is common in posterior column and wall fractures. Local soft tissues are frequently compromised and are carefully inspected before determining the timing of surgery and the approach.

Initial Management

Similar to pelvic ring injuries, acetabular fractures frequently occur with injuries to other organ systems. During resuscitation, an anteroposterior pelvis film will show most acetabular pathology. When hemodynamic stability is achieved, Judet views and a CT scan are obtained to determine whether traction is necessary. Distal femoral skeletal traction is applied in the emergency room or on the floor. Twenty to thirty pounds of skeletal traction will suffice to partially reduce the femoral head and disimpact the joint.

A dislocated femoral head is reduced as though there were no acetabular fracture. If necessary, skeletal traction is applied while the reduction is held manually. Open reduction is necessary for the rare irreducible dislocation.

Definitive Management

Goals of surgery include reduction of the articular surface, removal of debris from the joint, and stable fixation, which will allow non-weight-bearing ambulation and range of motion. The primary relative indication for nonoperative management is a congruous joint that is stable without traction. Posterior wall fractures that involve up to one-half of the posterior articular surface may be stable. If posterior stability is documented, nonoperative management is considered. However, if the fragment is large enough to obtain stable fixation, internal fixation will decrease the chance of late loss of reduction. Very low, transverse T-shaped and anterior column fractures can be managed nonoperatively if the weight-bearing portion of the joint is stable and congruous.

Surgical approaches are divided into two categories: limited and extensile. The term *limited* implies visualization of one column. The term *extensile* implies exposure of part or all of both columns through one incision. Occasionally, two limited incisions are used to achieve the exposure of both columns. The approach used depends on the type of fracture and the surgeon's experience.

The **limited** approaches are the Kocher–Langenbeck and ilioinguinal approaches. The **Kocher–Langenbeck** approach exposes the posterior column and posterior one-half of the superior dome. Fractures that can be exposed through this approach include posterior wall, posterior column, and associated posterior column–posterior wall. Transverse and transverse with posterior wall fractures can be reduced and stabilized with this approach if the anterior fracture does not require fixation, or if it can be stabilized with a percutaneous lag screw.

The **ilioinguinal** approach affords exposure of the anterior column from inside the pelvis. Exposure from the anterior sacroiliac joint around the inner pelvic brim and down to the pubic symphysis is possible. This exposure is demanding but extremely valuable for certain fractures. Fractures routinely exposed through this approach include anterior wall and anterior column fractures. Like the Kocher–Langenbeck approach, other fractures can be stabilized through this approach including transverse, anterior column with posterior hemitransverse, and, occasionally, both-column fractures. When the ilioinguinal approach is used for a transverse or associated fracture, the posterior fracture must either not require fixation or be secured with an image-guided posterior column lag screw.

The two **extensile** approaches are the triradiate and the extended iliofemoral. The advantage of these approaches are that they expose both columns and the articular surface. The disadvantage is the increased soft tissue dissection and resultant propensity for heterotopic bone formation.

The **triradiate** approach combines the posterior Kocher–Langenbeck approach with an anterior limb designed to expose the inferior one-half of the ilium and the proximal one-half of the anterior column.

The **extended iliofemoral** approach provides exposure of the two columns similar to the triradiate approach but greater exposure of the proximal one-half of the ilium.

The indication for an extensile approach is a fracture that cannot be satisfactorily reduced and stabilized via a limited approach.

Complications

Complications of acetabular fractures are similar to those of hip dislocation and are covered in the section Dislocations of the Hip.

DISLOCATIONS OF THE HIP

Classification

Dislocations of the hip are classified according to the location of the femoral head as being posterior, anterior, or obturator. **Posterior** dislocations are by far the most common type of dislocation. The mechanism of injury is an axial load applied to the flexed adducted hip, such as would occur when the knee strikes a dashboard. **Anterior and obturator** dislocations are caused by hyperabduction of the hip. The greater trochanter impinges on the acetabular rim and levers the head out of the acetabulum. Extension and external rotation force the hip anteriorly, resulting in an anterior dislocation. Flexion and internal rotation force the hip inferiorly, resulting in an obturator dislocation.

Associated Injuries

Multisystem injuries, sciatic nerve injury, and fracture of the femur, knee, acetabulum, femoral head, and neck are associated with hip dislocations. Multisystem injuries reflect the high-energy trauma required to dislocate a hip. The presence of injuries to other systems is determined by adhering to the assessment guidelines outlined in Chapter 1. Sciatic nerve injury follows posterior dislocation of the hip and is the result of the femoral head impacting and stretching the nerve. The injury is almost always a neurapraxia and is manifested by partial loss of function, most frequently peroneal nerve function. The most accurate method of determining whether the femoral head and acetabulum are fractured is CT. Fractures about the knee are ruled out by a focused examination and radiographs.

Diagnosis and Initial Management

History and Physical Examination

The patient has severe pain. When the hip is dislocated posteriorly, there is a history of significant trauma. The leg is shortened. The hip is flexed approximately 30° and internally rotated. Anterior dislocations are often the result of less significant trauma and are characterized by external rotation and different degrees of abduction. Obturator dislocations are caused by significant trauma and are characterized by at least 45° of fixed abduction of the hip.

Radiographic Examination

The diagnosis is confirmed by an anteroposterior radiograph of the pelvis. Spot anteroposterior and lateral radiographs of the hip are also obtained to evaluate the femoral head and acetabulum. Radiographs of the femoral neck, femoral diaphysis, and knee are examined to rule out fracture. After reduction, new films are obtained to assess whether the reduction is concentric. In equivocal cases, a CT scan is obtained.

Initial Management

Initial management is reduction. The patient is sedated. Posterior dislocations are reduced by flexing the patient's knee, applying traction in line with the femur, and adducting the hip. Anterior and obturator dislocations are reduced by pulling in line with the femur, while an assistant pulls the thigh laterally. For anterior dislocations, the hip is also internally rotated. Straight traction is safe in the reduction of hip dislocations. Internal and external rotation must be performed very gently because of the risk of fracturing the femoral neck. If reduction is not possible with intravenous sedation, the patient is anesthetized in the operating room, and reduction with the aid of fluoroscopy is performed. Interposition of the capsule and external rotators in the acetabulum may prevent closed reduction, necessitating open reduction.

Definitive Management

Definitive management is skeletal traction until pain and muscle spasm have resolved (usually 7–14 days). Non-weight-bearing is maintained an additional 6 weeks. Surgical intervention is necessary for irreducible dislocations and to debride the joint when the reduction is not concentric. The joint is approached posteriorly. If the dislocation is posterior, very little dissection is necessary once the gluteus maximus has been split. The acetabulum is cleared of debris, and the femoral head is reduced. Postoperative management is as described in the section Initial Management.

Complications

Complications of acetabular fractures and hip dislocation are posttraumatic arthritis, heterotopic ossification, avascular necrosis, and instability. **Arthritis** is characterized clinically by pain with motion and radiographically by loss of joint space and formation of osteophytes. Management is conservative with nonsteroidal antiinflammatory drugs. If conservative management fails, older patients are managed with an arthroplasty. Patients younger than age 50 years are managed with arthrodesis. **Heterotopic ossification** is more common following an extensile surgical approach and when there is concomitant head injury. Indocin decreases the severity of heterotopic ossification and is administered to patients who are not threatened by a prolonged bleeding time. Once heterotopic ossification has been diagnosed, passive range-of-motion exercises are stopped for a minimum of 8 weeks, or until the bony mass shows radiographic signs of maturing. The position of the hip is determined. If it is not in a position of function (i.e., 0° of abduction, 10–20° of flexion, and neutral rotation), the patient is placed in skeletal traction to improve the alignment because there is a high probability of ankylosis. The bony mass may be excised after it matures. Maturity is indicated by normal serum alkaline phosphatase levels and a cold bone scan. **Avascular necrosis** of the femoral head is rare after acetabular fracture or hip dislocation. Its diagnosis and management are covered in Chapter 17. **Chronic instability** is extremely rare after dislocation without fracture, if it has been successfully managed with imbrication of the posterior capsule of the hip joint. Chronic instability after acetabular fracture is managed with reduction, stabilization, and bone grafting of the nonunion if there are no signs of posttraumatic arthritis. If there is arthritis, an arthroplasty or arthrodesis is performed.

SELECTED READINGS

Fractures and Dislocations of the Pelvis

Bucholz RW: The pathological anatomy of malgaigne fracture–dislocations of the pelvis. *J Bone Joint Surg* 63A:400–404, 1981.

Hanson PB, Milne JC, Chapman MW: Open fractures of the pelvis: review of 43 cases. *J Bone Joint Surg* 73B:325–329, 1991.

Moreno C, Moore EE, Rosenberger A, Cleveland HC: Hemorrhage associated with major pelvic fracture: A multispecialty challenge. *J Trauma* 26:987–993, 1986.

Acetabular Fractures

Judet R, Judet J, Letournel E: Fractures of the acetabulum: classification and surgical approaches for open reduction: Preliminary report. *J Bone Joint Surg* 46A:1615, 1964.

Letournel E: *Fractures of the acetabulum*. New York, Springer-Verlag, 1981.

Matta J, Anderson L, Epstein H, Hendricks P: Fractures of the acetabulum: a retrospective analysis. *Clin Orthop* 205:230–240, 1986.

Dislocations of the Hip

Epstein HC: *Traumatic dislocations of the hip*. Baltimore, Williams & Wilkins, 1980.

17

Intracapsular Fractures of the Proximal Femur

Clayton R. Perry

Intracapsular fractures of the proximal femur are low-energy fractures of the femoral neck, high-energy fractures of the femoral neck, and fractures of the femoral head.

HISTORICAL PERSPECTIVE OF THE MANAGEMENT OF LOW-ENERGY FRACTURES

The evolution of the management of these fractures reflects the evolution of fracture surgery. Femoral neck fractures and their complications were defined, classified, and then reclassified. Alterations in management were based on the refinements of the classification system, and as the management evolved, the incidence of complications decreased.

In 1823, Cooper described the physical and anatomical findings of femoral neck fractures and observed that they were frequently complicated by nonunion and avascular necrosis. Following the advent of radiographs in the early 1900s, low-energy fractures were further classified as being either abduction or adduction fractures. Abduction fractures correspond to Garden stages I and II. Adduction fractures correspond to Garden stages III and IV. The significance of this classification was that patients with abduction fractures had a better prognosis, in that their fractures would heal with prolonged bedrest.

In 1911, Cotton modified the management of femoral neck fractures based on whether the fracture were the abduction or adduction type. He reasoned that, if patients with abduction fractures had a better prognosis, then converting an adduction fracture to an abduction fracture should improve the prognosis. He did this by closed manipulation. Traction was applied to the extremity, and the fracture was impacted by striking the padded greater trochanter with a mallet. Manipulation was followed with bed rest and casting. Leadbetter improved on this method by describing a less traumatic reduction maneuver (hip flexion followed by abduction and internal rotation).

Loss of reduction and the complications of prolonged bed rest and casting still contributed to morbidity. To counter these problems, surgeons attempted internal fixation. Isolated reports of these attempts appear in the literature. However, the technique was not in general use until Smith-Petersen, in 1937, reported his method and results of open reduction and fixation with a triflanged nail. Johansson, Thornton, and Jewett improved upon Smith-Petersen's concept by introducing a cannulated triflange nail, thus making closed nailing practical; adding a sideplate; and increasing the strength of the nail–side–plate combination by manufacturing it in one piece.

The management of selected femoral neck fractures with hemi-arthroplasty further decreased the postoperative morbidity due to loss of fixation and avascular necrosis. In 1943, Moore described a stainless steel prosthesis that was used to replace a proximal femur. He subsequently developed a standardized prosthesis that was inserted through a posterior approach. Independently of Moore, the Judet brothers developed an acrylic hip prosthesis. In 1950, they described 300 cases in which their prosthesis had been used. Garden further classified femoral neck fractures and found that certain fractures had an extremely high incidence of avascular necrosis. His classification system is used as the basis for determining whether to treat the fracture with fixation or hemiarthroplasty. Hemiarthroplasties were further modified by adding a second bearing surface. These bipolar prostheses may decrease the incidence of acetabular protrusion, but there have been no controlled studies to demonstrate this.

ANATOMY

The three important anatomic considerations of femoral head and neck fractures are the intracapsular location of the fracture, the degree of osteopenia, and the vascular supply of the femoral head.

The **intracapsular location** means that the fracture site is bathed in synovial fluid that lyses the fracture hematoma, thus decreasing healing potential. The neck is covered with synovium and the head with articular cartilage. Therefore, healing is endosteal; periosteal healing does not occur. Intracapsular hematoma increases intracapsular pressure, resulting in avascular necrosis.

Osteopenia leads to loss of fixation and, therefore, is a relative indication for hemiarthroplasty. The Singh index correlates the degree of osteopenia with the trabecular systems remaining (Fig. 17-1). There are six grades of osteopenia. Grade VI indicates normal bone with all trabecular systems present. Grade I indicates extreme osteopenia with all trabecular systems absent, except the principal compressive trabeculae, of which only a few remain.

Disruption of the **vascular supply to the femoral head** results in avascular necrosis. The three groups of vessels that supply the femoral head are the ascending cervical or retinacular vessels, the intramedullary vessels, and the artery of the ligamentum teres (Fig. 17-2). Of these three, the retinacular vessels are the most important. They arise from the extracapsular arterial ring formed by the medial and lateral circumflex arteries and run along the femoral neck beneath the synovium, piercing the femoral neck just distal to the margin of the articular cartilage. A second arterial ring, which is intraarticular and subsynovial, is formed by terminal branches of the retinacular vessels at the margin of

FIG. 17-1 The Singh index. Numbers 1, 2, and 3 indicate secondary trabecular systems that disappear in the early stages of osteoporosis (grades V and VI). Number 4 indicates the principal tensile trabeculae. This system is reduced in grades III and IV and absent in grade II osteoporosis. Number 5 indicates the principal compressive trabeculae. This system is the last to disappear.

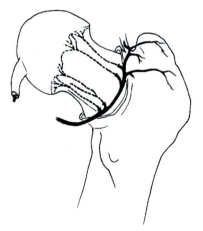

FIG. 17-2 Retinacular arteries and artery of the ligamentum teres.

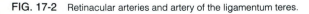

the articular cartilage of the femoral head. This ring also gives off branches that supply the femoral head.

Descending intramedullary metaphyseal arteries anastomose with ascending branches from the nutrient artery system of the femoral shaft. The intramedullary vessels are disrupted in all displaced femoral neck fractures.

The artery of the ligamentum teres takes origin from the obturator artery. It supplies the area around the fovea but is not adequate to supply the entire femoral head. Fractures of the femoral head occurring distal to the fovea have a high incidence of avascular necrosis of the fragment because the vascular supply from the artery of the ligamentum teres is disrupted.

LOW-ENERGY FEMORAL NECK FRACTURES

Classification

Low-energy femoral neck fractures are classified according to a system described by Garden (Fig. 17-3). Stage I is an incomplete fracture frequently in slight valgus. Stage II is a complete but undisplaced fracture. Stage III is a complete fracture partially displaced, but with an intact posterior retinacular attachment (ligament of Whitebrecht). Stage IV fractures are completely displaced with tearing of all retinacular vessels.

Diagnosis and Initial Management

History and Physical Examination

There is hip, groin, or thigh pain. If the fracture is not displaced, pain is the only physical finding. If the fracture is displaced, the leg is externally rotated; however, unlike intertrochanteric fractures, there is minimal shortening.

Radiographic Examination

Anteroposterior and lateral radiographs of the hip and an anteroposterior radiograph of the pelvis confirm the diagnosis and estimate the degree of osteopenia.

Initial Management

Prior to surgery the injured extremity is prevented from rotating externally with Buck's traction and pillows. Patients with undisplaced fractures (i.e., Garden stages I and II) are moved carefully to prevent displacement.

Associated Injuries

These low-energy fractures are usually not associated with other injuries; however, many patients with femoral neck fractures have med-

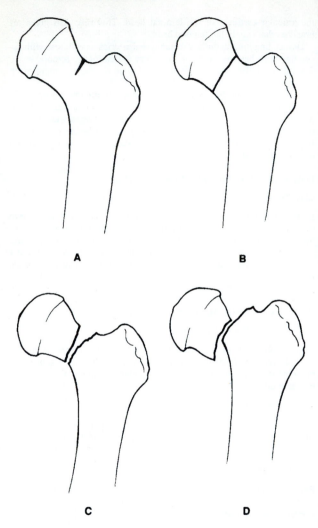

FIG. 17-3 The Garden classification system: *(A)* stage I, *(B)* stage II, *(C)* stage III, and *(D)* stage IV.

ical problems. Cardiovascular and pulmonary systems are addressed specifically. Infections of the genitourinary system are common, and, if present, treatment is initiated.

Definitive Management

The definitive management is either **pinning** or **hemiarthroplasty.** The procedure is based on Garden's classification system, the age of the patient, and the degree of osteopenia. Osteoarthritis is an indication for arthroplasty, but is uncommon in patients with low-energy femoral neck fractures.

Surgical Technique

Stage I and II fractures are stabilized with screws or pins. Reduction is not necessary for these undisplaced fractures. Two to four screws are inserted percutaneously. They must be parallel with each other and with the long axis of the neck so that with weight-bearing the fracture will collapse along the axis of the screws. The most dense bone in the femoral head is subchondral; therefore, the screws must penetrate to within 0.5 cm of the subchondral bone. The threads should not cross the fracture or they will prevent collapse.

Garden stage III fractures have an intact vascular supply, and potentially the femoral head can be salvaged. If the patient is younger than 75 years or extremely ill and cannot undergo a significant operation, the fracture is reduced and fixed. If the patient is older than 75 years, not a high-demand user, and can withstand a significant operative procedure, a hemiarthroplasty is performed. The fracture is reduced by separating the fragments by externally rotating the leg. Traction is then applied to bring the fracture out to length and the leg is internally rotated, thereby reducing the fracture and preventing apex anterior angulation. An absolutely anatomic reduction is mandatory. There is a high incidence of avascular necrosis with fractures stabilized in more than 20° of valgus (an anteroposterior alignment index of 180°) and a high incidence of nonunion in fractures stabilized in varus or with more than 20° of apex anterior angulation (lateral alignment index of 160°; Fig. 17-4). If reduction within these limits is not possible, a hemiarthroplasty is performed. Inability to achieve reduction is most frequently due to incorrect staging of the fracture (i.e., the fracture is stage IV).

Garden stage IV fractures are managed with a hemiarthroplasty (Figs. 17-5 and 17-6). The decision to use cement is made at the time of surgery. We use an anterolateral approach that is a modification of the approach described by Hardinge (1983). The anterolateral approach

FIG. 17-4   The anteroposterior index is the angle formed by the primary compressive trabeculae and the medial cortex of the femoral diaphysis. The lateral index is the angle formed by the primary compressive trabeculae and the axis of the neck.

FIG. 17-5   Garden stage IV fracture.

minimizes wound problems associated with posterior approaches and provides better exposure than a straight anterior approach.

Postoperatively, weight-bearing as tolerated is allowed. Posterior precautions, including an abduction pillow between the legs while the patient is sleeping, are enforced for 3 weeks.

Complications

Low-energy femoral neck fractures are frequently the beginning of the end for debilitated patients. The incidence of **mortality** at 1 year approaches 30%. The incidence of postoperative infection is high, presumably because of decreased resistance, other foci of **infection** (e.g., the urinary tract and decubiti), and incontinence leading to contamination of the incision. Infection can be managed by two-stage revision or by chronic suppression with oral antibiotics. Avascular necrosis and nonunion are best managed by hemiarthroplasty.

FIG. 17-6   Hemiarthroplasty for Garden stage IV fracture.

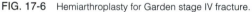

HIGH-ENERGY FEMORAL NECK FRACTURES

Classification

High-energy femoral neck fractures have a worse prognosis and occur in younger patients than low-energy fractures.

We classify high-energy fractures into four groups: type I, undisplaced fractures; type II, simple displaced fractures; type III, comminuted displaced fractures; and type IV, fractures with associated fracture of the acetabulum or femur (Fig. 17-7). In addition to the displacement and the presence of associated injuries, verticality of the fracture line is assessed according to the classification system described by Pauwels (Fig. 17-8). More vertical fractures (i.e., Pauwels' type III) have a higher incidence of nonunion secondary to increased shear and decreased compression across the fracture.

FIG. 17-7 The classification of high-energy femoral neck fractures: (*A*) type I, (*B*) type II, (*C*) type III, and (*D*) type IV.

type I
<30°

type II
>30° <50°

type III
>50°

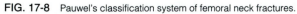

FIG. 17-8 Pauwel's classification system of femoral neck fractures.

Diagnosis and Initial Management

History and Physical Examination

Pain and external rotation are usually present; associated injuries may mask these findings.

Radiographic Examination

Anteroposterior and lateral radiographs of the hip and an anteroposterior radiograph of the pelvis confirm the diagnosis.

Initial Management

During the initial evaluation, skeletal or Buck's traction is applied.

Associated Injuries

There is a high incidence of other associated system injuries (e.g., chest contusion) and of associated injuries to the musculoskeletal system (e.g., pelvic fractures or ipsilateral knee injuries).

Definitive Management

Patients with high-energy fractures are usually young. Salvage of the femoral head is of paramount importance, and hemiarthroplasty is acceptable only as a last resort.

Type I (undisplaced) fractures are stabilized with percutaneous screws.

Type II (simple displaced) fractures are reduced closed. If there is any doubt as to the adequacy of reduction, the femoral neck is reduced under direct vision with the Watson–Jones approach. This approach uses the interval between the tensor fascia lata and the gluteus medius and can be extended distally and laterally for the placement of a lag screw and sideplate.

Type III (comminuted) fractures are exposed through a posterolateral approach, with the patient in the lateral decubitus position on a fracture table. The neck is reduced and stabilized with a lag screw and sideplate. Cancellous bone graft from the distal femur or iliac crest is used to augment the fixation.

In type IV (associated with fracture of the acetabulum or femur) fractures, stabilization of the fractured femoral neck is the primary goal. If there is a posterior fracture of the acetabulum or hip dislocation, the femoral neck is approached posterolaterally. Management of femoral neck fractures associated with a diaphyseal femoral fracture is dependent on the type of femoral neck fracture. In undisplaced neck fractures, a reconstruction locked nail is used for both fractures. Displaced fractures are managed with the patient supine on the fracture table. An open reduction of the femoral neck is performed, and fixation is done with screws. The femoral shaft fracture is stabilized with a plate or retrograde nail.

Complications

The complications unique to high-energy intracapsular femoral neck fractures are nonunion and avascular necrosis. Risk factors for these complications include the degree of initial displacement, time to reduction and stabilization, bone density, and quality of reduction and stabilization. Theoretically, core decompression is of value in the management of **avascular necrosis** if done before arthritic changes. When symptomatic segmental collapse occurs, there are two options: osteotomy or fusion. Osteotomies are designed to move the involved portion of the femoral head from under the weight-bearing surface of the acetabulum and to replace it with healthy bone. Osteotomies are either rotational about the long axis of the femur or varus/valgus. If an osteotomy is not possible (i.e., the avascular portion is too large), a hip fusion is performed. In patients with **nonunion**, an intertrochanteric osteotomy designed to make the plane of the nonunion more horizontal, thereby decreasing shear stresses across the nonunion, is performed. In addition, the nonunion is bone grafted.

FRACTURES OF THE FEMORAL HEAD

Classification

The third type of intracapsular fracture of the femur is fracture of the femoral head. Although femoral head fractures are invariably associated with a dislocation of the hip joint, we include them in this chapter because their anatomy, pathology, and management are very similar to those of high-energy femoral neck fractures.

Femoral head fractures are classified into four types. In type I fractures, the fracture is below the fovea. In type II fractures, the fracture line extends above the fovea. Type III and IV fractures are type I or II injuries associated with a fracture of the femoral neck or acetabular rim, respectively (Fig. 17-9).

Diagnosis and Initial Management

History and Physical Examination

The physical findings are those of a posterior dislocation of the hip. The hip is flexed and adducted, and the extremity is shortened.

Radiographic Examination

Anteroposterior and lateral radiographs of the hip indicate a dislocation of the hip, with a retained fragment of the femoral head in the acetabulum (Fig. 17-10). Computed tomography (CT) and tomography confirm the diagnosis.

Initial Management

Initial management is reduction of the dislocation. Type I, II, and IV fractures are reduced closed, without any specific precautions. In gen-

FIG. 17-9   Classification of femoral head fractures: (A) type I, (B) type II, (C) type III, and (D) type IV.

FIG. 17-10   Type II fracture of the femoral head.

eral, the easier the reduction, the less stable it is. Type III fractures are reduced while being monitored with fluoroscopy. If the femoral neck fracture is being displaced, the closed reduction is abandoned and open reduction is performed emergently. Unstable reductions are maintained with skeletal traction and abduction of the hip.

Associated Injuries

Sciatic nerve injury is associated with these dislocations. Frequently, there are associated multisystem injuries.

Definitive Management

Definitive management is surgical. The goals of surgery are to obtain a stable concentric reduction of the hip joint, and either to reduce anatomically and fix the femoral head fracture or to excise nonessential fragments. Type I and II injuries are exposed through a posterolateral (Kocher–Langenbeck) approach to the hip. The external rotators and capsule are invariably torn posteriorly; therefore, as the fibers of the gluteus maximus are split, the hip joint is exposed. The hip is dislocated posteriorly, and internal rotation of the femur affords limited exposure of the medial fragment and the hip joint. The medial fragment has synovial attachments called the *retinacular leash*.

Type II fractures also have the ligamentum teres attached to the medial fragment. The dislocation is reduced, and the head fracture is stabilized with screws placed in the lateral aspect of the head and neck and directed medially toward the fragment.

Type III injuries have an associated femoral neck fracture. The Kocher–Langenbeck approach is used to expose both fractures. The head fracture is reduced and stabilized first. The neck fracture is reduced and stabilized with screws under fluoroscopic control. Older patients are managed with a hemiarthroplasty.

Type IV injuries have an associated acetabular fracture, usually a posterior lip fracture. When it does not require stabilization, the head fracture is approached as if it were a type I or II injury. If the acetabulum requires stabilization, the Kocher–Langenbeck approach is used to expose the hip joint. The hip is dislocated, and the joint and fractures are debrided of bone fragments and hematoma. The hip is reduced, the femoral head fracture is stabilized with screws, and the acetabulum is stabilized according to its fracture pattern.

Postoperatively, the extremity is placed in balanced suspension with the hip abducted 30°. At 4 weeks, the patient is allowed to ambulate nonweight-bearing on the affected side. At 12 weeks, full weight-bearing is allowed.

Complications

Long-term complications include **posttraumatic arthritis** and **avascular necrosis.** Nonunion has not been reported. Arthritis and symptomatic avascular necrosis are managed with hip fusion in younger patients or with hip replacement in older patients.

SELECTED READINGS

Low-Energy Femoral Neck Fractures
Cooper AP: *A treatise on dislocations and on fractures of the joints*, 2d ed. London, Longman, Hurst, 1823, pp 570–576.
Cotton FJ: Artificial impaction in hip fracture. *Am J Orthop Surg* 8:680, 1911.
Davis GG: An operation for ununited fractures of the neck of the femur. *Univ Med Mag Philadelphia* 13:507, 1900.
Garden RS: Low-angle fixation in fractures of the femoral neck. *J Bone Joint Surg* 43B:647–661, 1961.
Jewett EL: One-piece angle nail for trochanteric fractures. *J Bone Joint Surg* 23:803–810, 1941.
Johansson S: On operative treatment of medial fractures of neck of femur. *Acta Orthop Scand* 3:362–392, 1932.
Judet J, Judet R: The use of an artificial femoral head for arthroplasty of the hip joint. *J Bone Joint Surg* 32B:166–173, 1950.
Kocher T: *Text-book of operative surgery* [English translation from 4th German ed]. London, A & C Black, 1911.
Leadbetter GW: A treatment for fracture of the neck of the femur. *J Bone Joint Surg* 15:931–940, 1933.

Moore AT: The self-locking metal hip prosthesis. *J Bone Joint Surg* 39A:811–827, 1957.

Niemann KMW, Mankin HJ: Fractures about the hip in an institutionalized patient population. *J Bone Joint Surg* 50A:1327–1340, 1968.

Pauwels F: Biomechanics of the normal and diseased hip. Berlin, Heidelberg, New York, Springer-Verlag, 1976, pp 83–86.

Smith-Petersen MN: Treatment of fractures of the neck of the femur by internal fixation. *Surg Gynecol Obstet* 64:287–294, 1937.

Whitman R: A new treatment for fracture of the neck of the femur. *Med Rec* 65:441–447, 1904.

Zuckerman JD, Skovron ML, Koval KJ, Aharonoff G, Frankel VH: Postoperative complications and mortality associated with operative delay in older patients who have a fracture of the hip: *J Bone Joint Surg* 77A: 1551–1556, 1995.

High-Energy Femoral Neck Fractures

Protzman RF, Burkhalter WE: Femoral neck fractures in young adults. *J Bone Joint Surg* 58A:689–695, 1976.

Swiontkowski MF, Winquist RA, Hansen ST: Fractures of the femoral neck in patients between the ages of twelve and forty-nine years. *J Bone Joint Surg* 66A:837–846, 1984.

Fractures of the Femoral Head

Butler JE: Pipkin type II fractures of the femoral head. *J Bone Joint Surg* 63A:1292–1296, 1981.

Pipkin G: Treatment of grade IV fracture–dislocation of the hip. A review. *J Bone Joint Surg* 39A:1027–1042, 1957.

General

Chung SMK: The arterial supply of the developing proximal end of the human femur. *J Bone Joint Surg* 58A:961–970, 1976.

Hardinge K: The direct lateral approach to the hip. *J Bone Joint Surg* 64B:17–19, 1983.

Singh M, Nagrath AR, Maini PS: Changes in trabecular pattern of the upper end of the femur as an index of osteoporosis. *J Bone Joint Surg* 52A:457–467, 1970.

18

Intertrochanteric Fractures

Enes Kanlic   Clayton R. Perry

This chapter covers intertrochanteric fractures and isolated fractures of the greater and lesser trochanters. Intertrochanteric fractures are extracapsular fractures of the proximal femur. The major fracture lines are located between the base of the femoral neck and the lesser trochanter.

ANATOMY

The proximal extent of the intertrochanteric region of the **femur** is the intertrochanteric line anteriorly and the intertrochanteric crest posteriorly. The distal extent of the intertrochanteric region is the lesser trochanter. The osseous tissue in this region is cancellous bone surrounded by a thin shell of cortical bone. The cancellous bone forms the secondary compressive, secondary tensile, and greater trochanteric trabeculae (see Singh index: intracapsular fractures of the proximal femur). The calcar is a thick plate of bone underlying the lesser trochanter. As the calcar extends proximally, it fuses with the cortex of the posterior medial femoral neck. The linea aspera, a thickened ridge of cortical bone on the posterior aspect of the femur, extends from the greater trochanter distally down the diaphysis.

Numerous **muscles** insert on, or originate from, the intertrochanteric region. The gluteus medius and minimus, the piriformis, and short external rotators insert on the greater trochanter. The iliopsoas inserts on the lesser trochanter. Because of the muscular insertions and origins, the intertrochanteric region has an extremely rich vascular supply. Posttraumatic avascular necrosis of the femoral head is very rare following an intertrochanteric fracture, in contrast to intracapsular fractures of the proximal femur. In addition, the muscular attachments tend to prevent displacement of the fragments following fracture. The rich vascular supply and the broad surfaces of cancellous bone will lead to rapid healing if the fracture is reduced and stabilized appropriately.

Classification

We classify intertrochanteric fractures according to the degree of osteopenia and the configuration of the fracture.

The Singh index is used to estimate the **degree of osteopenia.** Osteopenia plays an important role in the configuration of the fracture, its healing potential, and its management.

The **fracture configuration** is classified into one of four groups: type 1, undisplaced; type 2, stable displaced; type 3, unstable displaced; and type 4, reverse obliquity (Fig. 18-1). **Undisplaced fractures** (type 1) are usually simple fractures along a line between the greater and lesser trochanters.

FIG. 18-1   Types of intertrochanteric fractures: (*A*) undisplaced, (*B*) displaced stable, (*C*) displaced unstable, and (*D*) reverse obliquity.

Stable displaced fractures (type 2) are those fractures, which when reduced, are stable. The sine qua non of stability is bone-to-bone contact across the fracture along the medial cortex of the femur. Fracture of the lesser trochanter does not always indicate an unstable fracture (i.e., there may be enough intact medial cortex for adequate bone-to-bone contact).

Unstable displaced fractures (type 3) are those fractures that have posteromedial comminution that is so extensive that it prevents bone-to-bone contact across the fracture. This comminution is usually a single large fragment that includes the lesser trochanter. Frequently, there is an associated fracture of the greater trochanter.

Reverse obliquity fractures (type 4) are those fractures in which the fracture line runs parallel to the long axis of the femoral neck (i.e., from lateral inferior to medial superior). This fracture pattern is unstable because the gluteus medius and minimus and piriformis externally rotate and abduct the proximal fragment while the adductors displace the distal fragment medially.

Diagnosis and Initial Management

History and Physical Examination

There is pain and inability to bear weight. There is usually a history of a minor fall. The injured leg is completely externally rotated, with the lateral part of the foot often touching the surface of the bed. In addition to external rotation, there is shortening. Occasionally, there is ecchymosis of the proximal thigh. Patients with femoral neck fractures usually do not have these physical findings because extreme external rotation is prevented by a partly intact hip capsule, and fracture hematoma is contained by the capsule minimizing ecchymosis.

Radiographic Examination

The clinical diagnosis is confirmed by the radiographic examination. A radiograph of the pelvis in the anteroposterior projection is of most use. The contralateral hip should be internally rotated 20° to profile the femoral neck to determine the Singh index. In addition to the anteroposterior pelvic radiograph, anteroposterior and lateral radiographs centered on the injured hip help to determine the fracture configuration. The lateral projection is obtained with the patient in the Danelius–Miller position (the patient is supine with the uninjured hip flexed). The film is placed lateral to the injured hip and the x-ray beam is directed through the hip. Other radiographic examinations (e.g., tomograms and CAT scans) are rarely useful in the evaluation.

Initial Management

The two goals of initial management are to make the patient as comfortable as possible and to prepare the patient for surgery as expeditiously as possible. Early stabilization of the fracture allows mobilization of the patient and minimizes the incidence of problems associated with prolonged recumbency (e.g., pneumonia, urinary tract infections, and decubiti).

The patient is made as comfortable as possible by positioning the injured extremity. This is accomplished by applying skin traction with the knee flexed between 10° and 20° over a pillow. External rotation is prevented by placing pillows laterally at the knee and foot. Because many patients with intertrochanteric fractures have fragile skin, the skin traction must be applied carefully to avoid skin breakdown. The malleoli and other bony prominences are carefully padded, and no more than 5 to 10 lbs. of weight is used. Skeletal traction is applied through a distal femoral traction pin if skin breakdown is present or if surgery will be delayed more than 2 days.

Associated Injuries

The most frequently associated injuries are due to the patient's osteopenia and other areas of the body. They are sustained at the same time as the intertrochanteric fracture. The patient must be carefully examined for any signs of wrist fracture or head injury. Radiographs of the femur and knee in addition to those of the pelvis are obtained.

Before surgery, the patient's medical status is optimized. These patients are frequently dehydrated. Dehydration coupled with the blood loss associated with fracture results in severe volume restriction, which must be corrected. In addition, patients who have sustained an intertrochanteric fracture are likely to have other medical problems. Patients' cardiac, pulmonary, genitourinary, and neurologic systems are carefully assessed.

Definitive Management

The definitive management of intertrochanteric fractures is operative reduction and stabilization. The most important factors affecting the eventual outcome are the age and general health of the patient, the degree of osteopenia, the configuration of the fracture, the quality of reduction, and the stability of fixation. Of these factors, the surgeon controls two: the quality of reduction and the stability of fixation.

The goals of **reduction** are to obtain bone-to-bone contact along the medial cortex, realign the fracture fragments, and in particular avoid varus angulation. The anesthetized patient is placed on the fracture table. The reduction and stabilization are monitored with fluoroscopy. Reduction is accomplished by gently, externally rotating the extremity to "unlock" the fragments and then applying axial traction. After the fracture is out to length, the extremity is internally rotated to align the fragments. The exact amount of internal rotation is determined by fluoroscopy (usually about 30°). The reduction is assessed fluoroscopically in the anteroposterior and lateral planes. In the anteroposterior plane, the fracture should be out to length and the neck shaft angle should be at least 130°. If there is shortening or varus angulation, the reduction maneuver of external rotation, more traction, and internal rotation is repeated. Slight abduction of the extremity may help reduce the fracture. Two bits of information are obtained from the lateral fluoroscopic projection: the direction of the axis of the femoral neck and the relative position of the diaphysis of the femur to the femoral neck. Knowing the direction of the axis of the femoral neck will help in the accurate placement of the implant. The relative position of the femoral diaphysis to the femoral neck is important because, if the diaphyseal fragment is posterior to the neck, further reduction may be necessary after the fracture is exposed. The distal fragment can be reduced by supporting it with a crutch positioned under the thigh or by levering it into place and maintaining reduction with a broad periosteal elevator while the plate is applied (i.e., the femoral shaft will have to be lifted anteriorly).

There are two basic types of implants that are used to **stabilize** intertrochanteric fractures: sliding screw-and-plate assemblies and intramedullary devices.

The **sliding screw-plate** allows controlled collapse and impaction of the fracture fragments, thus making an osteotomy unnecessary and minimizing shortening (Fig. 18-2). There are a few important points of technique: the screw is located inferiorly in the femoral head, and it should extend to within 0.5 cm of the subchondral bone to prevent cut-out; the barrel of the sideplate should not extend across the fracture, or it may prevent postoperative impaction across the fracture; two-thirds of the barrel should be occupied by the lag screw to prevent disengagement or binding of the lag screw in the barrel; and the traction should be released intraoperatively to assess the amount of shortening that will occur.

Intramedullary devices are used most frequently to stabilize type 3 (displaced unstable) and type 4 (reverse obliquity) fractures. The two types of intramedullary devices used to stabilize intertrochanteric fractures are antegrade nails with one or more locking screws inserted into the femoral head and retrograde nails. The intramedullary location of both devices prevents medial displacement of the distal fragment and has a mechanical advantage over the sliding screw-plate. Antegrade intramedullary hip screws are often shorter than standard intramedullary nails and have the associated complication of fracture of the femur at their distal tip. Flexible retrograde intramedullary nails (e.g., Ender's nails) are inserted by a closed technique; thus, there is minimal blood loss. This technique has the disadvantage of insertion site symptoms if the nails back out. Important points regarding technique are: the medullary canal must be "stacked" or filled with nails to prevent them from backing out; at least two nails must be inserted to within 1 cm of the subchondral bone to stabilize the fracture adequately; and the nails must have an anteversion bend to prevent an external rotation deformity.

The technique or method of stabilization depends on the configuration of the fracture. Type 1 (undisplaced) and type 2 (displaced stable)

FIG. 18-2 Stable displaced intertrochanteric fracture stabilized with a sliding screw-plate device. An expanding dome has been substituted for the lag screw.

fractures are stabilized with a sliding screw-plate device. If the fracture is type 3 (displaced unstable), there are two options: to restore bone-to-bone contact along the medial cortex or to impact the fragments into a more stable configuration. Bone-to-bone contact can be restored if there is a single large fragment postero medially that can be reduced and held in place with lag screws or cerclage wires. The advantage of this option is that leg length is maintained. The disadvantage is that it is very difficult to stabilize the posteromedial fragment; if fixation fails, uncontrolled shortening of the fracture with loss of fixation will occur. Impaction of the fragments into a more stable configuration is done by displacing the distal fragment medially and placing the medial cortex of the proximal fragment into the medullary canal of the distal fragment. The fracture is purposefully aligned in valgus, and a "high angle" (e.g., 145°) screw-plate assembly is used to stabilize it. The advantages of this option are that fixation is extremely stable and loss of reduction is rare.

The disadvantage is that the extremity is shortened 2 to 4 cm. Type 4 (reverse obliquity) fractures cannot be stabilized with a screw-plate assembly because they will shorten and displace (Fig. 18-3). Either a 95° screw-plate device or an intramedullary device (Figs. 18-4 and 18-5) is used to stabilize reverse obliquity fractures.

If there is severe osteopenia (i.e., Singh grade 1 or 2), fixation is augmented with polymethylmethacrylate. Care is taken to avoid placing cement between bone fragments and thus inhibit bone healing.

Complications

Complications following intertrochanteric fracture include loss of reduction with cutting out of the fixation and infection. Other complications such as nonunion and avascular necrosis are extremely rare.

Loss of reduction with cutting out of the fixation is the most frequently encountered complication. It is more common in patients with

FIG. 18-3 Reverse obliquity intertrochanteric fracture stabilized with a sliding screw-plate device. Uncontrolled shortening has occurred.

FIG. 18-4   Anteroposterior radiograph of a hip showing one of the alternative methods of stabilization of reverse obliquity fractures: a 95° screw-sideplate device.

severe osteopenia (i.e., Singh index of 1 or 2) who have sustained displaced unstable or reverse obliquity fractures. It is best managed operatively by removing the fixation device, revising the reduction to a more stable configuration, and reinserting the fixation device. Polymethylmethacrylate is used to increase the stability of fixation. If the articular surface of the femoral head and acetabulum have been damaged, an arthroplasty with a calcar replacement prosthesis is performed.

Infection is more common after open reduction and internal fixation of intertrochanteric fractures than after other closed fractures because the patients are debilitated. Implants that provide stability are left in place until healing of the fracture has occurred. Antibiotics, based on the sensitivities of the pathogenic organisms, are administered as long as necessary to control the infection. Once the fracture has healed, the

FIG. 18-5   Anteroposterior radiograph of a hip showing one of the alternative methods of stabilization of reverse obliquity fractures: flexible intramedullary nails.

implants are removed, the area is debrided of avascular tissue, and antibiotics are administered for 6 weeks.

ISOLATED FRACTURES OF THE GREATER AND LESSER TROCHANTERS

Isolated fractures of the greater trochanter are the result of a direct blow or an avulsion. When they are minimally displaced, they will heal. If they are displaced, nonunions frequently develop but are usually asymptomatic. Fractures of the lesser trochanter are rare injuries. They are the result of an avulsion of the iliopsoas tendon and are treated conservatively. The primary importance of isolated fractures of the trochanters is that they may signal an undisplaced intertrochanteric fracture. Radiographs should be carefully examined to rule out this possibility.

SELECTED READINGS

Baumgaertner MR, Curtin SL, Lindskog DM, Keggi JM: The value of the tip-apex distance in predicting failure of fixation of peritrochanteric fractures of the hip. *J Bone Joint Surg* 77-A:1058–1064, 1995.

Boyd HB, Griffen LL: Classification and treatment of trochanteric fracture. *Arch Surg* 58:853–866, 1949.

Bridle SH, Patel AD, Bircher M, Calvert PR: Fixation of intertrochanteric fractures of the femur. A randomized prospective comparison of the Gamma nail and the dynamic hip screw. *J Bone Joint Surg* 73B:330–334, 1991.

Kenzora EJ, McCarthy ER, Lowell JD, Sledge BC: Hip fracture mortality. *Clin Orthop* 186:45–56, 1984.

Miller WC: Survival and ambulation following hip fracture. *J Bone Joint Surg* 60A:930–933, 1978.

19

Fractures of the Femoral Shaft

Kenneth A. Davenport

The femoral diaphysis is the tubular section extending from the intertrochanteric region to the supracondylar region.

ANATOMY

The important anatomical features of the femoral diaphysis are its shape, vascular supply, surrounding muscles, and neighboring neurovascular structures.

The femur has an **anterior bow** that differs widely from patient to patient but averages 12–15°. Posteriorly, the cortex thickens into a ridge called the **linea aspera,** which is the origin of the medial and lateral intermuscular septa.

The **blood supply** flows through endosteal and periosteal vessels. Endosteal vessels originate from one or two nutrient arteries that enter the proximal third of the femur through foramina in the linea aspera. These nutrient arteries originate from the profunda femoris artery and supply the inner two-thirds of the diaphyseal cortex. Periosteal vessels supply the outer one-third and originate from arteries supplying the surrounding muscles. Following fracture, the periosteal vessels become the dominant vascular supply.

The muscles of the thigh form three **compartments** separated by intermuscular septa. The anterior compartment contains the knee extensors. The posterior compartment contains the knee flexors. The medial compartment contains the hip adductors.

Unopposed action of muscles results in predictable displacement dependent on the level of the fracture. In fractures proximal to the isthmus of the medullary canal, the proximal fragment is abducted (gluteus), flexed, and internally rotated (iliopsoas). Fractures distal to the isthmus are in varus (adductors) and angulated posteriorly (knee extensors and gastrocnemius).

Neurovascular structures of the thigh are the sciatic nerve, the femoral nerve, the superficial femoral artery, and the deep femoral artery. The sciatic nerve is cushioned from the femur by muscles; therefore, it is seldom injured in association with fractures of the femur. The femoral nerve enervates the quadriceps femoris. The superficial femoral artery enters the posterior compartment of the thigh from the medial compartment through the adductor hiatus, or Hunter's canal, located just proximal to the distal metaphyseal flare of the femur. The artery is tethered by the intermuscular septum, and a fracture at this level is likely to result in its injury. The deep femoral artery gives off approximately four perforating branches prior to ending proximal to the knee. The perforators enter the anterior compartment from the posterior compartment through the lateral intermuscular septum. Their clinical significance is that, when they are cut, they retract beneath the lateral intermuscular septum and are a source of uncontrolled bleeding.

Classification

Fractures of the femoral diaphysis are classified according to location and stability. The location is defined as being proximal, middle, or distal third. Fractures of the proximal third are subtrochanteric fractures, and fractures of the distal third merge with supracondylar fractures.

The key to classifying fractures of the femoral diaphysis is the concept of **stability** (Fig. 19-1). Stability is defined in terms of the percentage of the circumference of the cortex that is intact and the obliquity of the fracture. Fractures with at least 50% of the cortex intact and an obliquity of less than 30° are stable. When reduced, stable fractures have intrinsic axial and rotational stability; unstable fractures will shorten or rotate. Type I fractures are simple transverse or oblique fractures with no comminution. Type II fractures are comminuted, but greater than 50% of their cortex is intact. Type III fractures have greater than 50% of their cortex comminuted, but there is some cortical contact between the proximal and distal fragments. Type IV fractures have segmental comminution. Type V fractures have a long oblique pattern.

Diagnosis and Initial Management

History and Physical Examination

A history of injury, pain, swelling, and obvious deformity are present.

Radiographic Examination

Anteroposterior and lateral radiographs are obtained and examined to rule out undisplaced comminution. Radiographs of the knee and pelvis rule out associated injuries.

Initial Management

Initial management makes the patient as comfortable as possible and optimizes the patient's condition for surgery. If surgery is to be performed within 12 h of admission, 5–10 lbs. of skin traction is applied with the thigh resting on a pillow. If surgery is delayed, 10–20 lbs. of skeletal traction is applied through a tibial pin to minimize the chance of contaminating the distal femur. Ligamentous injury of the knee is ruled out prior to applying traction through a tibial pin. Initially with traction, the hip and knee are flexed 30°, and the calf is supported in a sling. Radiographs are obtained in traction, and traction is adjusted accordingly. Ideally, the fracture is aligned and distracted 0.5 cm.

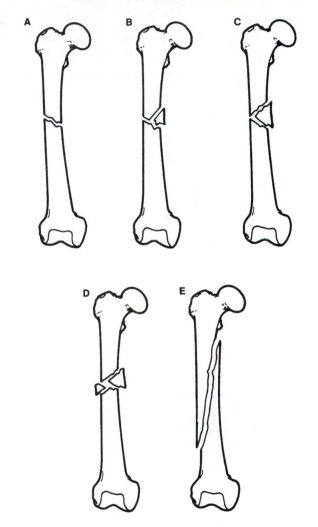

FIG. 19-1 Classification of diaphyseal fractures of the femur: (*A*) type I, (*B*) type II, (*C*) type III, (*D*) type IV, and (*E*) type V.

Associated Injuries

Neurovascular injuries and compartment syndrome of the thigh and buttock are ruled out by a focused examination of the injured extremity.

Skeletal injuries associated with fractures of the femoral diaphysis are **fracture of the femoral neck, hip dislocation, pelvic ring injury, and ligamentous injury of the knee.** The presence of a femoral neck fracture, hip dislocation, or pelvic ring injury is determined by radiographs of the hip and pelvis. Anteroposterior and lateral radiographs of the knee are obtained, and the knee is carefully examined for an effusion and pain with palpation of the patellar tendon and medial– and lateral–collateral ligaments. When it is not possible to rule out ligamentous injury, the patient is reexamined after fracture fixation.

Definitive Management

Fractures of the femoral diaphysis are managed with open reduction and plating, reduction and application of an external fixater, or closed reduction and intramedullary nailing.

Relative indications for **plating** are inability (usually due to other injuries) to place the patient on the fracture table, a grade III open fracture, fractures around other implants (e.g., the femoral stem of a total hip arthroplasty), an associated fracture of the femoral neck or intercondylar fracture of the distal femur, and obliteration of the medullary canal (usually due to a previous fracture). The disadvantages of plating fractures of the femoral diaphysis are a higher risk of infection and the prolonged postoperative non–weight-bearing. Surgical exposure is from a lateral approach through the interval between vastus lateralis and the lateral intermuscular septum. The vastus lateralis is elevated subperiosteally from the femur. Fracture fragments are identified and anatomically reduced. A broad dynamic compression plate on the lateral side of the femur is used to stabilize the fracture. A minimum of eight cortices of fixation proximal and distal to the fracture are required for adequate fixation. Medial cortical defects are grafted with autogenous cancellous bone to stimulate healing and decrease the incidence of plate failure. Postoperatively, motion of the hip and knee is encouraged. Strict non–weight-bearing is maintained until bony trabeculae cross the fracture, usually at 10 to 12 weeks after fixation.

The primary indication for **external fixation** is a grade III open fracture. The advantages of external fixation are that it is quick; it stabilizes the fracture but does not place a foreign body in a contaminated wound; and it allows access to the wound. The disadvantages are that stability is not absolute; the pins placed through the lateral muscles of the thigh "tack" these muscles to the femur, resulting in loss of knee motion; and there is a high incidence of nonunion.

The fracture is reduced through the open wound after debridement and irrigation. A lateral frame is applied with two to four half-pins proximal and distal to the fracture. If possible, the pins are located outside the zone of injury. The fascia lata and underlying muscles around each pin are incised proximally and distally to minimize irritation and loss of knee motion. The postoperative management is tailored to the patient. In general, toe-touch weight-bearing is maintained until the fracture has healed. Knee and hip motion are encouraged. After the soft tissue has healed, the incidence of nonunion is minimized by grafting the fracture with autogenous cancellous bone or by removing the fixater and stabilizing the fracture with an intramedullary nail. An intramedullary nail is inserted only if there have been no signs of infection of the fracture or pin sites.

The majority of fractures of the femoral diaphysis are managed with **intramedullary nailing.** The advantages are a low incidence of infection, a high incidence of healing, the ability to bear weight postoperatively, and the avoidance of soft tissue devascularization of fracture fragments.

Nails are inserted through the proximal femur and driven distally (i.e., antegrade nailing) or through the distal femur and driven proximally (i.e., retrograde nailing). **Antegrade nails** are rigid, and the femur is always reamed prior to their insertion. **Retrograde nails** are rigid and flexible, and the femur is not necessarily reamed before insertion. Type I and type II fractures of the femoral diaphysis are managed with either type of intramedullary nail. Type III, IV, and V fractures of the femoral diaphysis are managed with antegrade or retrograde statically locked nails.

Antegrade intramedullary nailing (Figs. 19-2 and 19-3) is performed with the patient supine or in the lateral decubitus position on the fracture table. The fluoroscopy machine is positioned at the medial side of the thigh if the patient is supine and at the anterior side if the patient is in the lateral decubitus position. The fracture is reduced. The nail is inserted through the piriformis fossae at the superior aspect of the base of the femoral neck. The cortex is perforated with a drill, and a guide-wire is inserted into the proximal fragment and driven across the reduced fracture. The femur is sequentially reamed. The appropriate size nail is driven across the fracture over the guide-wire. In type I and II fractures, the nail is locked dynamically. If the fracture is in the distal third of the femur, the nail is locked distally. When the fracture is in the proximal two-thirds of the femur, the nail is locked proximally. In type III, IV, and V fractures, the nail is locked statically by placing proximal and distal locking screws. Postoperatively, patients with stable fractures are allowed to bear weight as tolerated. Patients with statically locked nails bear weight 50% on the injured side. If radiographic healing progresses over the first 3 to 4 months, weight-bearing is advanced as tolerated. If radiographic signs of healing are delayed, full weight-bearing is delayed; then at 4 to 6 months the fracture is grafted with autogenous cancellous bone. Alternatively, the nail is dynamized by removing either proximal or distal locking screws. If the nail is dynamized, the patient is followed carefully for signs of shortening or rotation. If these occur, the nail is relocked statically and then bone grafted.

FIG. 19-2 Fracture of the femoral diaphysis. This is a type II fracture because there is comminution involving less than 50% of the cortex. In the addition, the fracture is open with a grade II soft tissue injury.

Retrograde flexible nailing of the femoral diaphysis is performed with the patient supine on the fracture table. The fluoroscopy machine is positioned at the lateral side of the thigh. The fracture is reduced. The medial and lateral metaphyseal cortices are perforated with a ¼-inch drill bit, and the hole is enlarged with an awl. The appropriate length nail is selected, and nails are driven from the medial and lateral portals simultaneously across the fracture. The lateral nail is driven into the greater trochanter. The medial nail is driven into the base of the femoral neck. The nails can be locked dynamically by placement of screws through the eyelets of the flexible nails into underlying bone. Postoperatively, knee flexion is encouraged when incisional pain allows, and weight-bearing is as tolerated when radiographic signs of healing are noted.

Retrograde rigid nailing (Fig. 19-4) is performed with the patient supine on a radiolucent operating room table. A roll is placed under the ipsilateral hip to prevent external rotation from developing. The leg is prepped and draped sterilely, and the knee is placed over a sterile

FIG. 19-3   Stabilization with a reamed antegrade statically locked nail.

bloster. Manual traction is applied to effect a reduction that is confirmed flouroscopically by bringing the C-arm in from the opposite side of the table. Intraarticular fractures should be stabilized at this point, before nailing. The patellar tendon is split longitudinally, allowing access to the knee; an entry portal is established, which is centered in the antero-posterior plane and in line with the medullary canal on the lateral x-ray view. This corresponds to the superior aspect of the femoral notch. The entry portal is enlarged to the chosen nail diameter, and a guidewire is placed. Reaming over the guide-wire may or may not be required. The nail is inserted until it lies just below the articular surface, so it will not interfere with knee motion. Distal locking is performed with a jig system and is followed by proximal locking done in a freehand manner. The post-operative course is similar to that described above.

Complications

The complications of fractures of the femoral diaphysis include malunion, nonunion, and infection.

FIG. 19-4   Stabilization with a reamed rigid retrograde nail.

Rotational and angular malunion is managed by osteotomy, realignment, and stabilization of the femur. A statically locked nail or plate is used for stabilization. Fractures that have healed with significant shortening are a difficult problem. Significant shortening is defined as greater than 3 cm or as resulting in gait disturbance or back pain not relieved by a shoe lift. Management options include lengthening the involved femur, lengthening the ipsilateral tibia, or shortening the contralateral femur. Lengthening the involved femur is the most attractive option because it corrects the deformity. Lengthening is achieved by applying an external fixator, osteotomizing the femur, and lengthening the femur in 1-mm increments per day. This procedure requires exceptional patient compliance. Lengthening the tibia is a simpler procedure, but the patient's knees are at different heights. Shortening of the contralateral femur is done closed; it has the lowest morbidity but results in overall loss of height.

Nonunion is managed by stabilizing the fragments and autogenous bone grafting or by dynamic compression applied with an external fixator. Intramedullary nails are usually the best method of stabilization, but plates are occasionally indicated (e.g., if there is a fragment of a broken nail in the canal which cannot be retrieved). If dynamic compression is used, a fixator is used to compress the ends of the nonunion together, usually at the rate of 0.25 mm per day. This technique can be combined with lengthening techniques to manage nonunions associated with a segmental defect or shortening.

Infection is managed with debridement, stabilization, and administration of antibiotics. When there is an associated nonunion, delayed grafting with autogenous cancellous bone or dynamic compression with an external fixator is performed.

SELECTED READINGS

Brumback RJ, Reilly JP, Poka A, Lakatos RP, Bathon GH, Bugess AR: Intramedullary nailing of femoral shaft fractures. Part I: Decision-making errors with interlocking fixation. *J Bone Joint Surg* 70A:1441–1452, 1988.

Kempf I, Grosse A, Beck G: Closed locked intramedullary nailing. Its application to comminuted fractures of the femur. *J Bone Joint Surg* 67A:709–719, 1985.

Moed BR, Watson JT: Retrograde intramedullary nailing, without reaming, of fractures of the femoral shaft in multiply injured patients. *J Bone Joint Surg* 77A:1520–1527, 1995.

Pankovich AM, Goldflies ML, Pearson RL: Closed ender nailing of femoral-shaft fractures. *J Bone Joint Surg* 61A:222–232, 1979.

Winquist RA, Hansen ST Jr: Comminuted fractures of the femoral shaft treated by intramedullary nailing. *Orthop Clin North Am* 11:633–648, 1980.

This chapter reviews fractures of the distal femur (supracondylar, intracondylar, and medial and lateral condyles); fractures of the proximal tibia (the tibial spines and medial and lateral condyles); injuries of the extensor mechanism (the tibial tubercle, ruptures of the patellar or quadriceps tendon, and fractures of the patella); and dislocations of the knee.

ANATOMY

The knee is a compound joint consisting of a sellar joint between the condyles of the femur and the patella and two condylar joints between the condyles of the femur and the tibial plateaus.

The **distal femur** consists of condyles and epicondyles. Medial and lateral condyles form the articular surface. They are narrower anteriorly, and the **medial condyle projects further distally than the lateral condyle,** which results in the distal articular surface forming an angle of 7° with the diaphysis. The **lateral condyle projects *farther* anteriorly (preventing lateral patellar subluxation) and posteriorly than the medial *condyle*.** The distal and posterior surfaces of both condyles are convex and articulate with the corresponding tibial plateau. The anterior surface of the distal femur is the coalescence of medial and lateral condyles. Its concave surface corresponds to the articular surface of the patella.

The **proximal tibia** expands to form the medial and lateral condyles, or plateaus, and tibial tuberosity. The articular surface of the tibia is the cartilage-covered medial and lateral plateaus, which match the corresponding articular surfaces of the femur. Congruency is further increased by the medial and lateral menisci. The two plateaus are separated by the anterior and posterior tibial spines (i.e., the intercondylar eminence). The anterior tibial spine is the insertion of the anterior cruciate ligament and the attachment of the anterior and posterior horns of the lateral meniscus and anterior horn of the medial meniscus. The posterior tibial spine is the attachment of the posterior horn of the medial meniscus. The posterior intercondylar areas are the insertion of the posterior cruciate ligament. The fibular facet on the lateral condyle faces laterally, distally, and posteriorly.

The **tibial tuberosity** is the anterior projection of the tibia into which the patellar ligament inserts. It is 2 cm distal to the articular surface of the tibia. Its upper surface is directly behind the patellar ligament and is an insertion site for intramedullary nailing.

The **patella** is the largest sesamoid bone of the body. It increases the lever arm of the quadriceps and protects the anterior articular surface of the distal femur. It is located 2 cm proximal to the articular surface of the tibia when the knee is extended. A more proximal location is referred to as *patella alta* and a more distal location as *patella baja.* With the exception of the apex, or lower pole, the posterior surface of the patella is covered with articular cartilage. The lower pole serves as the origin of the patellar ligament. The articular surface of the patella is convex and is divided into smaller medial and larger lateral sections by a vertical ridge. The medial and lateral halves are further divided into two or three pairs of facets by faint horizontal ridges in the articular surface. The lateral facets are more distinct than the medial, and the upper lateral facet is slightly concave. In addition, there is a single facet on the extreme medial border of the patella that runs the length of the patella and articulates with the medial femoral condyle when the knee is flexed.

FRACTURES OF THE DISTAL FEMUR

Fractures of the distal femur involve the distal metaphysis and articular surface of the femur.

Classification

Distal femoral fractures are classified according to whether there is intraarticular extension and whether one or both condyles are fractured into three types: type I, extraarticular fractures; type II, intraarticular fractures in which both condyles are involved; and type III, fractures of a single condyle.

Extraarticular fractures (type I), also known as supracondylar fractures, are divided into simple fractures and those with supracondylar comminution (Figs. 20-1 and 20-2).

Intraarticular fractures (type II), or intracondylar fractures, are divided into four subtypes based on the presence of intraarticular displacement and metaphyseal comminution. The subtypes are simple metaphyseal fractures with undisplaced intraarticular component, simple metaphyseal fractures with displaced intraarticular component, comminuted metaphyseal fractures with undisplaced intraarticular component, and comminuted metaphyseal fractures with displaced intraarticular component (Figs. 20-3 through 20-8).

Fractures of a single condyle (type III) are further divided into four subtypes based on the plane of the fracture and the condyle involved. The subtypes are fractures in the coronal plane of the medial or lateral condyles and fractures in the sagittal plane of the medial or lateral condyles (Figs. 20-9 and 20-10).

Associated Injuries

Injuries associated with supracondylar fractures of the femur are fractures and dislocations of the proximal femur and pelvis, ligamentous disruption of the knee, injury of the popliteal artery, and injury of the

FIGS. 20-1 and 20-2   Type I supracondylar fractures.

peroneal and tibial nerves. These injuries are more likely to occur in association with high-energy fractures.

Associated **fractures and dislocations of the proximal femur and pelvis** are most likely to occur in an automobile accident as part of the "dashboard injury" complex. They are ruled out by physical examination and review of radiographs of the proximal femur and entire pelvis.

The most frequently disrupted **ligament** is the patellar ligament. Disruption of the collaterals and cruciates also occurs. Accurate physical examination of the ligaments is usually not possible before fracture fixation. Radiographic signs of ligamentous injury are loss of parallelism between the articular surfaces of the femoral condyles and tibial plateaus and bony avulsion of the cruciates (Figs. 20-7 and 20-8). After stabilization of the fracture, all ligaments are examined and repaired if injured.

Early identification of an associated **popliteal artery** injury is key. The cardinal finding is decreased dorsalis pedis and posterior tibial pulses. This may be due to torsion or traction of the vessels. If aligning the fracture does not result in the return of pulses within 5 min, assume that the popliteal artery is injured and obtain an angiogram. Once the location of the vascular injury is determined, surgery to stabilize the fracture and restore circulation is performed emergently. Occasionally, the popliteal artery injury is an intimal tear, and pulses that are initially present will suddenly disappear with artery thromboses. For this reason, vascular checks are performed every 2 h for the first 36 h after injury.

FIGS. 20-3 through 20-6   Type II intraarticular or intracondylar fractures.

Management of the normal vascular examination (arteriogram vs. clinical checks) is controversial. Some centers use vascular Doppler studies and ankle–arm indices, whereas others rely on arteriograms. In high-energy dislocations and in multiply traumatized patients, an arteriogram will quickly and clearly define the integrity of the artery.

Injuries of the **peroneal and tibial nerves** are identified by assessing sensation and the ability to plantarflex and dorsiflex the ankle. These

FIGS. 20-7 and 20-8   Type II fracture stabilized with a retrograde nail after the condyles had been lagged together. The tibial spines are avulsed, indicating a cruciate injury.

injuries are managed with range-of-motion exercises of the ankle and foot and splinting in a functional position.

Diagnosis and Initial Management

History and Physical Examination

There is pain and a history of injury. Obvious instability and deformity are present with type I and II fractures but may not be present with fractures of a single condyle.

Radiographic Examination

Radiographs in the anteroposterior and lateral projections are sufficient to evaluate the injury. The tunnel view of the distal femur in which the anteroposterior radiograph is obtained with the knee flexed to 30° is helpful but painful for the patient. Radiographs of the pelvis, hip, femur, and tibia are examined for associated injuries.

Initial Management

The key factor in the initial management is evaluation of the vascular status of the leg. If a vascular injury has not occurred, the leg is immobilized in a toe-to-groin splint and iced. If splinting does not adequately immobilize the fracture, skeletal traction is used. A proximal tibial pin is inserted, the knee is placed on pillows, the calf is supported in a sling, and 10 to 20 lbs. of traction is applied. Posttraction radiographs are obtained to assess alignment and to determine whether the knee joint is being distracted because of ligamentous disruption.

Definitive Management

The definitive management of supracondylar fractures is surgery. The surgical approach, stabilization device, and whether bone graft is used are based on the type of fracture.

We stabilize fractures without intraarticular extension with an antegrade or retrograde intramedullary nail. **Antegrade locked nailing** of a supracondylar fracture is performed as described in Chapter 19. To decrease the incidence of nail breakage through a distal locking hole, there should be at least 5 cm of intact bone proximal to the distal screw holes; therefore, this method can be used only for very proximal supracondylar fractures.

FIGS. 20-9 and 20-10 Fractures of a single condyle in the coronal and sagittal planes.

The fracture can be stabilized with a **rigid retrograde nail** inserted through the intercondylar notch. The objections to this technique are the intraarticular insertion portal, possible synovial metalosis, and the potential difficulty of removing the nail (Figs. 20-7 and 20-8).

Intracondylar fractures (type II) are managed with a plate and screws. Intramedullary nails are not an option unless the intraarticular fracture can be reduced and stabilized in such a way that the fixation will not interfere with nail insertion and that redisplacement of the intraarticular fracture will not occur during reaming or insertion of the nail. Intercondylar fractures with a simple metaphyseal component and undisplaced condyles are stabilized with a 95° sideplate and lag screw. To minimize the potential that the undisplaced condyles will displace during lag screw insertion, they are stabilized with two large cancellous screws before reaming for the lag screw. Fractures with metaphyseal comminution and an undisplaced intracondylar component are managed similarly; however, the medial side of the metaphysis is grafted with autogenous cancellous bone. Anatomic reduction of comminuted metaphyseal fragments is not mandatory as long as the relationship of the condyles to the distal diaphysis is restored.

The management of intracondylar fractures with a simple metaphyseal component and displaced condyles is more complex. The condyles must be reduced; therefore, a useful option is to use a surgical approach that exposes the distal articular surface. A straight anterior incision is made. The quadriceps tendon is split in line with its fibers; this incision is continued distally as a lateral parapatellar incision. If necessary, the tibial tuberosity is predrilled, osteotomized, and reflected proximally for better exposure. The condyles are reduced and held in place with Kirschner wires and screws. The fixation of the intercondylar fracture is planned so that it does not interfere with placement of the device used to fix the condyles to the femur (e.g., a side-plate and lag screw). Fractures with metaphyseal comminution and a displaced intracondylar component are managed similarly; however, the medial side of the metaphysis is grafted with autogenous cancellous bone. In fractures with segmental comminution, the medial side of the metaphysis is plated through the same incision. The medial plate functions as a buttress and is fastened to the bone with unicortical screws.

Supracondylar and intracondylar fractures that are complicated by osteopenia are stabilized as described, but polymethylmethacrylate (PMMA) can be used to provide more stable fixation. After the fragments have been reduced, PMMA while in its doughy state is inserted into the medullary cavity across the fracture. This is done through a cortical window at the level of the fracture. After the PMMA has hardened, the fracture is stabilized with plates and screws. If PMMA is used, it is mandatory to graft the medial side with autogenous bone.

Fractures of the medial or lateral condyles in the sagittal plane are exposed through a medial or lateral parapatellar surgical approach. The condyle is reduced and held in place with lag screws or a buttress plate. Fractures in the coronal plane involve the posterior portion of the condyle. They are exposed through a midmedial or midlateral incision. The surface of the fragment is covered with articular cartilage and is stabilized with countersunk screws.

After stabilization of supracondylar, intracondylar, and single condyle fractures, early motion is encouraged as soon as incisional pain becomes tolerable. The duration of nonweight-bearing is dependent on the stability of the fracture, the stability of fixation, and the rate of healing.

Complications

Complications are nonunion, malunion, and posttraumatic arthritis. **Nonunion** is managed with autogenous bone graft and rigid stabilization. Revision of the internal fixation device is frequently necessary, depending on the time from initial injury and surgery. A stiff knee worsens the prognosis. In cases in which the knee is stiff or in which stabilization of the distal fragment is impossible because of its small size or osteopenia, arthrodesis is performed. If there is no prior history of infection, an intramedullary rod is used. If there is a history of infection, an external fixater is used.

Varus and valgus **malunions** are invariably symptomatic and eventually result in arthritis. Extension and flexion malunions are better tolerated. Symptomatic malunion is managed with corrective osteotomy of the femur.

Posttraumatic arthritis is managed with nonsteroidal antiinflammatory drugs and local injection of steroids. Arthroscopic debridement provides short-term relief of symptoms. The last resort is arthroplasty or arthrodesis. Arthroplasty is reserved for low-demand elderly patients.

FRACTURES OF THE TIBIAL PLATEAU

Fractures of the tibial plateau involve the proximal articular surface of the tibia.

Classification

Tibial plateau fractures have been classified by many systems, but the system described by Schatzker et al. (1979) is currently most commonly used. It is as follows: type I, split fracture of the lateral plateau; type II, split and depressed fracture of the lateral plateau; type III, depressed fracture of the lateral plateau, frequently osteoporotic; type IV, fracture of the medial plateau; type V, bicondylar fracture of the proximal tibia; and type VI, bicondylar plateau fracture and associated metaphyseal fracture (Figs. 20-11 through 20-17). Types I to III are low-energy fractures. Types IV to VI are high-energy injuries. In addition, we include a low-energy fracture of the medial tibial plateau.

Split fractures (Schatzker type I) of the lateral plateau occur in young patients with dense bone. The mechanism of injury is usually a blow to the lateral side of the knee. The fracture, which is best seen on the anteroposterior projection, is vertical and seldom displaced more than 3 mm. The lateral meniscus may be torn peripherally and dislocated into the fracture site (Fig. 20-11).

Split-depressed fractures (Schatzker type II) are the most common type of tibial plateau fracture. The mechanism of injury is a valgus stress that impacts the lateral femoral condyle against the plateau, fracturing the lateral portion of the plateau from the proximal tibia. As the femoral condyle continues to impact the remaining portion of the lateral plateau, it drives a segment of articular surface into the metaphysis. This depressed segment is always on the medial side of the fracture, not on the split fragment. Whether the depressed segment is anterior or posterior depends on the degree of flexion at the time of injury (extension is associated with anterior depression, flexion with posterior depression; Figs. 20-13, 20-18, and 20-19).

Depressed fractures (Schatzker type III) occur in osteopenic bone. The mechanism of injury is a low-energy valgus stress: the lateral femoral condyle sinks into and depresses the lateral plateau. The lateral plateau, including the metaphyseal cortex, is tilted laterally (Fig. 20-12).

Low-energy medial plateau fractures are similar to depressed fractures of the lateral plateau but are the result of a varus force across the knee. The entire medial plateau is tilted medially (Fig. 20-14).

High-energy medial plateau (Schatzker type IV) fractures are fracture dislocations frequently associated with neurovascular injuries. They are caused by axial and valgus forces across the knee, resulting in

FIGS. 20-11 through 20-17   Types of tibial plateau fractures.

FIGS. 20-11 through 20-17 *Continued.*

the lateral femoral condyle impacting the tibial spines along a vector directed medially and distally. The medial tibial condyle and the tibial spines are fractured and driven along this vector. The lateral–collateral ligament is ruptured; the cruciates and medial–collateral ligaments are intact (Fig. 20-15).

Bicondylar plateau fractures (Schatzker type V) involve both condyles and are the result of complex high-energy trauma. Associated neurovascular and ligamentous injuries and compartment syndrome are common (Fig. 20-16).

Plateau fractures associated with a fracture of the proximal metaphysis (Schatzker type VI) are similar to bicondylar fractures in that they are the result of high-energy trauma and frequently have associated neurovascular injuries. There is a high incidence of nonunion and postoperative infection due to the magnitude of the injury and the extensive surgical exposure necessary to reduce and stabilize the fracture (Fig. 20-17).

Associated Injuries

Injuries frequently associated with fractures of the tibial plateaus are ruptures of the collateral ligaments, occlusion of the popliteal artery or trifurcation, compartment syndrome, and injury of the posterior tibial or common peroneal nerve.

Fracture of the medial or lateral plateau may be associated with a rupture of the **contralateral–collateral ligament.** Apparent ligamentous laxity may be a misinterpretation of motion occurring through the fracture site. To determine definitively if there is a ligamentous injury, the knee is stressed under fluoroscopy.

Injuries of the **popliteal artery or trifurcation** are most likely to occur with high-energy medial–tibial plateau and bicondylar fractures. If distal pulses are absent, an arteriogram is obtained.

Compartment syndrome is indicated by the presence of the classic signs of increased intracompartmental pressure: pain at rest, pain with passive stretch of muscles, tense compartments, and numbness in the first web space.

Injuries of the **posterior tibial and peroneal nerves** are identified by assessing sensation on the plantar aspect of the foot and in the first web space and by assessing active contraction of the flexor and extensor hallucis longus.

Diagnosis and Initial Management

History and Physical Examination

There is pain, swelling, and a history of injury. There may be no discernible deformity, but there is a large knee effusion, which, when aspirated, has blood with fat in it, indicating an intraarticular fracture.

Radiographic Examination

Radiographs in the anteroposterior and lateral planes are of most use. Tilting the beam 10° caudally so that it profiles the articular surface provides more accurate information regarding the amount of depression. Tomography and CAT scans are helpful.

Initial Management

A long leg splint with the knee in 20° of flexion is applied. The knee is iced.

Definitive Management

The goals of management of tibial plateau fractures are to decrease the risk of posttraumatic osteoarthritis and provide a stable knee with a normal axis of alignment. Indications for operative management are reducible intraarticular incongruity, intraarticular displacement (i.e., a gap without a step-off) of 3 mm or more, ligamentous instability, or a deviation in the alignment of the knee. Indications for nonoperative management are a fracture that cannot be satisfactorily reduced and stabilized, usually due to extensive comminution, blisters, and preexisting arthritis.

The **nonoperative management** of tibial plateau fractures that are minimally displaced or in which there is preexisting osteoarthritis consists of 4 to 8 weeks of immobilization in a long leg cast, followed by 4 to 8 weeks of nonweight-bearing and protected mobilization in an orthosis. Displaced fractures that are managed nonoperatively are placed in balanced skeletal suspension with the knee at 45°. A sling supports the calf, and 10 to 20 lbs. of traction is applied through a distal tibial pin. Alignment of the fracture is assessed radiographically every 2 to 3 days for the first 2 weeks, and traction is adjusted accordingly. At 2 to 3 weeks, passive motion in traction is initiated. At 4 to 6 weeks, there is usually enough healing clinically and radiographically that balanced suspension can be discontinued and a long leg cast can be applied. The cast is continued 8 to 10 weeks from injury. Nonweight-bearing is continued 12 weeks from injury. Minimally displaced plateau fractures are best evaluated with a careful examination (frequently under anesthesia) to look at varus and valgus stability in full knee extension. Less than 10° of valgus instability is a clinical finding that indicates good potential for nonoperative management. This finding was described initially by Rasmussen (1973).

The goal of **operative management** is anatomic alignment of the joint surface and stabilization adequate to allow early motion. The surgical exposure and method of stabilization are based on the type of fracture.

Split fractures are reduced closed under fluoroscopy and stabilized with percutaneous screws. To reduce the fracture, the knee is flexed to 30° and a varus stress is applied. At the same time, the lateral plateau is pushed medially toward the proximal tibia. If this maneuver does not result in reduction, the fracture is exposed through a lateral parapatellar approach. The block to reduction (frequently the lateral meniscus) is identified and removed. Postoperatively, the extremity is placed in a continuous passive motion machine and moved from 10° to 30°. When the patient can perform active range of motion, the continuous passive motion is discontinued. Nonweight-bearing is maintained for 6 to 8 weeks.

Split-depressed fractures are exposed through a straight anterior incision. The anterior horn of the lateral meniscus is incised and the fracture is "booked open" through the split component, thereby exposing the depressed segment. The depressed segment is elevated and bone grafted, and the split fragment is reduced and stabilized with a plate (Figs. 20-18 and 20-19).

FIG. 20-18   Split-depressed tibial plateau fracture.

FIG. 20-19 Split-depressed tibial plateau fracture seen in Fig. 20–18 reduced and stabilized with a plate.

Depressed fractures are managed operatively through a straight anterior skin incision. The lateral plateau is elevated with a bone tamp inserted through a window in the lateral metaphysis. The tibial attachment of the meniscus is incised, and the meniscus is retracted superiorly to expose the plateau. The resulting defect is packed with autogenous bone graft. A plate is applied laterally with two large cancellous screws within 5 mm of subchondral bone. These screws function to support the articular surface.

Medial plateau fractures are managed operatively through a straight anterior incision or a posteromedial incision. Depending on the location of the fracture, the anterior horn of the medial or lateral meniscus can be incised. There may be minimal compression with high-energy fractures in which case bone grafting is not necessary. A plate is required for stabilization because simple cannulated screws do not provide adequate stability to prevent displacement.

Bicondylar fractures are exposed by incising one or both anterior horns of the menisci. The tibial tubercle can be osteotomized and the patellar tendon reflected. Fragments are reduced, bone graft is used to fill defects, and medial and lateral plates are applied. High-energy injuries have significant risks associated with postoperative soft tissue complications.

Plateau fractures with an associated metaphyseal fracture are managed by first addressing the intraarticular fracture and then the metaphyseal fracture. Articular reduction is mandatory and usually internally fixed with cannulated screws. Metaphyseal reduction and fixation is either with a plate or, more commonly, hybrid external fixation with small wire fixation of the proximal tibial component. Prolonged casting of the metaphyseal fracture is not an option because a stiff knee will result.

Early postoperative motion is encouraged. With the exception of split fractures, nonweight-bearing is maintained for 12 weeks. Patients with split fractures can bear weight as tolerated at 6 weeks.

Complications

Complications of tibial plateau fractures are arthritis, nonunion, infection, and late subsidence of a reduced plateau. **Arthritis** results from articular incongruity or injury to the articular cartilage that occurred at the time of fracture. Patients younger than age 50 years are managed with nonsteroidal antiinflammatory drugs and local steroid injections. If the symptoms warrant, an arthrodesis or a varus or valgus high tibial osteotomy designed to "unload" the involved condyle is performed. Patients older than age 50 years with arthritis are managed with an arthroplasty.

Nonunion of tibial plateau fractures is rare; when it occurs, it is often accompanied by infection. In evaluating the nonunion, it is important to determine whether it is infected, whether the knee joint is arthritic, and how much motion is occurring through the knee as opposed to through the nonunion. If there is no evidence of infection and there is severe arthritis, the nonunion is managed with an arthroplasty in patients older than age 50 years. In patients younger than age 50 years, the nonunion is managed with an arthrodesis by using an intramedullary nail. Management of aseptic nonunions without arthritis consists of rigid stabilization in the form of plates and screws and autogenous cancellous bone grafting. Restricted knee motion is associated with a high incidence of failure of fixation. The principles of management of **infected nonunions** of tibial plateau fractures are debridement of necrotic tissue and foreign bodies, stabilization of the nonunion with screws and plates, management of dead space with antibiotic impregnated beads or muscle flaps, soft tissue coverage with local or free tissue transfer, and antibiotic coverage based on the sensitivities of the pathogenic organisms. Septic nonunion of the tibial plateau is frequently associated with destruction of the joint. In these cases, knee arthrodesis is performed with an external fixater.

Late subsidence of a reduced tibial plateau occurs in osteopenic patients who have sustained a depressed fracture of the lateral plateau or a low-energy fracture of the medial plateau. At-risk patients are followed closely after weight-bearing has been initiated. If subsidence is suspected, weight-bearing is discontinued, and aggressive physical therapy, in particular strengthening and active range of motion, is instituted. After 2 to 4 weeks, partial weight-bearing in a varus (lateral plateau) or valgus (medial plateau) orthosis is reinstituted and gradually increased. Radiographs are obtained weekly until the patient is full weight-bearing. If subsidence has occurred and instability or alteration in the axis of the knee is symptomatic, management is osteotomy or arthroplasty.

INJURIES OF THE EXTENSOR MECHANISM

This section reviews fractures of the patella and injuries of the quadriceps tendon and patellar ligament.

FRACTURES OF THE PATELLA

Classification

Fractures of the patella are undisplaced or displaced, simple or comminuted, and transverse or vertical (Figs. 20-20 through 20-23). **Undisplaced** fractures are all fractures with less than 3 mm of displacement and no step-off. The patient has active knee extension or at a minimum

FIG. 20-20   Undisplaced comminuted patellar fracture.

FIG. 20-21   Displaced simple transverse patellar fracture.

FIG. 20-22   Displaced comminuted patellar fracture.

FIG. 20-23   Displaced vertical patellar fracture.

can perform a straight leg raise. **Displaced** fractures are simple or comminuted and transverse or vertical. Fragments are displaced more than 3 mm, or there is a step-off involving the articular surface. Frequently, active knee extension is absent.

Associated Injuries

Fractures of the proximal femur and acetabulum are associated with patellar fractures sustained during high-energy trauma (i.e., the dashboard injury). The treating physician should recognize long-term articular injury, which can occur and result in debilitating symptoms. Radiographs of the hip, femur, and tibia are obtained and examined. The knee is carefully stressed to detect any injury of the stabilizing ligaments. The hip is put through a range of motion to rule out associated fracture or dislocation.

Diagnosis and Initial Management

History and Physical Examination

There is pain and a history of direct trauma to the knee or forceful flexion of the knee (e.g., during a fall). There may be a palpable soft tissue defect gap at the fracture site. A large hemarthrosis with fat is present. After aspiration, local anesthetic is injected. When some degree of anesthesia has been achieved, the patient's ability to extend the knee actively is determined. Loss of active extension is an indication for surgery.

Radiographic Examination

Anteroposterior and lateral radiographs are useful. A "skyline" view determines the presence of an intraarticular step-off but may not be possible because of discomfort. This view is obtained by flexing the knee 45°, placing the cassette at midcalf, and directing the beam from proximal to distal through the anterior aspect of the knee. Tomography and computed tomography are not helpful.

Initial Management

The knee is splinted in full extension and iced.

Definitive Management

Management is based on the type of fracture. Undisplaced transverse or comminuted fractures that can be raised as a straight leg raise are managed by immobilizing the knee in extension, in a cylinder cast, or in a knee immobilizer. Partial weight-bearing is maintained for at least 3 weeks, during which time radiographs are obtained at weekly intervals. If displacement occurs, open reduction and internal fixation is necessary. At 6 weeks, immobilization is discontinued, and active range of motion is initiated. Undisplaced vertical fractures are managed similarly, but the period of immobilization is only 4 weeks.

Displaced fractures are managed with open reduction and fixation. The fracture is approached through a straight and midline anterior incision, extending from 4 cm proximal to the patella to 2 cm distal to the tibial tubercle. Transverse incisions have been recommended in the past but can interfere with future knee exposures. Fractures are reduced and stabilized with screws or Kirschner wires, or the comminuted segment is excised and the quadriceps tendon or patellar ligament is sutured to the remaining patella. The retinaculum is repaired with nonabsorbable braided sutures. The repair can be protected with a load-sharing cable extending from the tibial tubercle to the proximal patella (Figs. 20-24 and 20-25). This is especially useful for avulsion-type fractures of the distal pole of the patellar.

Complications

Complications of patellar fractures include posttraumatic arthritis and loss of fixation. **Posttraumatic arthritis** is managed conservatively with nonsteroidal antiinflammatory drugs and steroid injections. If this is not successful in managing the symptoms, a patellectomy is performed. Patellectomy has significant functional deficits, especially loss of power, and should be weighed in patient counseling. **Loss of fixation** is managed with revision of the fixation.

FIGS. 20-24 and 20-25 Simple transverse fracture before and after fixation.

INJURIES OF THE QUADRICEPS TENDON AND PATELLAR LIGAMENT

Classification

Disruption of the quadriceps tendon and patellar ligament is classified as either a bony avulsion or midsubstance tear.

Associated Injuries

There are no specific injuries associated with rupture of the quadriceps tendon. The patellar ligament rupture is frequently associated with long-term patellar tendonitis, knee hyperextension, and jumping (i.e., basketball) injuries.

Diagnosis and Initial Management

History and Physical Examination

There is a history of the knee giving away, usually preceded by a forceful contraction of the quadriceps. There is pain and a palpable gap in the tendon or ligament. If active extension is present, the rupture is partial. Loss of active extension indicates a complete rupture and means that surgical repair is necessary.

Radiographic Examination

The radiographic signs are subtle and may consist only of an effusion. A bony avulsion from the patella or tibial tubercle and patella alta (patellar tendon avulsion) or patella baja (quadriceps tendon rupture) may be present.

Initial Management

The knee is splinted in full extension and iced.

Definitive Management

Partial rupture of the quadriceps tendon and patellar ligament is managed nonoperatively. The knee is immobilized in extension for 4 to 6 weeks, after which gentle active and passive motion is initiated.

Complete ruptures are managed operatively. The surgical exposure is through a midline longitudinal incision centered over the site of injury. The type of repair depends on whether the injury is an avulsion or a midsubstance tear. Avulsions are reattached through drill holes in the patella or tibial tuberosity. Midsubstance tears are repaired by end-to-end repair with a Kessler suture or locking whip stitch, as described by Krackow et al. (1988). Associated tears in the retinaculum are repaired with braided nonabsorbable figure of eight sutures. Patellar ligament repairs are protected with a load-bearing wire or cable loop extending from the proximal pole of the patella to the tibial tubercle.

Postoperatively, quadriceps tendon repairs are protected 4 to 6 weeks in a splint. Weight-bearing is as tolerated on crutches. At 4 to 6 weeks, the splint is removed daily for active range-of-motion exercises. At 8 weeks, the splint and crutches are discontinued. When the patellar tendon has been repaired and a load-bearing cable or wire has been used, postoperative immobilization is not necessary. Intraoperative flexion of the knee to 90° gives the clinician an estimation of the construct strength. Active range of motion is usually initiated 2 weeks after surgery. Crutches are used for 4 weeks.

Complications

The complications of quadriceps tendon and patellar ligament rupture are primarily failure of the repair and infection. **Failure of the repair** is a serious complication. In the rare instance when it is caught early, the repair can be redone; however, the duration of immobilization must be extended. Usually, failure of the repair is caught later, and a more extensive surgical procedure is required. V-Y advancement of the quadriceps, tendon grafts using the fascia lata, or transfer of semitendinous and gracilis muscles is performed to restore the continuity. **Infection** of the repair is relatively common because of its subcutaneous location. When infection occurs, it is treated aggressively with antibiotics. Surgical management of the infected repair is usually not necessary. The indications for surgery are a septic knee requiring drainage and loss of tissue over the patellar tendon requiring a soft tissue transfer (e.g., gastrocnemius flap).

LIGAMENTOUS INJURIES OF THE KNEE

This section describes the diagnosis and management of knee dislocations.

Classification

We classify knee dislocations according to which ligaments are disrupted.

There are four ligaments that may be disrupted: the anterior cruciate (ACL), posterior cruciate (PCL), lateral–collateral (LCL) and corner, and medial–collateral (MCL) and corner. The determination of which ligaments are disrupted is based on the physical examination either immediately after the injury or later under anesthesia.

For many years, the sine qua non of knee dislocations was complete disruption of both cruciate ligaments. Recently, it has become clear that the PCL is occasionally intact. This is a key point: a functioning PCL directs surgical management to the treatment of the torn ACL. In contrast, the dislocation in which both cruciate ligaments are torn is a much more complicated and unstable pattern requiring treatment of both cruciate ligaments.

One or both of the collateral ligaments may be disrupted during a knee dislocation. Disruption of a collateral ligament implies disruption of underlying capsular structures and directs the surgical approach to ligamentous repair.

Associated Injuries

Injuries associated with knee dislocations are vascular, neurologic, or skeletal.

Roughly one-third of all knee dislocations have an associated **popliteal artery** injury. The presence of pedal pulses does not rule out an arterial injury (e.g., an intimal tear). Therefore, arteriography, even in the presence of palpable postreduction pulses, is justifiable. Disruption of the popliteal artery is a surgical emergency. Circulation must be reestablished within 8 h or the chance of salvaging the leg is minimal. Stabilization of the knee with external fixation is the most effective means of protecting the vascular repair. The external fixator can be left in place and used to manage the ligamentous injury.

The **peroneal and tibial nerves** are at risk. The peroneal nerve is injured more frequently than the tibial nerve, with an incidence of about 20%. The peroneal nerve is most commonly injured in association with the lateral ligamentous complex (e.g., adduction injury to the knee ACL/PCL/LCL/PLC torn, MCL intact). It is usually a traction injury that cannot be repaired. The differential diagnosis of peroneal and tibial nerve deficit includes compartment syndrome.

Bony avulsions of ligamentous origins and insertions are distinct from fracture–dislocations of the knee in which ligamentous injury is associated with a fracture of the tibial or femoral condyles. Frequently, a bony avulsion facilitates ligamentous repair. The PCL is avulsed in approximately 80% and the ACL in approximately 50% of complete bicruciate knee dislocations.

Diagnosis and Initial Management

History and Physical Examination

The mechanism of injury is important because the incidence of associated injuries, in particular popliteal artery disruption, is less with low-energy (e.g., sports-related) injuries.

The diagnosis of a displaced knee dislocation is obvious because of the gross deformity. However, frequently, the dislocation has been reduced at the site of the injury, and swelling may be the only obvious physical finding. Lacerations are assumed to communicate with the joint unless proven otherwise. A medial skin furrow may indicate that the dislocation is complex or irreducible with closed methods.

A focused vascular evaluation includes palpation of pedal pulses, examination of leg and foot compartments, and assessment of skin color and capillary refill. A focused neurologic evaluation includes examination of the peroneal nerve (i.e., sensation on the dorsum of the foot and ability to dorsiflex the ankle) and tibial nerve (i.e., sensation on the plantar aspect of the foot and ability to plantarflex the ankle, foot, and toes).

The initial ligamentous evaluation is performed in a standardized manner with reference made to the contralateral knee for comparison. The knee is stressed in full extension in varus and valgus; knee opening in full extension indicates an injury to both cruciates and the associated collateral. Instability in 30° of flexion indicates a torn MCL (valgus) or LCL (varus) (Fig. 20-26). Hyperextension indicates a torn ACL and posterolateral corner (a positive hyperextension recurvatum test). A positive Lachman test indicates a torn ACL. A Lachman test is performed by flexing the knee to 25°. One hand stabilizes the thigh and the other stresses the tibia to displace the knee anteriorly and posteriorly (Fig. 20-27). If there is an abnormal amount of motion, the test is positive. Anterior and posterior drawer tests are performed by flexing the knee to 90° and applying anterior and posterior stresses, respectively. Instability indicates a torn ACL and capsule or PCL and capsule, respectively. Posterior cruciate injury is best evaluated clinically with a posterior drawer test.

Radiographic Examination

The neurovascular and radiographic examinations are performed prior to reduction. Anteroposterior and lateral radiographs aid in classifying the injury by the position of the tibia on the femur and determining

FIG. 20-26   Stressing the MCL.

FIG. 20-27   Lachman test.

whether there are associated fractures. After the initial closed reduction, the injury is further evaluated with magnetic resonance imaging (MRI). MRI identifies which ligaments are disrupted and distinguishes midsubstance tears from avulsions. This is particularly useful in planning the management of a PCL disrupted knee dislocation.

Radiographs are obtained while the patient is anesthetized. The extended knee is stressed in varus and valgus. Joint line opening indicates complete disruption of both cruciate ligaments and of either the MCL or LCL.

Thus, with the initial evaluation, pre- and postreduction radiographs, MRI, examination under anesthesia, and stress radiographs, an accurate preincision prediction of the damaged structures is made.

Initial Management

Reduction is usually straightforward and accomplished with longitudinal traction and manipulation. Once the joint is reduced, the vascular and neurologic examinations are repeated. The knee is splinted and iced. Postsplinting radiographs are obtained to ensure maintenance of reduction. The onus is on the physician to identify an associated vascular injury as early as possible. At a minimum, the patient is admitted for observation. In most cases, ankle–arm indices or arteriography are performed to rule out an associated arterial injury. Frequently, ankle–arm indices are used in low-energy or sporting dislocations, and arteriography is used in multitrauma patients.

Definitive Management

With the recent advances in ligament reconstruction and repair, it makes intuitive sense to perform acute (within 3 to 5 days) ligamentous repairs.

Furthermore, surgical repair allows early range of motion. Associated injuries to the posterolateral corner are best treated surgically early rather than reconstructed late. Occasionally, closed management of knee dislocations is required because of associated injuries (soft tissue, multiple trauma, infection).

Closed management consists of immobilization of the knee in extension for 6 weeks, followed by manipulation under anesthesia and arthroscopy and range-of-motion exercises. This length of time frequently allows for satisfactory healing of the PCL. Frequently, manipulation under epidural anesthesia is required to regain full motion. Early range of motion as currently used to manage combined isolated ACL/MCL injuries results in laxity or complete bicruciate injuries, with involvement of the ligamentous corner.

Surgical Management

There are fundamental techniques and principles of surgical management. **Midline incisions** are used whenever possible to minimize the incidence of wound-healing problems if other surgical procedures are performed in the future. Repair of midsubstance ligament tears can be accomplished with the **looping suture** technique, as described by Marshall et al. (1991), or the **locking whip stitch,** as described by Krackow et al. (1988). Midsubstance cruciate tears are reconstructed. Midsubstance collateral and corner ligamentous injuries are repaired. Ligaments avulsed from their insertions or origins are **reattached with a screw and spiked washer.** Fixation of an autograft or allograft is accomplished by **fixing the graft in bony tunnels** in the femur and tibia. The key to reconstruction of the dislocated knee is first **repairing the PCL.**

Acute simultaneous PCL/ACL surgery is not recommended, and ACL reconstruction is usually delayed. The exception to this rule is an ACL avulsion in which reattachment increases the stability of the knee without increasing the complexity or duration of surgery. Repair of collateral injuries adds to stability and is especially useful in the treatment of the posterolateral corner. **Arthroscopy** of the acute knee dislocation (within 14 days of injury) is contraindicated because of the risk of fluid extravasation due to the capsular disruption. Simultaneous PCL/ACL reconstructions are preferred but usually on a delayed basis (2 to 6 weeks), after motion has been started and the capsule has healed (unsealed), to allow for arthroscopy.

Specific Surgical Techniques

The following descriptions of surgical management of the dislocated knee are based on the ligaments involved.

Type I ACL/MCL/LCL torn, PCL intact: PCL integrity directs the treatment of this type of dislocation to the anterior cruciate ligament.

Repair of the ACL is performed either immediately or until range of motion is restored and collateral healing has occurred.

Type II ACL/PCL torn, MCL/LCL intact: This injury pattern is rare, and the management is simplified by the intact collaterals. The key to successful management is repair of the PCL and ACL.

Type III ACL/PCL/MCL torn, LCL/PLC intact: The primary goal is repair of the PCL and MCL. Through a straight midline or paramedian incision, the knee joint is exposed and the menisci is inspected. Gentle dissection medially exposes the MCL, which is repaired. The PCL, if avulsed, can be reattached to the femur or tibia through this same incision. Midsubstance PCL tears are repaired by using an autograft obtained from the patellar ligament or an allograft. Final tensioning and fixation of PCL and MCL repairs are performed with the knee flexed 20° and with the hip externally rotated, thereby reducing the medial tibiofemoral compartment. The presence of a functioning posterolateral corner simplifies the treatment of this type of knee dislocation. Simultaneous or staged ACL reconstruction is required for functional stability. Simultaneous ACL/PCL reconstruction is best performed on a subacute basis (3 to 6 weeks postinjury) to avoid stiffness.

Type IV ACL/PCL/LCL/PLC torn, MCL intact: The torn LCL and PLC complicates treatment. It is important to reestablish the posterolateral corner and associated tendinous structures (i.e., biceps femoris and/or iliotibial band) in addition to the PCL. The incision is posterolateral. The peroneal nerve is isolated and retracted, and the knee is inspected by subluxing the tibiofemoral joint. The locking-whip stitch is used to reattach or repair the LCL and associated posterolateral structures if torn. Tibial avulsions of the PCL are reattached through the posterolateral incision. A medial incision is used to reattach the PCL when it has been avulsed from the femur or if a femoral tunnel is required for reconstruction. ACL reattachment is performed acutely if present. Eventual ACL reconstruction will be required to allow for functional knee stability.

Type V ACL/PCL/MCL/LCL/PLC torn: This pattern is most frequently a high-energy injury characterized by gross instability and frequently accompanied by neurovascular compromise. Repair of the PCL and posterolateral corner is the primary goal. By using a posterolateral incision, these two structures are explored and repaired. A medial incision may be required to reattach the PCL to the femur or to reconstruct it with an autograft or allograft. ACL reconstruction, simultaneous or staged, allows for functional knee stability. The presence of multitrauma complicates management.

Complications

Complications unique to a dislocation of the knee are arthrofibrosis, residual laxity, and incompetent lateral structures.

Arthrofibrosis results in loss of motion. It is best avoided by following the surgical repair with rigorous physical therapy. If 90° of flexion has not been obtained by 6 weeks postsurgery, manipulation under epidural anesthesia and arthroscopic scar excision are performed. Epidural anesthesia is continued postoperatively 2 to 3 days to maintain motion.

Residual laxity is frequently due to reattachment of a stretched PCL. Residual laxity is best avoided by reconstructing the stretched PCL with autograft or allograft at the initial repair.

Incompetent lateral structures result in **posterolateral rotary instability** (PLRI). Repair of the lateral structures can be difficult (midsubstance tears of the LCL are particularly difficult) but should be attempted. Unlike combined ACL/LCL injuries in which the LCL is frequently treated nonoperatively, the LCL in a knee dislocation is repaired or reconstructed to promote lateral stability. Biceps tenodesis can be used to augment an LCL injury. The ACL reconstruction is necessary after initial LCL/PCL surgery (ACL functioning as an internal collateral) to provide stability in extension.

SELECTED READINGS

Supracondylar Fractures of the Femur
Giles JB, DeLee JC, Heckman JD, Keever JE: Supracondylar–intercondylar fractures of the femur treated with a supracondylar plate and lag screw. *J Bone Joint Surg* 66A:864–870, 1982.
Ker NB, Maempel FZ, Paton DF: Bone cement as an adjunct to medullary nailing in fractures of the distal third of the femur in elderly patients. *Injury* 16(2):102–7, 1984.
Mize RD, Bucholz RW, Grogan DP: Surgical treatment of displaced, comminuted fractures of the distal end of the femur. *J Bone Joint Surg* 64A:871–879, 1982.

Fractures of the Tibial Plateau
Fernandez D: Anterior approach to the knee with osteotomy of the tibial tubercle for bicondylar tibial fractures. *J Bone Joint Surg* 70A: 208–219, 1988.
Perry CR, Evans LG, Rice S, Fogarty J, Burdge RE: A new surgical approach to fractures of the lateral tibial plateau. *J Bone Joint Surg* 66A:1236–1240, 1984.
Rasmussen PS: Tibial condylar fractures. *J Bone Joint Surg* 55-A:1331–1350, 1973.
Schatzker J, McBroom R, Bruce D: The tibial plateau fracture. The Toronto experience 1968–1975. *Clin Orthop* 138:94–104, 1979.

Injuries of the Extensor Mechanism
Levy M, Goldstein J, Rosner M: A method of repair for quadriceps tendon or patellar ligament (tendon) ruptures without cast immobilization. *Clin Orthop* 218:297–301, 1987.

Patellar Fractures
Levack B, Flannagan JP, Hobbs S: Results of surgical treatment of patellar fractures. *J Bone Joint Surg* 67B:416–419, 1985.
Perry CR, McCarthy JA, Kain CC, Pearson RL: Patellar fixation protected with a load-sharing cable: A mechanical and clinical study. *J Orthop Trauma* 2:234–240, 1988.

Dislocations of the Knee

Frassica FS, Franklin HS, Staeheli JW, Pairolero PC: Dislocation of the knee. *Clin Orthop* 263:200–205, 1992.

Green NE, Allen BL: Vascular injuries associated with dislocation of the knee. *J Bone Joint Surg* 59A:236–239, 1977.

Krackow KA, Thomas SC, Jones LC: Ligament–tendon fixation: Analysis of a new stitch and comparison with standard techniques. *Orthopaedics* 11:909–917, 1988.

Marshall JL, Warren RF, Wickiewicz TL, Reider B: The anterior cruciate ligament: A technique of repair and reconstruction. *Clin Orthop* 143:97–106, 1979.

Schenck RC, Burke RL: The dislocated knee. *Perspect Orthop Surg* 2(2):119–34, 1991.

Schenck RC, Burke R, Walker D: The dislocated knee: A new classification system. *South Med* 85(9):3S–61S, 1992.

21 | Fractures of the Tibial Shaft

C.M. Court-Brown

This chapter reviews fractures of the tibial and fibular diaphysis.

HISTORY

Fractures of the tibial shaft are common wartime injuries; thus, management of these injuries has concerned surgeons for centuries. Until recently, the prognosis for open tibial fractures was very poor, and amputation rates and mortality were high. The first major advance in the management of tibial fractures was the introduction of Plaster of Paris casts in 1800 or so. This permitted ambulant fracture treatment. Cast treatment was modified in the 20th century to allow knee and ankle motion, but brace management of tibial fractures was popularized by Sarmiento in the 1960s.

Operative management of tibial shaft fractures was first used in the second half of the 19th century, with external fixators and bone plates being introduced. Intramedullary tibial nailing started in the 1940s, and locking intramedullary nails were introduced in the 1970s. The management of open fractures has always presented surgeons with a challenge. Until the introduction of asepsis and effective anesthesia, management methods of tibial shaft fractures were crude. The advent of antibiotics, the first of which were the sulphonamides, also improved results by lowering both morbidity and mortality. However, adequate management of open tibial fractures was not really feasible until the 1970s, when coverage with free and local soft tissue transfers was introduced. The cooperation between orthopedic surgeons and plastic surgeons has been a major factor responsible for the improvement in the management of these difficult injuries.

ANATOMY

The proximal and distal 5 cm of the tibia are metaphyseal. The diaphysis of the tibia is triangular in cross-section, having medial, lateral, and posterior surfaces separated by anterior, medial, and lateral borders. The anterior border is sharp proximally, but distally it becomes blunt and runs into the medial malleolus. The medial border is blunt proximally but sharpens distally as it runs into the posterior border of the medial malleolus. The lateral border of the tibia is also blunt proximally, but it sharpens as it runs distally into the lateral side of the inferior tibial metaphysis. The medial surface of the tibial diaphysis is subcutaneous, accounting for the high incidence of open tibial fractures. The lateral surface is hollowed proximally for the tibialis anterior muscle. The posterior surface is bounded by the medial and lateral borders and is crossed proximally by the soleal line. This ridge gives rise to the soleus muscle.

The shaft of the fibula is long and slender and has anterior, posterior, and lateral surfaces separated by anterior, posterior, and medial borders. It has a slight spiral twist.

A major function of the tibia is to anchor the musculature that controls the movement of the ankle and foot. There are four myofascial compartments in the leg. These compartments are of considerable importance in tibial diaphyseal fractures.

The anterior compartment is bounded by the lateral border of the tibia, the interosseous membrane, the anterior fibula, and the deep fascia. It contains four muscles: tibialis anterior, extensor hallucis longus, extensor digitorum longus, and peroneus tertius. The muscles are supplied by the deep peroneal nerve and the anterior tibial artery that runs through the anterior compartment and continues below the ankle joint as the dorsalis pedis artery.

The lateral compartment is contained by the lateral border of the fibula, the deep fascia, and fascial connections between the fibula and deep fascia. It contains the peroneus longus and brevis muscles, which are supplied by the superficial peroneal nerve.

There are two posterior compartments: deep and superficial. The deep posterior compartment, in addition to the anterior compartment, is most often involved in compartment syndrome. It is bounded by the posterior surface of the tibia, the medial and posterior borders of the fibula, the interosseous membrane, and the fascia, which separates it from the superficial posterior compartment. It contains four muscles: popliteus, flexor hallucis longus, tibialis posterior, and flexor digitorum longus. All these muscles are supplied by the posterior tibial nerve and the main neurovascular bundle containing the posterior tibial nerve and artery that runs through the compartment.

The superficial posterior compartment is bounded by fascia and contains gastrocnemius and soleus muscles in addition to the plantaris muscle. These are supplied by branches from the posterior tibial nerve.

The sural and saphenous nerves run between the skin and deep fascia.

Classification

Tibia fractures are classified according to the mechanism of injury, location, fracture configuration, and whether the fracture is open.

The **three mechanisms of injury** are excessive loading, pathologic fractures, and stress fractures. When considering the mechanism of injury, it is vital to distinguish between low- and high-energy injuries. The ultimate prognosis of tibial fractures is governed by the extent of associated soft-tissue injury, which is much greater in motor-vehicle accidents and gunshot injuries than it is in minor falls or sports-related injuries. The worst prognosis is seen in tibial fractures caused by prolonged crushing because this destroys the soft tissue vasculature and frequently leads to muscle death. The most common mechanism of injury is **excessive loading of normal bone.** The force, or applied load, may be indirect (i.e., torsional), causing a spiral fracture in the weakest part of the diaphysis at the junction of the middle and distal thirds of the bone. Fracture may be due to a direct force such as a direct blow. These injuries usually involve a bending or shearing component and are usually higher energy than the torsional injuries.

Occasionally, the fracture is **pathologic** in that it occurs in abnormal bone as a result of a relatively minor force. The most common cause for a pathologic fracture is senile osteoporosis. The tibia may also be affected by metabolic bone diseases, such as Paget's disease or osteomalacia, or it may be the site of metastatic deposits from carcinomata or multiple myeloma.

Stress fractures of the tibial diaphysis are due to repeated submaximal loading of normal bone, usually in young people. In military recruits, the majority of stress fractures occur in the upper third. With athletes, the involvement is lower in the tibia, most frequently at the junction of the middle and lower thirds. In ballet dancers, most stress fractures are found in the middle third of the tibia. Stress fractures of the fibula are prone to occur just above the ankle in runners.

Location of the fracture is described as being in the proximal, middle, or distal third. Fracture **configuration** is described as transverse, oblique, or spiral. In addition, there may be a loose fragment that does not involve the complete cortex, which is commonly referred to as a *butterfly fragment.* When the cortical fragmentation is circumferential, the fracture is referred to as comminuted. Segmental fractures have two separate fractures with an intervening intact cortical tube. Other factors used to determine the overall prognosis are the degree to initial displacement and the presence or absence of a segmental fibular fracture.

The classification of **open fractures** is presented in "Clinical Evaluation/Initial Management of Patients with Multiple Injuries" (Chap. 1). It has prognostic value in terms of the time to union and the patient's return to function. The type III subtypes are particularly important.

Diagnosis and Initial Management

History and Physical Examination

There is a history of trauma, and the patient complains of pain. There may be obvious deformity. The skin is examined for open wounds, and distal pulses and sensation are documented.

Radiographic Examination

Anteroposterior and lateral radiographs are diagnostic of fractures from excessive loading and pathologic fractures. Occasionally, oblique x-rays may be useful in visualizing the periosteal reaction associated with an occult stress fracture. Radiographs of the knee and ankle are examined to identify associated fractures. If a stress fracture is suspected, a technetium bone scan may be diagnostic.

Initial Management

Initial management is reduction of displaced fractures, application of a toe-to-groin splint, elevation, and application of ice. Reduction is accomplished by traction and manipulation while intravenous analgesia is administered (hematoma blocks are not used for tibial fractures).

Associated Injuries

Associated injuries include **compartment syndrome** and injuries of the knee and ankle. The term *compartment syndrome* is used to describe the collection of signs that occur when intracompartmental pressure rises beyond a critical point. The cardinal signs of compartment syndrome are pain, pain with passive stretch of muscles, tense compartments, and elevated pressures. The pathophysiology and diagnosis of compartment syndrome are described in detail in Chapter 1. Failure to diagnose a compartment syndrome has catastrophic consequences. Muscle necrosis leads to significant soft tissue resection or even amputation. Undetected deep posterior compartment syndromes lead to clawing of the foot and toes. A delay in undertaking a fasciotomy for compartment syndromes in adults after tibial fracture results in a high incidence of nonunion. Once a diagnosis of compartment syndrome is made, the treatment is fasciotomy. This is a straightforward procedure and is best carried out through two incisions: one medial and one lateral. The medial incision allows for decompression of the superficial and deep posterior compartments, and the lateral incision permits decompression of the anterior and lateral compartments.

Injuries of the knee and ankle are ruled out by physical examination and radiographs.

Definitive Management

There are five methods used to manage tibial fractures: casts or braces, plating, intramedullary nailing, external fixation, and amputation.

The advantage of **cast management** is the low incidence of infection; however, there is a high incidence of joint stiffness, malunion, nonunion, and muscle wasting. The method is very labor intensive and relies on frequent outpatient visits for radiographic monitoring of fracture position and cast or brace adjustment.

The incidence of malunion and joint stiffness is much less with **plating** than with casts or braces. The infection rate associated with plating of closed fractures is about 4%, but it rises when plating is used for more severe open fractures. Failure of fixation is more commonly seen with plating than with other fixation techniques.

The advantage of **closed intramedullary nailing** is that the fracture site remains closed (Fig. 21-1). The absence of a cast allows for early joint movement and increases patient mobility. Muscle tone is also preserved. The union rate is high, and nonunion can often be treated by repeating the nailing procedure, a process known as *exchange nailing*. The disadvantage of intramedullary nailing is knee pain secondary to the infrapatellar incision and prominence of the underlying nail. This occurs in up to 60% of patients. Infection rate in closed fractures is higher than the rate after cast management or external fixation but lower than the rate with plating.

Surgeons use both unreamed nails and reamed nails. Reamed nails require the intramedullary canal to be shaped into a tube to admit a larger nail, which is achieved with flexible reamers. There are theoretical concerns about damage to the intramedullary vasculature with reaming, but clinical evidence suggests the reaming is advantageous in most tibial

FIG. 21-1   Management with a statically locked nail.

fractures. The major breakthrough in intramedullary nailing was the introduction of locking with proximal and distal screws, which traverse both nail and bone cortices. This simple modification of the original intramedullary nail controls bone length, rotation, and angulation of even severely comminuted fractures.

The primary indication for **external fixation** is severe soft tissue injury. The disadvantages of external fixation are the high incidence of nonunion and pin tract infections and restriction of soft tissue access (Fig. 21-2). The types of external fixation devices are described in Chapter 2.

There is a high incidence of eventual **amputation** after type IIIC open fractures, with a lower but significant incidence after type IIIB open fractures. Other than the severity of the soft tissue injury, indications for amputation include damage of the posterior tibial nerve, multiple trauma, and elderly patients with preexisting diseases such as arteriosclerosis or diabetes. When amputation is considered, the decision is made by two experienced orthopedic traumatologists and the am-

FIG. 21-2   Management with an external fixator.

putation is carried out early in the patient's treatment to minimize medical, psychological, and social problems.

Choice of Method of Management

The choice of method of management is based on the type of patient and the type of fracture.

Casts or braces are used for **low-energy fractures** in young people, which only require about 3 months of immobilization. Under these conditions, joint stiffness is reduced to a minimum.

Other fractures are best managed with fixation. Intramedullary nailing provides the best results for fractures of the **middle and distal thirds** of the tibial diaphysis. Fractures of the **proximal third** of the diaphysis are technically difficult to nail. These usually are high-energy injuries and frequently are comminuted. Nailing does not adequately control this type of fracture, and closed external fixation using a unilateral or multiplanar frame or plating provides better fixation. Similarly, some distal metaphyseal fractures are difficult to nail, particularly if the fracture is oblique or spiral. These are to be managed with closed external fixation or plating. In the 5% of patients who present with a fracture of the tibia having a proximal or distal intraarticular fracture in addition to a diaphyseal fracture, fixation of both fractures is undertaken regardless of what the surgeon might choose to do for the equivalent isolated fractures. These are high-velocity injuries frequently associated with significant soft tissue damage, and fixation permits improved postoperative rehabilitation. The surgeon must select treatment methods appropriate for both fractures. The use of a proximal plate to stabilize a plateau fracture frequently renders nailing impossible, and closed external fixation is preferred for middle and distal third diaphyseal fractures. Plating is a good method of stabilizing a proximal diaphyseal fracture associated with a tibial plateau fracture. If there is an associated ankle fracture, it is managed in the conventional manner by using plates and screws, with a nail used to stabilize the diaphysis. In recent years, surgeons have begun to make more use of external fixation to stabilize proximal and distal tibial fractures.

The most important part of the management of **open fractures** is the surgery of the soft tissues. A thorough debridement is performed as soon as possible. All devitalized and dubiously vital tissue is removed. This includes skin and muscle as well as bone fragments. The skin wound is never closed, primarily because closing inevitably causes tension and may lead to infection. Rather, the soft tissue defect is closed with a delayed primary closure, split thickness skin graft, or flap. Stabilization of open fractures is with either external fixation or intramedullary nailing using either a reamed or unreamed nail.

Stress fractures are managed with a cast or brace. There is rarely any indication for internal fixation because these fractures are not associated with significant soft tissue damage and usually heal in a relatively short time.

Ideally, it is better to treat metastatic deposits in the tibia before the **pathologic fracture** occurs. The method of management depends on the overall prognosis of the patient. Unless the prognosis is very poor, the fracture should be stabilized. Because some of the bone will have been replaced by neoplastic tissue, these fractures are often unstable. Intramedullary nailing with filling of the bone defect with polymethylmethacrylate (PMMA) provides the best method of stabilization. The use of locked intramedullary nails has decreased the need for PMMA.

Complications

Complications of tibial diaphyseal fractures are infection, delayed union and nonunion, and malunion.

Infection following open tibial fractures is usually caused by severe soft tissue trauma and inadequate debridement. The most common pathogenic organism is *Staphylococcus aureus*. Posttraumatic osteomyelitis is difficult to treat if it has been present for a prolonged period. Management is relatively straightforward if the condition is detected early and treated adequately. Management involves stabilization of the fracture, drainage of abscess cavities, resection of devitalized and infected tissues, and antibiotic administration. Bone and soft tissue defects created by debridement are managed afterward with flap coverage and corticocancellous bone grafting, vascularized bone transfer, or bone transport techniques.

Delayed union is overdiagnosed. In the past, surgeons have failed to classify tibial fractures adequately in grouping all tibial fractures together and expecting them to heal in a similar time. In contrast, **nonunion** is a definite entity indicating failure to heal. There are two forms of nonunion: hypertrophic and atrophic. In hypertrophic nonunion, there are clear radiologic signs of an attempt to heal the fracture, and it is likely that the nonunion has occurred for mechanical reasons. Conversely, atrophic nonunions show no evidence of fracture union radiographically and occur because of impaired vascularity at the fracture site. These are common after severe open fractures.

The management of hypertrophic nonunion is to alter the biomechanical environment of the fracture. If the nonunion has followed cast or brace treatment, then the application of a plate, external fixator, or an intramedullary nail will stimulate union. If the hypertrophic nonunion has followed the use of a plate or external fixation device, then closed intramedullary nailing is the treatment of choice if the nonunion is well aligned.

Atrophic nonunions are managed with autogenous cancellous bone grafting. Should the nonunion persist, the surgeon will have to consider vascularized bone grafts or bone transport.

There is no definition of what constitutes **malunion;** however, 5° of angulation or rotational abnormality and 1 cm of shortening provide a reasonable working definition. If a patient presents with a malunion, care must be exercised in determining whether further surgery is worthwhile. Experience suggests that, if the patient presents with ankle osteoarthritis in conjunction with a tibial malunion, correction of the malunion may not lessen the degree of discomfort in the ankle joint, although it may slow down the deterioration of the joint. Management is corrective osteotomy and stabilization with any of the previously described methods.

FRACTURES OF THE FIBULAR SHAFT

Isolated fractures of the fibular diaphysis are usually the result of a direct blow and frequently occur during sporting activities. The most important diagnostic point relating to fractures of the diaphysis of the fibula is that the surgeon should exclude an associated ankle fracture. In suprasyndesmotic ankle fractures, the fibular fracture occurs in the diaphysis and may even occur as high as the fibular neck in the Maisonneuve fracture. If a fracture of the fibular diaphysis is encountered, it is important to check for the presence of an ankle injury.

If the fibular fracture is unrelated to an ankle injury, management is symptomatic. Usually the patient will manage with a light wrap, but if there is significant discomfort, the application of below-knee walking plaster is helpful.

SELECTED READINGS

Bone LB, Sucato D, Stegemann PM, Rohrbacher BJ: Displaced isolated fractures of the tibial shaft treated with a cast or intramedullary nailing: An outcome analysis of matched pairs of patients. *J Bone Joint Surg* 79A:1336–1341, 1997.

Court-Brown CM, Pennig D (eds): *Tibia and fibula.* Oxford, Butterworth Heinemann, 1997.

Court-Brown CM, Will E, Christie J, McQueen MM: Reamed or unreamed nailing for closed tibial fractures. A prospective study in Tscherne C1 fractures. *J Bone Joint Surg* 78B:580–583, 1996.

Sarmiento A, Gersten LM, Sobol PA, Shankwiler JA, Vangsness CT: Tibial fractures treated with functional braces. *J Bone Joint Surg* 71B:602–609, 1989.

Fractures and Dislocations of the Ankle

Clayton R. Perry

This chapter reviews injuries of the distal tibia, fibula, and talus and their ligaments and joint capsule. These are indirect fractures, direct fractures, and sprains.

ANATOMY

The ankle is a uniaxial joint. Articular surfaces are covered with hyaline cartilage. Range of motion of the talus in relation to the tibia is 10° of dorsiflexion and 20° of plantar flexion. The fibula moves laterally several millimeters and rotates externally as the talus dorsiflexes.

The **talus** consists of a head, body, and neck. The head articulates with the navicular, the body with the tibia (the superior articular surface of the body is called the *trochlea*) and the calcaneus. The neck extends between the body and head. In fractures of the ankle, we are primarily concerned with the relation between the body of the talus and the ankle mortise, composed of the medial malleolus, tibial plafond, and lateral malleolus. The trochlea of the talus is concave when viewed from the front and convex when viewed from the side. It fits perfectly in the ankle mortise, which is reciprocally shaped. In most cases, the body of the talus is wider anteriorly than posteriorly. This difference averages 2.4 mm, although it may be as much as 6 mm. Dorsiflexion of the talus results in the "close pack" position (i.e., there is maximal contact between joint surfaces and maximal ligamentous tension). The greater width between the malleoli required for this position is afforded by the slight external rotation and lateral movement of the fibula. To prevent loss of dorsiflexion, syndesmotic screws are inserted with the talus dorsiflexed.

The **distal tibia** consists of the plafond or weight-bearing surface, the medial malleolus, the anterior and posterior processes, and the lateral surface.

The **plafond** has a convex shape when viewed in the anteroposterior projection. This convexity corresponds to the concavity of the trochlea. A seemingly insignificant medial or lateral shift of the talus markedly decreases the area of contact between the bearing surfaces and increases the pressure per unit area, resulting in destruction of articular cartilage.

The **medial malleolus** is the medial process of the distal tibia and is formed by the anterior and the posterior colliculi, which are separated by the intercollicular groove. The superficial deltoid ligament is attached to the anterior colliculus, and the deep deltoid to the posterior colliculus. Tendons of the posterior tibialis and flexor digitorum longus lay in a sulcus on the posterior surface of the posterior colliculus, thus preventing its displacement when fractured.

The **anterior process** is the anterior edge of the distal tibia, which laterally forms the anterior tibial tubercle or tubercle of Chaput. The **posterior process** is the posterior edge of the distal tibia, which laterally forms the posterior tibial tubercle, often referred to as the *posterior malleolus* or *Volkmann's tubercle.*

The **lateral surface** of the tibia between the anterior and posterior tubercles is concave and articulates with the corresponding convex surface of the distal fibula. Hyalin cartilage extends 1 mm into the tibiofibular joint; the remainder is covered with fibrocartilage.

The medial surface of the **distal fibula** is covered with hyaline cartilage and articulates with the lateral side of the talar body. The anterior tubercle, or tubercle of LeFort, and the posterior tubercle are the insertion points of the anterior and posterior tibiofibular ligaments, respectively. The posterior surface of the distal fibula has a sulcus for the peroneal tendons.

The three ligament complexes that stabilize the ankle are the **deltoid, syndesmotic, and lateral–collateral** (Figs. 22-1 and 22-2). These may be disrupted in the substance of the ligament or avulsed with a fragment of bone from either insertion. A *sprain* is an injury of a ligamentous complex and is a grade I-rupture of intraligamentous fibers without damage to surrounding tissues and without lengthening of the ligament; grade II-partial rupture of the ligament with enough intraligamentous fibers ruptured results in lengthening of the ligament and damage of surrounding soft tissue; and grade III rupture, or avulsion of the ligament, results in significant damage of surrounding soft tissue.

The **deltoid ligament** consists of superficial (attaching to the anterior colliculus) and deep (attaching to the posterior colliculus) parts and runs between the medial malleolus and the talus, os calcis, and navicular. It resists external rotation and lateral displacement of the talus.

The **syndesmosis complex** consists of the interosseous membrane, anterior tibiofibular ligament, posterior tibiofibular ligament, inferior transverse ligament, and interosseous ligament. Anterior and posterior ligaments are attached to the corresponding tubercles of the tibia and the fibula. The inferior transverse ligament reinforces the posterior tibiofibular ligament. The interosseous ligament is a strong and short band located at the distal extent of the interosseous membrane. In addition, the interosseous membrane extends from just above the interosseous ligament through the entire length of the tibia and fibula.

Collateral ankle ligaments run from the fibula to the talus and calcaneus. They resist medial tilt (adduction) and anterior or posterior displacement of the talus. There are three ligaments: anterior talofibular,

FIG. 22-1   Ligaments of the ankle: (*A*) the deep deltoid, (*B*) the anterior talofibular, (*C*) the anterior tibiofibular, and (*D*) the interosseous membrane and the interosseous ligament.

FIG. 22-2   The lateral–collateral ligaments of the ankle: (*A*) the anterior talofibular, (*B*) the calcaneofibular, and (*C*) the posterior talofibular.

calcaneofibular, and posterior talofibular. The latter two ligaments lay under the peroneal tendons.

INDIRECT ANKLE FRACTURES

Indirect ankle fractures are caused by indirect torsional forces applied to the ankle. These forces result in motion of the talus in relation to the distal tibia and fibula. As these motions become pathologic, ligament complexes are disrupted, and fractures occur, resulting in predictable injury patterns on which the classification system is based. Before describing the classification system, the individual components of these injuries are reviewed.

In the majority of cases, the obliquity of the **fibular fracture** indicates the mechanism of injury, and the location of the fracture in relation to the syndesmosis (above, at, or below the syndesmosis) indicates the severity of the injury. The higher the fibular fracture, the more severe the injury.

The **anterior tibiofibular ligament complex injury** is an avulsion of the tubercle of Chaput, rupture of the ligament itself, or avulsion of the anterior tubercle of the fibula.

The **deltoid ligament complex injury** is a fracture of the medial malleolus, rupture of the deep deltoid ligament complex, or fracture of the anterior and posterior colliculi. Rupture of the deep deltoid ligament results in loss of stability of the ankle. The deltoid ligament complex normally allows only 2 mm of lateral shift of the talus. When the talus is grossly displaced, rupture of the deep deltoid ligament is obvious. When the talar shift is more subtle, the precise amount of the talar shift is determined by stress radiographs. When the medial malleolus has been fractured, the superficial and deep deltoid ligaments remain attached to the fractured fragment. These injuries always result in loss of ankle stability.

Classification

Indirect ankle fractures are classified according to the position of the foot at the time of the injury and the direction of the injuring force (Table 22-1). Thus, two words are used: the first word indicates the position of the foot (supination/pronation), and the second word indicates the direction of the force applied to the foot (adduction/abduction or external/internal rotation). Adduction and abduction occur around the long axis of the talus and result in medial and lateral, respectively, tilts of the talus. Internal and external rotation occur around the long axis of the tibia. Occasionally, injuries that do not fit this "extended Lauge-Hansen" classification occur. These "atypical injuries" are the result of other factors (e.g., ligamentous laxity or osteopenia) overriding the primary determinants.

TABLE 22-1 Extended Lauge-Hansen Classification of Indirect Ankle Fractures

1. Supination–external rotation
   a. Stage 1—anterior tibiofibular complex disruption
   b. Stage 2—fracture of fibula at or above the syndesmosis
   c. Stage 3—posterior tibiofibular complex disruption
   d. Stage 4—deltoid ligament complex disruption
2. Pronation–abduction at syndesmosis
   a. Stage 1—deltoid ligament complex disruption
   b. Stage 2—fracture of fibula at syndesmosis
3. Pronation–abduction above syndesmosis
   a. Stage 1—deltoid ligament complex disruption
   b. Stage 2—anterior and posterior tibiofibular ligament complex disruption
   c. Stage 3—fracture of the fibula above the syndesmosis
4. Pronation–external rotation
   a. Stage 1—deltoid ligament complex disruption
   b. Stage 2—anterior tibiofibular ligament complex disruption
   c. Stage 3—fracture of the fibula above the syndesmosis
   d. Stage 4—posterior tibiofibular ligament disruption
5. Supination–adduction
   a. Stage 1—lateral–collateral ligament complex disruption
   b. Stage 2—vertical fracture of the medial malleolus

Two hints regarding this classification: supination injuries always start on the lateral side and pronation injuries on the medial side. The sequence in which structures are injured follows the direction of the force (e.g., adduction and abduction injuries proceed from lateral to medial or from medial to lateral, respectively).

Supination–external rotation (SE) fractures of the ankle are the most common type of indirect ankle fracture (Figs. 22-3 to 22-5). They are characterized by the typical SE fibular fracture and, in complete injuries, a disrupted deltoid ligament complex. The fibula fracture is oblique and extends from anterior distal to posterior proximal. If the medial malleolus is fractured, it has an oblique pattern. The first stage of the injury is either disruption of the anterior tibiofibular ligament complex or fracture of the fibula below the anterior tibiofibular complex. If the anterior tibiofibular ligament is disrupted, the second stage is fracture of the fibula at or above the syndesmosis. Subsequent stages are the same regardless of where the fibula is fractured. These stages are injury of posterior tibiofibular complex and injury of the deltoid ligament complex. When there is an SE fibular fracture, an intact medial malleolus, and no widening of the medial clear space, an external rotation stress radiograph is mandatory to determine whether the deep deltoid ligament is ruptured.

FIG. 22-3 Supination–external rotation injury.

FIG. 22-4 Anteropostero radiograph of a supination–external rotation injury.

FIG. 22-5   Lateral radiograph of a supination–external rotation injury.

Pronation–abduction (PA) fractures occur at two levels, at and above the syndesmosis, and are frequently complicated by compression of the lateral surface of the tibial plafond. The first stage of injury is rupture of the deltoid complex. The second stage is simultaneous rupture of the anterior and posterior tibiofibular complexes. If the interosseous ligament and membrane are not injured, diastasis does not occur, and the third stage of injury is the characteristic PA fracture of the fibula at the level of the syndesmosis. This fracture is comminuted laterally (Figs. 22-6 to 22-8). Occasionally, the interosseous ligament ruptures, the interosseous membrane also tears, and the fibula fractures 2–3 cm above the syndesmosis. The fracture characteristically has a lateral butterfly.

In atypical PA fractures, the anterior tibiofibular and interosseous complexes are disrupted, with fractures below the syndesmosis.

Pronation–external rotation (PE) fractures are characterized by the typical PE fibular fracture, which is 2–4 cm above the syndesmosis and has a short oblique pattern that runs from the anterior edge of the fibula posteriorly and inferiorly (i.e., opposite an SE fibular fracture). The first stage is rupture of the deltoid ligament or transverse fracture of the medial malleolus. The second stage is rupture of the anterior tibiofibular and interosseous ligament. The final stage of injury is rupture of the posterior tibiofibular ligament (Fig. 22-9). Because the PE lesion starts with injury of the deltoid ligament, there is no need for stress radi-

FIG. 22-6   Pronation–abduction injury at the level of the syndesmosis.

FIG. 22-7   Anteroposterior radiograph of a pronation–abduction injury.

FIG. 22-8   Lateral radiograph of a pronation–abduction injury.

FIG. 22-9   Pronation–external rotation injury of the ankle.

ographs even if the talus is reduced and a fracture of the medial malleolus is not present.

Supination–adduction (SA) fractures are characterized by a vertical fracture of the medial malleolus and disruption of the lateral–collateral ligaments (Fig. 22-10). The first stage is disruption of the lateral–collateral ligament complex, usually an avulsion fracture of the fibula distal to the syndesmosis. The second stage is a vertical fracture of the medial malleolus. The medial corner of the plafond is frequently compressed.

Atypical Indirect Injuries

In addition to the SE, PA, PE, and SA lesions, there are several atypical lesions. Although the same forces are applied to the ankle, the usual patterns of injury do not occur. The reason for this is not clear, although variability in the size and strength of ligament complexes plays a role.

The stages of a **Maisonneuve fracture** are: (1) injury of the anterior tibiofibular and interosseous ligament complexes, (2) injury of the posterior tibiofibular ligament complex of the syndesmosis, (3) rupture or avulsion of the anteromedial joint capsule, (4) PE- or SE-type fracture of the proximal fibula, and (5) injury of the deltoid ligament complex. The significance of this injury is that failure to recognize the diastasis and stabilize the syndesmosis results in loss of reduction, widening of the mortise, and eventual arthritis.

FIG. 22-10   Supination–adduction injury of the ankle.

The mechanism of the **Bosworth fracture,** or posterior dislocation of the fibula behind the tibia, is external rotation on the supinated foot. There are seven stages of injury: (1) injury of the anterior tibiofibular complex, (2) rupture of the posterior tibiofibular complex, (3) rupture or stretching of the anteromedial capsule, (4) partial tear of the interosseous membrane, (5) dislocation of the fibula behind the tibia, (6) an oblique fracture of the fibula (SE-type) at the level of the syndesmosis (if the fracture occurs above the syndesmosis, the proximal fragment of the fibula is too short to reach the tibia and be locked behind it), and (7) injury of the deltoid ligament complex.

Fracture–dislocation of the ankle with translocation of the medial structures into the tibiofibular space is a distinct lesion. The talus, in a PA lesion, displaces the fibula sufficiently laterally to allow for translocation of the medial structures, which include tendons, posterior tibial artery and nerve, into the interosseous space. These structures become trapped, thus resulting in an irreducible fracture–dislocation.

Diagnosis and Initial Management

History and Physical Examination

The history of injury is rarely helpful because the patient seldom can describe the direction of the injuring force. On physical examination, areas of ecchymosis, swelling, and tenderness are examined over the anteromedial and posteromedial joint line and laterally over the entire length of the fibula. The condition of the skin is noted. Frequently, the skin will be badly contused or damaged. Gentle manipulation of the ankle may show gross instability.

Radiographic Examination

The standard radiographic examination consists of anteroposterior, lateral, and mortise views. The mortise view or true anteroposterior view of the ankle is obtained with the foot in 20° of internal rotation. The radiographs are examined with the following six points in mind. (1) Is there a fracture of the medial malleolus, and, if so, what type is it? This information is important for planning a method of fixation. If there is compression of the medial plafond, bone grafting is anticipated. (2) The direction and location of the fibula fracture are noted. The direction is the mirror of the mechanism of injury. The location or level at which the fracture occurs is an approximate indicator of the extent of the injury. Thus, an SE fracture above the syndesmosis indicates, at the very least, rupture of the anterior tibiofibular ligament. If there is a fracture of the medial malleolus, a complete lesion is present, with all syndesmosis ligaments ruptured. (3) Is there a rupture of the deltoid ligament complex? The answer may be obvious if the injury is a pronation lesion. The initial stage of pronation injuries is rupture of the deltoid ligament complex. Therefore, if the medial malleolus is intact in association with a PA or PE fibular fracture, there is no need for stress films to demonstrate widening of the mortise. However, an SE lesion in which the medial malleolus is intact and the mortise appears normal will require a stress radiograph if there is any tenderness over the medial side. (4) When there is an injury of the medial ligament complex, without a fracture of the fibula at the ankle, the entire length of the fibula is radiographed to determine whether there is a high-fibular fracture. (5) Other associated fractures should be recognized, such as those involving the posterior tibial process (Volkmann), anterior tibial tubercle (Chaput), and fibular tubercle (Wagstaffe). (6) The dome of the talus is examined for osteochondral fractures.

External rotation stress radiographs are obtained when there is an indication that the deltoid ligament may be ruptured despite the fact that the mortise is reduced. The foot is gently externally rotated, and a mortise view of the ankle is obtained. The width of the clear space between the lateral tibial plafond and the lateral talus is determined. Likewise, the width of the clear space at the corner where the tibial plafond joins the medial malleolus and the medial corner of the talus is determined. A difference greater than 3 mm between these two measurements indicates a ruptured deltoid ligament (Figs. 22-11 and 22-12).

Tomography, computed tomography (CT), and arthrography are not necessary to evaluate indirect fractures of the ankle.

Initial Management

Subluxations or frank dislocations are reduced by pulling in line with the deformity. The ankle is splinted, elevated, and iced. Excessive swelling, ecchymosis, and blisters usually improve sufficiently with this regimen for surgery in 4–7 days.

Associated Injuries

Associated injuries of neurovascular structures are rare, but they should be ruled out with a careful focused examination of the extremity. Compartment syndrome is occasionally associated with indirect fractures of the ankle; if suspected on the basis of the clinical examination, compartment pressures are measured.

Definitive Management

Definitive management is by surgical or closed methods. The primary indications for surgery are unstable injuries and fractures of the medial malleolus. Surgery is rarely indicated for an isolated fibular fracture without ligamentous injuries.

All injuries involving the medial and lateral sides of the ankle (bimalleolar) are unstable. An undisplaced fracture may be maintained in a

FIG. 22-11   A mortise view of an ankle indicating a fracture of the fibula slightly above the syndesmosis and a medial clear space measuring 3.5 mm. The width of the articular cartilage measures 3 mm laterally.

long leg cast, but the position of the fragments must be carefully monitored. A displaced bimalleolar fracture, even when anatomically reduced, tends to redisplace; therefore, it should be internally fixed.

Displaced fractures of the medial malleolus, which are treated conservatively, frequently do not heal. Therefore, these fractures are reduced and stabilized to minimize the incidence of nonunion. The high incidence of nonunion in conservatively treated fractures is attributed to the periosteum, which is invariably interposed between the fracture fragments, and to inhibition of healing by synovial fluid from the ankle.

Closed Reduction

Closed reduction is performed by reversing the mechanism of injury and the position of the foot (e.g., SE fractures are reduced by internally rotating and pronating the foot). A short leg cast is applied while the reduction is maintained. It is then extended to a long leg cast with 30° of

FIG. 22-12   External rotation stress radiograph of the ankle shown in Fig. 22-9. The increase in the width of the medial clear space indicates that the deltoid ligament has been ruptured and that this is an unstable ankle injury.

knee flexion. Cast immobilization is continued for 6 weeks. The position of the fragments is monitored with frequent radiographs.

Open Reduction

Under tourniquet control, an incision is made laterally over the fibula and extended distally and anteriorly directly over the distal syndesmosis. Exposure of the medial side is through a curved incision centered over the anterior medial corner of the mortise. The anterior skin bridge formed by these two incisions must be at least 6 cm wide. The skin is handled carefully to avoid injuring it further. The dome of the talus is examined, as are the anterior tibiofibular ligament complex and the anterior talofibular ligament. The fracture of the fibula and medial malleolus are reduced and stabilized. We use a one-third tubular plate posterolaterally on the fibula and two partially threaded cancellous screws in the medial malleolus. The presence of a diastasis is determined by distracting the fibula from the tibia after fixation. If a diastasis is present, a syndesmotic screw is inserted. If bone grafting of an impacted medial or lateral plafond is required, cancellous bone is obtained from the ipsilateral distal femur. If ruptured, the anterior tibiofibular ligament complex is repaired before closure. Postoperatively, a short leg cast is applied when the incisions are stable (usually at 2 days), and the cast is maintained for 2 weeks. At 2 weeks, the cast is taken off, the sutures are removed, and a removable cast is applied to facilitate skin care. At 6 weeks, range of motion of the ankle and partial weight bearing are initiated.

Complications

Complications of indirect ankle fractures include arthritis, infection, and nonunion. These complications are more frequent after direct ankle fractures; therefore, their management is covered at the end of the section Direct Ankle Fractures.

DIRECT ANKLE FRACTURES

Direct ankle fractures are usually caused by the talus being driven into the distal tibia, causing a pylon or burst fracture. Occasionally, they are caused by a direct impact (e.g., gunshots or crushing). These injuries are frequently open and associated with injuries of the foot, proximal tibia, and fibula. Fractures caused by direct impact will not be discussed further except to say that the rules to follow in their management are good wound care, reduction of the articular surfaces, maintenance of alignment, and early bone grafting, if necessary.

Classification

There are three types of pylon fractures: type I, the articular surface is not involved or is undisplaced; type II, a portion of the articular surface is displaced, but there is an undisplaced segment of the articular surface; and type III, the entire plafond is involved (Figs. 22-13 and 22-14). The severity of injury parallels these fracture types.

Diagnosis and Initial Management

History and Physical Examination

The diagnosis of pylon fractures is usually obvious. Typically, there is a history of a fall and severe pain localized to the ankle. There may be deformity of the ankle. A careful neurovascular examination is performed, with particular attention paid to the anterior and posterior tibial pulses and capillary refill. The skin is examined for lacerations or blisters.

A

B

C

D

FIG. 22-13 Classification of direct fractures of the ankle: (*A–B*) type I fracture, (*C–D*) type II fracture, and (*E–F*) type III fracture.

FIG. 22-13 *Continued.*

FIG. 22-14 Mortise radiograph of a type II direct fracture of the ankle. Although there is intraarticular involvement, a portion of the articular surface is undisplaced.

Radiographic Examination

The standard anteroposterior, lateral, and mortise views are of most value. Tomograms and CT scans help in determining the extent of articular damage and the degree of comminution.

Initial Management

Initial management consists of aligning the ankle by traction. These injuries are usually unstable and thus easily aligned. The ankle is splinted, elevated, and iced.

Associated Injuries

Lumbar spine fractures are the injuries most frequently associated with pylon fractures due to a fall. They are ruled out with physical examination and radiographs. Neurovascular injuries are ruled out with a careful physical examination.

Definitive Management

Management of pylon fractures must be individualized. Ultimately, the severity of injury and the adequacy of reduction of the articular surfaces will determine the outcome. The extended surgical procedures necessary to reduce and stabilize displaced fractures are fraught with complications; therefore, attenuated soft tissue is a relative contraindication to an extended surgical procedure. Likewise, vascularity and sensation must be assessed. The presence of lymphedema, venous stasis, or peripheral neuropathy are relative contraindications to open reduction. Most importantly, the surgeon must decide if he or she is capable of reducing and stabilizing the fracture. Some fractures are so comminuted, with such extensive destruction of the articular surface, that open reduction and internal fixation is not an option. In these cases, closed management, early fusion, or external fixation should be used to produce a stable painless ankle.

Closed initial management with early fusion is used when the tibial plafond or dome of the talus is irrevocably injured. Initially, the fracture is managed with external immobilization, often with a period in calcaneal traction. When swelling and blisters have subsided, a cast or external fixator with pins in the calcaneus and talus is applied. Tibiotalar fusion with autogenous cancellous bone graft is performed when the condition of the skin permits.

The goal of **open reduction and internal fixation** is anatomic, stable reduction of the joint. Usually, medial and lateral incisions are made. The exact location and length of the incisions are based on the fracture pattern and are tailored to each case. Once the fragments have been identified, the fibula, if fractured, is plated, thus aligning the anterior tubercle of the tibia around which other fragments are reduced and held in place with screws and plates. Bone graft is packed beneath depressed segments. An extended period of elevation after surgery is required to decrease the incidence of postoperative wound problems. The duration of non–weight bearing depends on the severity of the fracture.

Complications

Complications are arthritis, infection, and nonunion.

Arthritis is due to an inadequate reduction of intraarticular fragments, varus or valgus malalignment of the entire articular surface, or damage to the articular cartilage that occurred at the time of the injury. If radiographically there is a joint space and clinically there is only minimal pain with motion, an osteotomy to realign the joint may help. If arthritic changes are advanced or the articular surface is aligned, the only option other than steroid injections and nonsteroidal antiinflammatory drugs is arthrodesis. The techniques that we use are excision of the distal fibula, removal of the remaining articular cartilage from the joint surfaces, autogenous cancellous bone graft to fill gaps, and stabilization with an external fixator. The pins of the external fixator are placed in the tibia proximally and in the talus and calcaneus distally.

Infection, especially of a pylon fracture, is a severe complication and often the precursor of amputation. If the infection is controlled (i.e., the patient is not systemically ill), the hardware is left in place, as long as it is providing stability, until the fracture has healed. Systemic antibiotics are used to control flare-ups of the infection. Once the fracture is healed, the hardware is removed and all necrotic bone is debrided. Frequently, a free flap is required for coverage. Six weeks of systemic antibiotics is administered.

Nonunion of the fibula or medial malleolus, if symptomatic, is treated with autogenous bone grafting and stabilization.

INJURIES OF THE LATERAL–COLLATERAL LIGAMENT COMPLEX

There are several facts concerning ankle sprains. (1) Rupture of the anterior talofibular ligament is usually an isolated injury. (2) Simultaneous rupture of all three collateral ligaments is very rare, the posterior talofibular ligament being the least vulnerable. (3) Rupture of the anterior talofibular ligament is usually a complete, or grade III, injury. This is not the case with the calcaneofibular ligament injury, which is frequently grade II. (4) Frequently, there are associated injuries of the anterior tibiofibular ligament.

Classification

Injuries of the lateral–collateral ligament complex of the ankle are classified into three groups. First degree: complete rupture of the anterior talofibular ligament only; the mechanism of injury is internal rotation of the pronated ankle. Second degree: complete rupture of the anterior talofibular and calcaneofibular ligaments but an intact posterior talofibular ligament; the mechanism of injury is internal rotation of the supinated foot. Third degree: all three lateral–collateral ligaments of the ankle are ruptured; the mechanism of injury is adduction of the supinated ankle.

Two patterns of medial malleolar fracture are associated with lateral–collateral ligament injuries: a vertical SA pattern and a supination–internal (SI) rotation fracture. This is a transverse or slightly oblique fracture of the medial malleolus and indicates a second-degree sprain.

Diagnosis and Initial Management

History and Physical Examination

The clinical evaluation is most important because radiographs frequently are of little help. Specifically, tenderness directly over the anterior tibiofibular ligament complex or over any of the three lateral–collateral ligaments is noted. In addition, stability of the talus in the coronal plane (adduction) and sagittal plane (anterior drawer) is assessed.

Radiographic Examination

Plain films are usually of little value and indicate only soft tissue swelling. An SA or SI medial malleolar fracture may be present on the mortise view.

Stress films are valuable. Stability in the coronal plane is assessed by adducting the midfoot while a mortise view is obtained. This view is compared with a stress film of the uninjured side. Varus tilt of the talus, which is 10° greater than that of the uninjured side, indicates a third-degree sprain. Stability in the sagittal plane is assessed with a lateral film of the ankle being taken while an anterior drawer test is performed. To perform the anterior drawer test, the heel is held in one hand while the other hand pushes the tibia posteriorly. Displacement anteriorly of greater than 3 mm when compared with the normal side indicates at least a first-degree sprain.

Initial Management

There is no dislocation or deformity to reduce; therefore, ice and elevation are adequate.

Definitive Management

A short leg walking cast is applied, with the ankle in neutral position. The cast is maintained for 4 weeks. A removable ankle splint is worn an additional 2 weeks.

If primary repair of the ligaments is indicated, the operative exposure is through an incision that parallels the peroneal tendons. The peroneal sheath is opened, and the tendons are retracted proximally to reach the posterior talofibular and calcaneofibular ligaments. The anterior talofibular ligament is the easiest to expose and repair. Postoperatively, the ankle is protected with a short leg cast for 4 weeks and a removable cast for 2 weeks.

Complications

The complication unique to this injury is laxity of the lateral–collateral ligament complex, resulting in "giving out" when a varus force is applied to the foot (e.g., when the patient walks on uneven ground). Management is conservative, with a lateral shoe wedge and peroneal strengthening exercises, or operative. Numerous operative techniques have been described. Most use the tendon of the peroneus brevis to replace the injured ligaments.

SELECTED READINGS

General

Vrahas M, Fu F, Veenis B. Intraarticular contact stresses with simulated ankle malunions. *J Orthop Trauma* 8:159–166, 1994.

Indirect Ankle Fractures

Ashhurst AP, Bromer RS: Classification and mechanism of fractures of the leg bones involving the ankle. *Arch Surg* 4:51–129, 1922.

Lauge-Hansen N: Fractures of the ankle. Combined experimental–surgical and experimental–roentgenologic investigations. *Arch Surg* 60:957–985, 1950.

Pankovich AM: Fracture of the fibula proximal to the distal tibiofibular syndesmosis. *J Bone Joint Surg* 60A:221–229, 1978.

Pankovich AM: Fractures of the fibula at the distal tibiofibular syndesmosis. *Clin Orthop* 143:138–147, 1979.

Phillips WA, Schwartz HS, Keller CS, Woodward HR, Rudd WS, Spiegel PG, Laros GS: A prospective, randomized study of the management of severe ankle fracture. *J Bone Joint Surg* 67A:67–78, 1985.

Direct Ankle Fractures

Ovadia DN, Beals RK: Fractures of the tibial plafond. *J Bone Joint Surg* 68A:543–551, 1986.

Ruedi TP, Allgower M: The operative treatment of intraarticular fractures of the lower end of the tibia. *Clin Orthop* 138:105–110, 1979.

Scheck M: Treatment of comminuted distal tibial fractures by combined dual-pin fixation and limited open reduction. *J Bone Joint Surg* 47A:1537–1553, 1965.

Tornetta P, Weiner L, Bergman M, Wtnik N, Steuer J, Kelley M, Yang E. Pilon fractures: treatment with combined internal and external fixation. *J Orthop Trauma* 7:489–496, 1993.

Injuries of the Lateral–Collateral Ligament Complex

Staples OS: Ruptures of the fibular collateral ligaments of the ankle. Result study of immediate surgical treatment. *J Bone Joint Surg* 57A:101–107, 1975.

Kitaoka HB, Lee MD, Morrey BF, Cass JR: Acute repair and delayed reconstruction for lateral ankle instability: twenty year follow-up study. *J Orthop Trauma* 11:530–535, 1997.

23 | Foot Injuries

Enes Kanlic   Clayton R. Perry

This chapter reviews injuries of the foot (i.e., distal to the ankle joint).

ANATOMY AND BIOMECHANICS

The foot is divided into the hindfoot, consisting of the Achilles tendon, talus, and calcaneus; the midfoot, consisting of the tarsal navicular, three cuneiforms, and cuboid; and the forefoot, consisting of the five metatarsals and corresponding phalanges.

The **talus** is unique in that no muscles insert on it, 60% of its surface is covered with articular cartilage, and its vascular supply is tenuous. Deltoid branches from the posterior tibial artery supply the medial talar body. The artery of the sinus tarsi is located in the sinus tarsi, plantar to the neck of the talus, and it gives off branches that enter the inferior neck. The dorsalis pedis gives off arterial branches that enter the superior neck. Most of the blood supply of the talus is through the talar neck; therefore, the body is susceptible to avascular necrosis following fracture.

The posterior portion of the **calcaneus** is the tuberosity and serves as the **Achilles tendon** insertion. The plantar fascia and the small muscles of the foot originate from the plantar surface of the calcaneus. The anterior process is the origin of the bifurcate ligament, which runs to the cuboid and navicular, stabilizing the midfoot. The superior aspect of the calcaneus has three facets that articulate with the talus. The posterior facet is more important than the middle and anterior. The talocalcaneal ligament runs from the superior surface of the calcaneus to the inferior surface of the talus. It lies in the sinus tarsi and is the primary stabilizer of the talocalcaneal articulation. The sustentaculum tali is on the medial side of the calcaneus. On its superior aspect is the middle facet, and on its inferior surface is the groove for the tendon of the flexor hallucis longus. The distal calcaneus articulates with the cuboid.

The **navicular** articulates with the head of the talus and the first and second cuneiforms. The posterior tibial tendon inserts on the tubercle of the navicular, supporting the medial longitudinal arch.

The bones of the foot form **longitudinal and transverse arches.** The longitudinal arch is higher medially than laterally. The medial segment (talus; navicular; cuneiform; and first, second, and third rays) is the dynamic portion of the foot and flattens during weight-bearing. The lateral segment (calcaneus, cuboid, and fourth and fifth rays) is flatter, more rigid, and contacts the ground first during weight-bearing. The transverse arch is due to the shape of the tarsals and bases of the metatarsals, which are broader on the dorsal than on the plantar aspect, forming a "Roman arch."

The bones of the foot are connected by fibrous structures (e.g., the plantar fascia), intrinsic muscles, and extrinsic muscles. The muscles and the tensioned plantar fascia act as a "tie" at the base of the longitudinal arch, which prevents it from flattening during weight-bearing.

The **subtalar joint** has four articulations: three between the anterior middle and posterior facets of the calcaneus and talus and one between the head of the talus and navicular. These articulations function as one multiaxial joint. Forty degrees of supination and pronation occur through the subtalar joint. The ankle and subtalar joints function together as a universal joint, with 45° of dorsal and plantar flexion.

The **Chopart joint,** or transverse tarsal joint, consists of talonavicular and calcaneocuboid articulations (Fig. 23-1). The amount of motion occurring through the Chopart joint is greater when the calcaneus is pronated. Thus, subtalar fusion is performed with the calcaneus in slight pronation.

The **Lisfranc joint,** or tarsometatarsal joint, is a series of plane joints. The greatest degree of motion occurs through the first metatarsal medial cuneiform articulation. Motion through the remainder of the joint is re-

FIG. 23-1   Chopart's, or transverse tarsal, joint, and a Lisfranc's, or tarsometatarsal, joint.

stricted by dorsal and volar ligaments and the bony architecture (i.e., the second metatarsal is inset between the first and third cuneiforms). The five metatarsal heads are connected with strong interosseous ligaments, but only the lateral four metatarsal bases have strong interosseous ligaments. In place of the interosseous ligament between the first and second metatarsal bases is the Lisfranc ligament, connecting the medial cuneiform and the base of the second metatarsal (Fig. 23-2). Because of this structural anomaly, dislocations of the Lisfranc joint are frequently limited to the lateral side (i.e., second through fifth metatarsals) or the medial side (i.e., first metatarsal).

The **metatarsophalangeal joints** function as hinge joints to tension the plantar aponeurosis.

The **interphalangeal joints** are hinge joints. They actively flex but extend actively only to neutral.

Classification

Injuries of the foot are classified according to the mechanism of injury: indirect, direct, or due to repetitive stress. They are further classified according to which structures are involved. These structures are the hindfoot (i.e., the Achilles tendon, the talus, the subtalar joint, and the calcaneus),

FIG. 23-2 The interosseous ligaments from the second through fifth metatarsals. In place of the ligament between the first and second metatarsal is the Lisfranc ligament, between the second metatarsal and the medial cuneiform.

the midfoot (i.e., navicular, cuneiforms, and the cuboid), and the forefoot (i.e., the tarsometatarsal joint, the metatarsals, and the phalanges).

DISRUPTION OF THE ACHILLES TENDON

Classification

Disruption of the Achilles tendon is due to direct (e.g., a laceration) or indirect (e.g., forced dorsiflexion of the ankle) injury. Direct injuries disrupt any part of the tendon and are open. Indirect injuries, or ruptures, occur at the musculotendinous junction or the insertion on the calcaneus. The younger the patient, the greater the chance that the injury is at the musculotendinous junction.

Diagnosis and Initial Management

History and Physical Examination

Pain is localized to the posterior ankle. Direct injuries have a laceration. Indirect injuries have a palpable defect at the site of injury. Active ankle plantar flexion is absent or weak. The Thompson test determines whether a complete rupture is present. The patient is prone, with the feet extending off the examining table. The calf musculature is compressed by the examiner; if the ankle plantarflexes, the tendon is partly intact. If not, there is complete disruption.

Radiographic Examination

Decrease in soft tissue density indicates the location of the rupture; however, this is a subtle finding. Magnetic resonance imaging (MRI) is useful in equivocal cases.

Initial Management

Initial management of a direct injury is debridement. If the tendon cannot be repaired within 12 h, the skin is closed. Indirect injuries are elevated and iced.

Associated Injuries

There are no injuries associated with an indirect injury of the Achilles tendon. Direct injuries are associated with injuries of surrounding tendons and neurovascular structures. Tendons frequently injured are the posterior tibialis, flexor hallucis longus, and flexor digitorum longus. The presence of tenodesis (i.e., flexion of the metatarsophalangeal and interphalangeal joints) with dorsiflexion of the ankle indicates that the long flexors are intact. The neurovascular structures at risk are the posterior tibial nerve and artery. Intact sensation on the plantar surface of the foot indicates that the posterior tibial nerve is intact. A palpable or Doppler posterior tibial pulse behind the medial malleolus indicates that the artery is intact.

Definitive Management

Definitive management is dependent on the type of disruption and the patient's age.

Direct injuries are managed with primary repair. Indirect injuries are managed with operative repair in young, healthy patients and with casting in older, less healthy patients. In comparison with a direct injury, the repair following an indirect injury is not as secure, and the incidence of complications is greater. The patient is positioned prone. The incision is over and parallel to the tendon. The peritendon is exposed and incised so that it can be repaired later. A Kessler-type suture approximates the ends. In indirect injuries, the ends are longitudinal strips, described as a "mop end," and it is key to place the Kessler suture in healthy tendon. If the disruption is extremely distal, the tendon is secured to the calcaneus by pull-through wires or suture anchors. Other lacerated tendons are repaired (direct injury). A short leg cast is applied, with the ankle plantar flexed 20°. At 3 weeks, the cast is changed, the sutures are removed, and another cast is applied, with the ankle in neutral. At 6 weeks, the cast is removed. If the repair is tenuous, immobilization is longer. A splint is prescribed, which is removed for active range-of-motion exercises and while sleeping. At 8 to 10 weeks, external immobilization is discontinued.

Nonoperative management of indirect injuries starts with application of a long leg cast. The knee is flexed 30° (to relax the gastrocnemius) and ankle plantar flexed 30°. At 4 weeks, a short leg cast is applied, with the ankle plantarflexed 30°. At 8 to 10 weeks, the ankle is positioned in neutral, and at 12 to 14 weeks, a removable splint is prescribed and active range of motion is initiated. Immobilization is discontinued at 16 to 20 weeks.

Complications

Complications of Achilles tendon disruption are failure of the repair and infection. Failure is managed with surgical revision. The plantaris tendon or strips of fascia lata are used to reinforce the repair. Infection is managed with administration of systemic antibiotics and debridement. Free tissue transfer or a split-thickness skin graft may be required for coverage.

FRACTURES OF THE TALUS

The four types of talar fractures are fractures of the neck, body, head, and lateral process.

Fractures of the **neck of the talus** are the most common talar fracture and are classified into four groups (Fig. 23-3). Type I is undisplaced. Type II is displaced with subluxation or dislocation of the talocalcaneal articulation. Type III is displaced with a talocalcaneal and a talotibial dislocation. Type IV is a type III fracture with a dislocation of the head

FIG. 23-3   The four types of talar neck fractures: (*A*) type I, (*B*) type II, (*C*) type III, and (*D*) type IV.

D

FIG. 23-3   *Continued.*

of the talus from the talonavicular joint. The incidence of avascular necrosis, delayed union, and nonunion is directly related to fracture displacement, length of time between injury and reduction, and quality of reduction. With early accurate reduction and stable fixation, the incidence of avascular necrosis and nonunion increases from approximately 10% in type I fractures to nearly 100% in type IV fractures.

Fifteen to twenty percent of talar fractures involve only the **talar body** (Fig. 23-4). Without an associated subtalar dislocation, the incidence of avascular necrosis is 25%. With an associated subtalar dislocation, the incidence of avascular necrosis is approximately 50%.

Fractures of the **head of the talus** comprise 5% to 10% of all talus fractures and frequently represent an injury of the Chopart joint (Fig. 23-5).

FIG. 23-4   Fracture of the talar body.

FIG. 23-5   Impaction fracture of the head of the talus.

Fractures of the **lateral process** are the second most common type of talar fracture (Fig. 23-6). They are caused by hyperextension of the supinated foot and are nondisplaced.

Osteochondral fractures involving the lateral side of the talar dome are usually traumatic in origin; those of the medial side are usually degenerative (Fig. 23-7).

Diagnosis and Initial Management

History and Physical Examination

There is pain distal to the ankle in the midfoot. There is obvious deformity in cases of talocalcaneal dislocation. Open wounds and skin tented over bone, which put the patient at risk for pressure necrosis, are noted. The neurovascular status distal to the injury is assessed.

Radiographic Examination

Anteroposterior, oblique, and lateral radiographs are adequate to evaluate talar neck and body fractures and talocalcaneal dislocation. Lateral process fractures are best seen on the lateral projection. The presence of osteochondral fragments in the talocalcaneal articulation is determined with coronal computed tomography (CT).

FIG. 23-6   Fracture of the lateral process of the talus.

FIG. 23-7   Medial and lateral osteochondral fractures of the dome of the talus.

The earliest signs of avascular necrosis are radiographic. The Hawkin sign is the appearance of a radiolucent line below the subchondral bone of the talar dome. This sign is best seen on a mortise view and appears between 6 and 8 weeks after injury. The Hawkin sign is due to resorption of subchondral bone, and its presence indicates that the talus is not avascular. MRI and radionuclide scans are useful in assessing vascularity.

Initial Management

Fractures without significant displacement and without an associated dislocation are splinted and iced. If there is displacement or a dislocation, time is crucial. The longer the delay to reduction, the higher the incidence of complications such as skin necrosis, nonunion, and avascular necrosis. Closed reduction is attempted in the emergency room. If unsuccessful, open reduction is indicated. Closed reduction of talar neck fractures with subtalar subluxation (type II) is accomplished by gentle plantar flexion of the foot and traction to the heel. Talar neck fractures with dislocation of the talocalcaneal, talocrural, or talonavicular joints are more difficult. Reduction is attempted by flexing the knee (thus relaxing the gastrocnemius) and applying traction through the heel.

Supination or pronation of the heel to increase the deformity as traction is applied frequently results in reduction. When reduction has been accomplished, it is usually stable. The foot and ankle are splinted, with the ankle in neutral, and iced.

Associated Injuries

Fracture of the head of the talus indicates injury to the Chopart joint; therefore, the calcaneocuboid joint is examined. Neurovascular injuries are rare and are ruled out with a careful examination. There are no other injuries specifically associated with fractures of the talus.

Definitive Management

Type I fractures are managed nonoperatively with a nonweight-bearing short leg cast until the fracture heals, usually 6 to 10 weeks. Radiographs obtained weekly for the first 3 weeks determine whether displacement of the fragments has occurred. **Fracture types II, III, and IV** are managed with open reduction and internal fixation (Figs. 23-8 and 23-9). Reduction of the talar neck fracture is not possible unless the subtalar joint is reduced. If closed manipulation does not result in reduction, the subtalar joint is exposed through a lateral incision over the sinus tarsi. Loose bodies and soft tissue that are blocking reduction of the talocalcaneal joint are removed, and the joint is reduced. The talar

FIG. 23-8 Lateral radiograph of the foot and ankle after a type II talar neck fracture. There is an associated supination–adduction-type fracture of the medial malleolus that is not evident on this projection.

FIG. 23-9 After reduction and fixation of the talar neck fracture with three screws. The fracture of the medial malleolus has been stabilized with two screws.

neck fracture is exposed through an incision medial to the extensor hallucis longus. Stabilization of the talar neck fracture is with screws inserted through the talar head and directed proximally. The screws are countersunk to minimize impingement on the navicular. Postoperatively, nonweight-bearing is maintained until the fracture is healed, at least 10 weeks.

Displaced fractures of the talar body are managed with open reduction and fixation. Exposure is through osteotomy of the medial malleolus. The fracture is reduced and stabilized with Kirschner wires, Herbert screws, or conventional screws. The fixation device cannot project above subchondral bone into the ankle joint or arthritis will result. If fixation is tenuous, an external fixator with pins in the tibia and the calcaneus neutralizes stresses across the fracture. Postoperatively, nonweight-bearing is maintained until healing occurs, at least 10 weeks. In most cases, immobilization is not necessary because fixation is stable.

Undisplaced **talar head fractures** are managed in a nonweight-bearing short leg cast for 6 weeks and with an arch support for an additional 3 to 6 months. Displaced fractures are managed with open reduction and fixation with screws or Kirschner wires. Small fragments are excised. An external fixator with pins in the calcaneus and first metatarsal neutralizes stresses across the fracture when fixation is tenuous.

Fractures of the **lateral process** of the talus are almost always undisplaced. They are managed symptomatically with immobilization in a cast for 4 to 6 weeks. If the fracture fails to heal, the fragment is excised.

Undisplaced **osteochondral fractures** of the talar dome are managed with nonweight-bearing in a short leg cast for 3 months. When conservative management fails or if the fragments are displaced, surgery is indicated. Lateral osteochondral fractures are located anteriorly on the talar dome and are exposed through an anterolateral approach. Osteotomy of the medial malleolus is required to expose medial osteochondral fractures. Small fragments are excised. Large fragments are pinned after curettage and drilling of their bed. Postoperatively, nonweight-bearing is maintained until healing is demonstrated radiographically. Alternatively, these injuries can be approached arthroscopically by a surgeon familiar with these techniques.

Complications

Complications of fractures of the talus are avascular necrosis, nonunion, and posttraumatic arthritis.

Avascular necrosis of the body of the talus is the complication unique to fractures and dislocations of the talus. It is most likely to occur following a displaced fracture of the talar neck or body. The diagnosis is based on the absence of the Hawkin sign. Once avascular necrosis has occurred, the goal is to prevent collapse of the talus by an extended period of nonweight-bearing in a patellar tendon bearing orthosis. Revascularization takes up to 36 months, and the orthosis is worn until there is radiographic evidence of revascularization.

The diagnostic sign of **posttraumatic arthritis** of the subtalar joint is pain with pronation and supination of the foot. The patient complains of pain induced by walking over uneven ground. Management is conservative with nonsteroidal antiinflammatory drugs and local injections of steroids. If this fails, the involved joints are arthrodesed. It is important to identify accurately the symptomatic joints to minimize the number of joints that are arthrodesed. The greater the number of joints that are arthrodesed, the more stress across remaining functional joints and the sooner they develop arthritis. Symptomatic joints are identified by injection with local anesthetic and observation of symptom-relief.

Nonunion is a complication of fractures of the talar neck and is associated with avascular necrosis of the body. Management is stabilization with screws and grafting with autogenous cancellous bone.

SUBTALAR DISLOCATION

The term *subtalar dislocation* denotes dislocation of both the talocalcaneal and talonavicular articulations.

Classification

Subtalar dislocations are classified according to the position of the forefoot in relation to the talus and whether there is an associated dislocation of the tibiotalar joint. The types of subtalar dislocation commonly encountered are medial, lateral, and pantalar. Medial dislocation is by far the most common type of dislocation and is caused by forefoot supination. Lateral subtalar dislocation is less common and is the result of forefoot pronation. Lateral dislocations are the result of greater force and have a worse prognosis than medial dislocation. Pantalar dislocations are most frequently a medial subtalar dislocation associated with a tibiotalar dislocation. They have a poor prognosis because of the high incidence of avascular necrosis and associated soft tissue injury. Plantar and rotary dislocations have also been reported but are uncommon.

Diagnosis and Initial Management

History and Physical Examination

The patient has pain localized to the foot. Deformity of the foot is obvious. The foot appears shortened and is in equinus. The head of the talus can be palpated anterior to the medial malleolus (lateral dislocation) or anterior to the lateral malleolus (medial dislocation). Fifteen percent of subtalar dislocations are open. In an even greater percentage of subtalar dislocations, the skin over the talus is injured and later sloughs.

Radiographic Examination

The diagnosis of subtalar dislocation is obvious radiographically. Anteroposterior, lateral, and oblique radiographs of the foot are obtained (Fig. 23-10). Other radiographic views and studies are not necessary to make the diagnosis. After closed reduction, coronal CT of the talocalcaneal joint determines the presence of osteochondral fragments in the joint and the congruity of reduction.

Initial Management

Once subtalar dislocation has been diagnosed, reduction is performed as quickly as possible to minimize the incidence of skin necrosis and avascular necrosis of the talus. The reduction maneuver is axial traction and pronation and supination of the heel. In addition, the head of the talus is relocated with digital pressure. Many subtalar dislocations cannot be reduced by closed means, and repeated forceful attempts at closed reduction are not indicated and jeopardize the viability of the skin over the head of the talus. If reduction is accomplished, a well-padded splint is applied, with the ankle in neutral.

Associated Injuries

Fracture of the neck of the talus and intraarticular osteochondral fractures of the talus and calcaneus are frequently associated with subtalar

FIG. 23-10   Lateral view of a foot after a lateral subtalar dislocation.

dislocation. Talar neck fractures are ruled out by careful assessment of the lateral radiograph of the foot. The presence of intraarticular osteochondral fragments is determined with coronal CT through the talocalcaneal articulation. There are no other injuries specifically associated with subtalar dislocation.

Definitive Management

The goal of management is a congruous reduction. If this is obtained with closed reduction and the skin is viable, a short leg cast is applied. Nonweight-bearing is maintained for 4 weeks. Skin necrosis precludes casting.

In cases in which a closed reduction cannot be accomplished, open reduction is performed. The most common obstacle to reduction of medial dislocations is "buttonholing" of the talar head through soft tissue laterally (i.e., the extensor retinaculum, extensor digitorum brevis, and bifurcate ligament). The most common cause of irreducible lateral dislocation is displacement of the posterior tibial tendon inferior to the neck of the talus. Occasionally, fractures of the head of the talus or interposed osteochondral fragments may block reduction. The surgical exposure for open reduction is through a longitudinal skin incision over the head of the talus. Interposed soft tissue is identified and incised or retracted, and osteochondral fragments are removed. If the posterior tibial tendon is disrupted, it is repaired after reduction. A pin is driven across the talonavicular joint. The foot is immobilized in a short leg cast, and nonweight-bearing is maintained for 6 weeks. Pantalar dislocations frequently must be reduced open. In addition to pinning of the talonavicular joint, the talocrural joint is also pinned. If the injury is open, an external fixator is used in place of a cast.

Complications

The complications of subtalar dislocation are avascular necrosis, subtalar arthritis, and infection secondary to an open injury or skin necrosis. Avascular necrosis and subtalar arthritis are managed as described in the section "Fractures of the Talus."

Infection is a devastating complication, particularly when it is coupled with avascular necrosis of the talus. The basic principles of debridement of necrotic tissue, early soft tissue coverage, stabilization of the foot and ankle, and appropriate antibiotic coverage must be followed. Debridement of necrotic tissue may result in a talectomy if the body of the talus is avascular. Stabilization is with an external fixator with pins in the tibia, metatarsals, and, if possible, calcaneus.

CALCANEUS

Classification

Fractures of the calcaneus are broadly classified as intraarticular or extraarticular. Intraarticular fractures involve the posterior facet. Extraarticular fractures involve the tuberosity, sustentaculum tali, and anterior process. In addition to being fractured, the calcaneus is occasionally dislocated.

Intraarticular fractures of the calcaneus are caused by axial loading of the talus, which is driven into the calcaneus. The talus acts as a wedge, producing the primary fracture. This fracture is in the sagittal plane, starting at the calcaneocuboid articulation and continuing posteriorly and medially through the posterior facet to the medial wall of the calcaneus. The primary fracture divides the calcaneus into an anterior medial half and a posterior lateral half (Fig. 23-11A). If the force of the axial load is not dissipated, the impact of the talus produces a compression fracture of the lateral portion of the posterior facet. There are variations of this basic fracture pattern due to the position of the foot (e.g., supination of the foot medializes the primary fracture; pronation lateralizes it; dorsiflexion results in a joint depression fracture (Fig. 23-11B); and plantar flexion results in a tongue-type fracture (Fig. 23-11C).

Extraarticular fractures of the calcaneus are caused by axial loading or by the avulsion of bony insertions and origins of ligaments and tendons. Isolated fractures of the tuberosity of the calcaneus are caused by direct impact or avulsion of the tendo-Achilles insertion. Fractures due to direct impact are minimally displaced; the plane of the fracture is sagittal (Fig. 23-12A). Avulsion fractures of the tendo-Achilles are displaced; the plane of the fracture is horizontal (Fig. 23-12B). Fractures of

A

B

C

FIG. 23-11 Intraarticular fractures of the calcaneus: (A) the primary fracture viewed from above, (B) joint depression fracture, and (C) tongue-type fracture.

FIG. 23-12   Extraarticular fractures of the calcaneus: (*A*) isolated fracture of the tuberosity caused by direct impact; the calcaneus is viewed from above; (*B*) isolated fracture of the tuberosity caused by an avulsion of the tendo-Achilles; and (*C*) fracture of the anterior process of the calcaneus.

the sustentaculum tali are caused by the medial side of the talus impacting the sustentaculum during axial loading of a supinated foot. Anterior process fractures are an avulsion of the origin of the bifurcate ligament caused by forefoot adduction and inversion (Fig. 23-12C). Dislocations of the calcaneus are extremely rare. There is usually a fracture of the calcaneus or cuboid at the calcaneocuboid articulation.

Diagnosis and Initial Management

History and Physical Examination

There is a history of an impact often caused by a fall or a twisting injury. Pain is localized to the hindfoot. When seen shortly after injury, prior to diffuse swelling, the exact location of the fracture can be determined by gentle palpation. Fracture of the sustentaculum tali is indicated by painful passive motion of the great toe (the flexor hallucis longus runs beneath the sustentaculum). An avulsion fracture of the tendo-Achilles is indicated by weakness of plantar flexion of the ankle. Loss of plantar flexion is not complete because the peroneal and posterior tibial muscles are intact.

Radiographic Examination

The four radiographic projections helpful in the evaluation of calcaneal fractures are the lateral, oblique, axial, and Broden views. The **lateral projection** is the most helpful and is diagnostic of posterior facet depression and tuberosity avulsion. The Bohler angle, or the tuber angle, and the crucial angle of Gissane, which indicate the extent of displacement and angulation, are determined from the lateral projection (Fig. 23-13). The loss of parallelism of the articular surface of the posterior facet of the calcaneus and talus is determined from the lateral projection.

The **oblique projection** is useful to assess the presence of a fracture of the anterior process of the calcaneus and to determine whether there is involvement of the calcaneal cuboid articulation.

The **axial projection,** or Harris or jumper's view, is obtained by placing the foot on the cassette with the ankle dorsiflexed and the beam angled 30° distally. The axial projection is useful in evaluating the tuberosity, the sustentaculum tali, and axial shortening.

The **Broden view** is used to assess the posterior and middle facets. To obtain this view, a lateral radiograph is obtained, with the foot passively dorsiflexed, supinated, and internally rotated. The beam is centered on the sinus tarsi.

Initial Management

Initial management is with a splint, ice, and elevation.

Associated Injuries

Forty percent of calcaneus fractures incurred in a fall is associated with a fracture of the lumbar spine, usually a stable compression fracture. Injury

FIG. 23-13   Lateral radiograph of the foot illustrating Bohler's (solid line) and Gissane's (dotted line) angles.

of the medial and lateral plantar nerves results in decreased sensation on the plantar aspect of the foot. Compartment syndrome is suspected if there is massive swelling and severe pain not relieved by ice, elevation, and customary amounts of analgesics. The diagnosis and management of compartment syndrome is covered in the section "Injuries of the Forefoot."

Definitive Management

Definitive management depends on the type of calcaneus fracture, the amount of displacement or angulation, and the presence of articular incongruity.

Intraarticular fractures of the calcaneus which are not significantly displaced are managed conservatively with nonweight-bearing for 4 weeks. Casting is counterproductive because it leads to stiffness of the subtalar joint.

Management of **displaced intraarticular fractures** is operative. Displacement is defined as loss of articular congruity of the posterior facet or at the calcaneal cuboid joint, loss of parallelism between the posterior facets of the calcaneus and talus, more than 4 mm of shortening of the tuberosity as seen on the axial projection, and a Bohler angle of 10° or less.

The surgical approach is through an extensile lateral incision or separate medial and lateral incisions. Because of flap necrosis, we reserve the extensile lateral approach for severely comminuted displaced fractures in young patients without a history of smoking or diabetes.

Surgery is delayed until swelling has decreased to the point that the skin on the dorsum of the foot wrinkles with ankle dorsiflexion (usually 10 to 14 days). The incision starts over the tendo-Achilles. It extends distally to the plantar skin, where it turns 90° and runs parallel with the plantar aspect of the foot. The incision is carried down to the calcaneus. A flap that includes the periosteum of the calcaneus is raised. The peroneal tendons and their sheath are elevated with the rest of the flap and reflected anteriorly, thereby exposing the entire lateral calcaneus, including the calcaneocuboid articulation and the posterior facet. Fragments are reduced and held in place with plates and screws.

In most cases, we prefer separate medial and lateral approaches. The goals of these surgical approaches are specific. The medial approach exposes the medial side of the calcaneus so that it can be brought out to length and its normal concavity can be restored. The lateral approach is designed to expose the posterior facet so that it can be reduced. These approaches have a low incidence of associated wound problems. The medial approach is through a skin incision that is parallel with the posterior medial border of the tibia. The incision starts proximal to the ankle joint and extends distally to the abductor hallucis brevis. The plantar branch of the posterior tibial nerve must be protected during the exposure. The medial wall of the calcaneus is reduced by disimpacting it with an elevator. The tuberosity fragment is stabilized with a staple or two-hole plate. The lateral approach is through a skin incision centered over the sinus tarsi. It starts at the lateral border of the extensor tendons and runs in a plantar direction posteriorly to the peroneal tendons. The fat in the sinus tarsi is excised, thereby exposing the posterior facet. This incision can be located slightly more anteriorly to expose fractures involving the calcaneocuboid articulation and fractures of the anterior process of the calcaneus. The posterior facet is reduced by elevating and rotating it posteriorly. If only the lateral part of the posterior facet is depressed, it is reduced and held in place with interfragmentary screws (i.e., the screws are inserted from the lateral fragment into the medial half of the facet). If the entire facet is depressed, it is held in its reduced position with Kirschner wires inserted through the fragment into the talus. Postoperatively, if the subtalar joint is not crossed by an implant, early motion is encouraged. Nonweight-bearing is maintained a minimum of 6 weeks. If the subtalar joint has been crossed with Kirschner wires, the extremity is immobilized in a short leg cast until the wires are removed at 6 weeks. At 8 weeks, partial weight-bearing is started and advanced.

Occasionally, tongue fractures can be reduced and stabilized with the Essex–Lopresti method of driving a large pin into the tongue fragment from posterior to anterior. The tongue fragment is then reduced under fluoroscopy by manipulating the pin, and the pin is advanced into the talus, thereby stabilizing the fracture. This technique seldom results in anatomic reduction but is of use when the patient has risk factors such as peripheral vascular disease or fracture blisters.

Isolated fractures of the **tuberosity caused by direct impact** are almost always minimally displaced and are managed with nonweight-bearing for 3 to 6 weeks. In the rare case of a displaced tuberosity fracture, the displaced fragment is on the medial side. The fracture is reduced and held in place with screws.

Isolated fractures of the **tuberosity caused by avulsion** of the tendo-Achilles are usually displaced. They are exposed through a medial approach, reduced, and stabilized with a large cancellous screw and washer. Postoperatively, if the fixation is adequate, immobilization is not required; however, nonweight-bearing is maintained for 4 to 6 weeks. In the rare case in which there is minimal displacement, an acceptable alternative form of management is a long leg cast, with the ankle plantar flexed 30° and the knee flexed 30°. At 3 to 4 weeks, the cast is changed to a short leg cast, with the ankle in neutral. Immobilization is continued a total of 6 weeks. Throughout this period, the fracture is followed radiographically. Displacement is an indication for open reduction and stabilization.

Fractures of the **sustentaculum tali** are managed in a short leg weight-bearing cast for 4 to 6 weeks.

Undisplaced fractures of the **anterior process** are managed in a short leg weight-bearing cast for 4 to 6 weeks. Displaced fractures are managed with open reduction and fixation. Excision of the fragment is not indicated as it is the origin of the bifurcate ligament. The fragment is small and fixation is not stable; therefore, the foot is maintained in neutral for 3 to 4 weeks with a short leg cast.

Dislocations of the calcaneus are managed in the same fashion as subtalar dislocations. An emergent closed reduction is performed. If closed reduction cannot be achieved, an open reduction is performed. After closed reduction, it is important to assess the talocalcaneal articulation for loose bodies; if present, these are removed. The reduction is usually stable and fixation not necessary. A short leg cast is maintained for 6 to 8 weeks.

Complications

Complications of fractures of the calcaneus are malunion, resulting in a widened heel and plantar fasciitis, subtalar arthritis, calcaneocuboid arthritis, and peroneal tendonitis.

A **widened heel and plantar fasciitis** are managed conservatively. Footwear is altered, and a heel cup may be necessary. Injections of local anesthetic and steroids may relieve symptoms for extended periods. Rarely, excision of a spike of bone is indicated.

Subtalar and calcaneocuboid arthritis are managed conservatively with nonsteroidal antiinflammatory drugs and local injections. Arthrodesis is a last resort.

Peroneal tendonitis is caused by impingement of the peroneal sheath. Local injections of anesthetic and steroids may help. The sheath must be explored and decompressed frequently.

INJURIES OF THE MIDFOOT

Injuries of the midfoot include fractures and dislocations of the navicular, cuneiform, and cuboid bones, and dislocations of the Chopart joint.

Classification

There are three types of fractures of the tarsal **navicular:** dorsal chip fractures, fractures of the tuberosity, and fractures of the body of the navicular. Dorsal chip fractures, the most common type of navicular fracture, are a capsular avulsion and are caused by plantar flexion and pronation of the foot. Fractures of the tuberosity are an avulsion of the posterior tibial tendon and occur during eversion of the foot. Fractures of the body of the navicular are the least common type of fracture of the navicular and are caused by forceful hyperextension and inversion.

Fractures of the **cuneiforms** are rare and are usually caused by direct trauma. Subluxation of the first cuneiform from its articulations with the navicular and the second cuneiform frequently occurs as part of a Lisfranc dislocation.

Fracture of the **cuboid** is due to direct trauma, capsular avulsion during inversion or eversion of the forefoot, or compression during abduction of the forefoot.

Chopart dislocation is a rare injury. There are three types: medial, lateral, and plantar. The mechanism of injury is, respectively, inversion, eversion, and plantar flexion of the forefoot. The bifurcate ligament ruptures and the talocalcaneal ligament remains intact; therefore, the talocalcaneal joint does not dislocate.

Diagnosis and Initial Management

History and Physical Examination

There is a history of either twisting or direct trauma to the midfoot and pain localized to the midfoot.

Radiographic Examination

The radiographic examination starts with anteroposterior, lateral, and oblique views of the foot. Stress views, obtained while inverting, everting, abducting, or adducting the forefoot, demonstrate instability of the Chopart joint. Other studies are seldom indicated.

Fracture of the navicular tuberosity can be confused with the os tibiale externum, an accessory ossicle. Distinguishing features are that the os tibiale externum is frequently bilateral and its edges are rounded.

Initial Management

Initial management consists of splinting, ice, and elevation. Dislocations of the Chopart joint are usually reduced by axial traction and manipulation of the forefoot under hematoma block. If closed reduction is not accomplished, immediate open reduction is indicated. Subluxations of the first cuneiform are usually not significantly displaced. In cases in which the soft tissue is not at risk, these injuries are splinted in situ.

Associated Injuries

There are no specific injuries associated with injuries of the midfoot.

Definitive Management

Dorsal chip fractures of the **navicular** are managed symptomatically with a short leg cast and weight-bearing as tolerated for approximately 4 weeks. Minimally displaced (2 mm or less) fractures of the tuberosity of the navicular are managed with a short leg cast with the forefoot inverted. At 4 weeks, the cast is changed and the foot is positioned in neutral; a short leg cast is applied and maintained an additional 2 weeks. Displaced fractures of the navicular are managed with open reduction and internal fixation. The surgical exposure is through an incision centered over the navicular, parallel to the anterior tibial tendon. The talonavicular joint is exposed and the navicular is reduced under direct vision when the joint is distracted with longitudinal traction. Interfragmentary screws or pins are used for fixation. Postoperatively, a short leg cast is applied. In cases in which the fixation is tenuous, an external fixater with pins in the calcaneus and first metatarsal is used to maintain length.

Fractures of the **cuneiforms** are usually managed with a short leg cast and weight-bearing as tolerated for 6 weeks. Indications for surgery include displacement, which threatens overlying soft tissue or intraarticular displacement that can be improved.

Subluxation of the first cuneiform is managed operatively. The articulations between the first cuneiform and the navicular and second cuneiform are involved. If there are associated fractures, the procedure is performed open, through a dorsal incision. Because the fragments are small, pins are used for fixation. If there are no associated fractures, the joints are reduced closed under fluoroscopy and pinned. It is important to stabilize both articulations. Postoperatively, a short leg cast is applied and nonweight-bearing is maintained for 6 weeks. At 6 weeks, the pins are removed and the patient is allowed to bear weight in a shoe with a stiff sole and an arch support.

Dislocations of the Chopart joint are managed operatively because reduction is unstable. Dislocations without associated fractures are stabilized with a minimum of two pins inserted under fluoroscopy. The first pin crosses the calcaneocuboid joint. The second pin crosses the talonavicular joint. A short leg cast is applied and nonweight-bearing is maintained for 6 weeks. At 6 weeks, the pins are removed and a stiff soled shoe and arch support are worn.

Complications

The complication of midfoot injuries is arthritis. Management is non-steroidal antiinflammatory drugs and alterations in footwear. If necessary, local injections of anesthetic agents and steroids are performed. Arthrodesis of an arthritic joint is a last resort.

INJURIES OF THE FOREFOOT

Injuries of the forefoot are the Lisfranc dislocation, fractures of the metatarsals and phalanges, and dislocations of the metatarsophalangeal joints and interphalangeal joints.

Classification

The mechanism of injury of the **Lisfranc dislocation** is hyperextension (Fig. 23-14). Lisfranc dislocations are classified into one of three groups:

FIG. 23-14 Mechanism of injury of a Lisfranc dislocation. The tarsometatarsal articulation is hyperextended, causing the weaker dorsal ligaments to rupture.

total incongruity, partial incongruity, and divergent (Fig. 23-15). **Total incongruity** is characterized by involvement of the entire joint and displacement in one direction (usually laterally). **Partial incongruity** is characterized by involvement of only part of the joint, usually either the first metatarsal or the second through fifth metatarsals. This break between the first and second metatarsals occurs because there is no stabilizing ligament between their bases, as there is between the bases of the other metatarsals. **Divergent** dislocations are characterized by involvement of the entire joint. Displacement is in two directions (usually the first metatarsal is displaced medially, the second through fifth metatarsals laterally).

Metatarsal fractures are classified as stress fractures or traumatic fractures. Two types of traumatic fractures bear special mention: the Jones fracture and avulsion fractures of the base of the fifth metatarsal. The **Jones fracture** is a transverse fracture of the fifth metatarsal at the junction of the proximal metaphysis and diaphysis (Fig. 23-16) and has characteristics of a stress fracture in that it may initially be incomplete, involving only the lateral cortex of the metatarsal. Jones fractures frequently fail to heal when managed nonoperatively. **Avulsion fractures of the base of the fifth metatarsal** occur when the insertion of the peroneus brevis is avulsed during forced inversion of the forefoot. This fracture is distinguished from the Jones fracture by its metaphyseal location and its tendency to heal when managed with immobilization (Fig. 23-17).

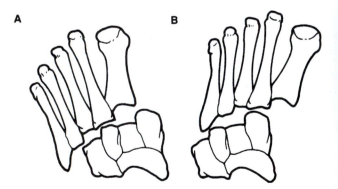

FIG. 23-15   Types of Lisfranc dislocations: (*A*) and (*B*) total incongruity of the Lisfranc joint, (*C*) and (*D*) partial incongruity of the Lisfranc joint, and (*E*) divergent dislocation of the Lisfranc joint.

C

D

E

FIG. 23-15 *Continued.*

Fractures of the **phalanges** are classified as intraarticular, extraarticular, or tuft fractures.

Dislocations of the metatarsal phalangeal and interphalangeal joints are classified according to the direction of displacement, as dorsal or volar.

FIG. 23-16   Jones fracture.

FIG. 23-17   Fracture of the base of the fifth metatarsal.

Diagnosis and Initial Management

History and Physical Examination

The patient complains of pain localized to the structure injured. The dorsum of the forefoot quickly becomes swollen and ecchymotic. Shortening of the forefoot indicates an unreduced Lisfranc dislocation or displaced fractures of all five metatarsals. Apparent hyperflexion or hyperextension of a metatarsophalangeal or interphalangeal joint indicates dislocation.

Radiographic Examination

Anteroposterior, oblique, and lateral radiographs are obtained. A fracture of the base of the second metatarsal indicates that the Lisfranc joint is disrupted. Loss of congruity between articular surfaces and double densities (i.e., one articular surface superimposed on another) indicates subluxation.

Stress radiographs assess the stability of the Lisfranc joint. Bone scans help diagnose stress fractures of the metatarsals prior to their radiographic appearance.

Initial Management

Initial management consists of alignment of severely displaced fractures, reduction of dislocations, immobilization, elevation, and ice.

Dislocations of the Lisfranc joint with an absent dorsalis pedis or posterior tibial pulse or compromised overlying skin are reduced closed emergently. A hematoma block is administered, and axial traction is applied to the involved rays by suspending the foot by the toes with finger traps. Inability to obtain a closed reduction is an indication for immediate open reduction.

Displaced fractures of the metatarsals are rare; when they occur, they are reduced with axial traction. If adequate reduction is achieved, the foot is immobilized in a short leg cast with a toe plate (i.e., the plantar surface of the cast extends distal to the toes). The cast is maintained 4 to 6 weeks. The Jones fracture and fracture of the base of the fifth metatarsal are seldom displaced and are casted. The Jones fracture may eventually require internal fixation. Stress fractures are managed with immobilization and nonweight-bearing.

Fractures of the phalanges are usually caused by direct trauma. Displaced fractures of proximal and middle phalanges are aligned with the aid of a digital block, and the toe is buddy taped to the neighboring toe. Nonweight-bearing is maintained until there is clinical and radiographic healing. Fractures of the distal phalanx are protected with a splint, and associated subungual hematomas are drained to relieve pain. Crushed open distal phalanges are managed with amputation in the operating room. Displaced intraarticular fractures of proximal and distal phalanges of the great toe are splinted and managed subsequently with open reduction and stabilization.

Dislocations of metatarsophalangeal and interphalangeal joints are managed with closed reduction under hematoma block. Simple axial traction and gently increasing of the deformity reduce the dislocation. Occasionally, an interphalangeal dislocation of the great toe is irreducible because of interposition of the long flexor tendon and requires open reduction. Isolated cases of irreducible metatarsophalangeal dislocations have been reported but are extremely rare. When reduction of a metatarsophalangeal or interphalangeal dislocation has been achieved, the toe is immobilized with a dorsal alumafoam splint and buddy taping. Immobilization is continued for 4 to 6 weeks.

Associated Injuries

Compartment syndrome of the foot is associated with forefoot injuries. Increased pain made worse by passive motion is the cardinal sign of compartment syndrome. The diagnosis is confirmed by measuring the compartment pressures and finding a value greater than 30 mmHg. Management is surgical release of the four osteofascial spaces of the foot. All four compartments are surgically released through two dorsal longitudinal incisions. The first is centered over the second interspace, and the second is centered over the fourth metatarsal. The dissection is made around each metatarsal, and the central compartment is opened between the first and second metatarsals.

Definitive Management

The definitive management of **Lisfranc dislocation** is reduction and stabilization with pins or screws. We prefer open reduction because we have been impressed with the amount of displacement and comminution that is routinely present (Figs. 23-18 and 23-19). The surgical exposure is through two longitudinal incisions: the first centered over the first interspace and the second over the third interspace. Only one incision is required for partial incongruity-type dislocations. The dorsalis pedis is at risk in the first interspace. The joint is debrided of free fragments of bone and cartilage, and intraarticular fractures are reduced and held in place with small-diameter Kirschner wires. The joint is reduced and stabilized with large-diameter Kirschner wires. The number and location of the Kirschner wires required to stabilize the reduction is dependent on the type of dislocation. Total incongruity dislocations require a minimum of two Kirschner wires: one in the first ray and the second in the fourth or fifth ray. Divergent dislocations require a minimum of three Kirschner wires: one in the first ray and the second and third wires in the second and fifth rays. Partial incongruity dislocations require a minimum of two Kirschner wires. The location of the wires is dictated by the rays involved. Postoperatively, the foot must be immo-

FIG. 23-18 Anteroposterior radiograph of a foot after a partial incongruity Lisfranc dislocation involving the bases of the second through fifth metatarsals. There are fractures of the second, third, and fifth metatarsal bases.

bilized in a short leg cast, and the patient is not allowed to bear weight until the wires are removed at 6 to 8 weeks. After the wires are removed, a short leg cast is reapplied and the patient is allowed to bear weight as tolerated. The cast is maintained for 2 to 4 weeks. After the cast is removed, the patient wears a stiff-soled shoe with an arch support for 6 months.

The definitive management of **metatarsal** fractures depends on the amount and direction of angulation and displacement. Dorsal or plantar angulation and displacement result in abnormal pressure on the plantar aspect of the foot and must be reduced and stabilized. Lateral displacement is usually not significant unless the first metatarsal is fractured. The closed management of metatarsal fractures is covered under "Initial Management" in this section. Open management consists of surgical exposure of the fracture through dorsal longitudinal incisions, reduction,

FIG. 23-19   Anteroposterior radiograph of the foot shown in Fig. 23-18 after open reduction of the Lisfranc joint and fixation with three Kirschner wires.

and stabilization with Kirschner wires. Small plates and screws are used to stabilize fractures of the first metatarsal. An intramedullary screw inserted from proximal to distal is used to stabilize the Jones fracture. Postoperative management is based on stability of fixation and quality of reduction and is tailored to the individual case.

Intraarticular fractures of the proximal and distal phalanges of the great toe are reduced and stabilized if displaced. The goal of surgery is to restore stability (frequently, these fractures are the result of a ligamentous, capsular, or tendinous avulsion) and to minimize the incidence of posttraumatic arthritis. Fractures of the metatarsophalangeal joint are approached through a straight dorsal incision. Fractures of the interphalangeal joint are approached through a midlateral incision. Fragments are reduced and held in place with small screws or small-diameter Kirschner wires. Postoperatively, the toe is splinted, and nonweight-bearing is maintained for 4 to 6 weeks.

Complications

Complications of forefoot injuries include posttraumatic arthritis of the Lisfranc joint and malunion of the metatarsals. **Posttraumatic arthritis of the Lisfranc joint** is managed with arch supports, nonsteroidal anti-inflammatory medication, and local injections of steroids. If these measures fail, the joint is arthrodesed. **Malunion of a metatarsal fracture** results in a localized area of increased pressure on the plantar aspect of the foot. A metatarsal bar or custom-molded shoe insert may compensate for the malunion and resolve the pain. If conservative measures are not acceptable, an osteotomy of the proximal metatarsal is performed. Fixation is not required, and the patient is encouraged to bear weight postoperatively so that the involved metatarsal head will heal in the proper location.

SELECTED READINGS

Injuries of the Hindfoot

Canale ST, Kelly FB Jr: Fractures of the neck of the talus. Long-term evaluation of seventy-one cases. *J Bone Joint Surg* 60A:143–156, 1978.

Comfort TH, Behrens F, Gaither DW, Denis F, Sigmond M: Long-term results of displaced talar neck fractures. *Clin Orthop* 199:81–87, 1985.

DeLee JC, Curtis R: Subtalar dislocation of the foot. *J Bone Joint Surg* 64A:433–437, 1982.

Hawkins LG: Fractures of the neck of the talus. *J Bone Joint Surg* 52A:991–1002, 1970.

Leung KS, Chan WS, Pak PPL, So WS, Leung PC: Operative treatment of intraarticular fractures of the os calcis—The role of rigid fixation and primary bone grafting: Preliminary results. *J Orthop Trauma* 3:232–240, 1989.

Miric A, Patterson BM: Pathoanatomy of intra-articular fractures of the calcaneus. *J Bone Joint Surg* 80A:207–212, 1995.

Sclamberg EL, Davenport K: Operative treatment of displaced intra-articular fractures of the calcaneus. *J Trauma* 28:510–516, 1988.

Injuries of the Midfoot

Main BJ, Jowett RL: Injuries of the midtarsal joint. *J Bone Joint Surg* 57B:89–97, 1975.

Tountas AA: Occult fracture subluxation of the midtarsal joint. *Clin Orthop* 243:195–199, 1989.

Injuries of the Forefoot

Arntz CT, Veith RG, Hansen ST Jr: Fractures and fracture–dislocations of the tarsometatarsal joint. *J Bone Joint Surg* 70A:173–181, 1988.

Hardcastle PH, Reschauer R, Kutscha-Lissberg E, Schoffmann W: Injuries to the tarsometatarsal joint. Incidence, classification and treatment. *J Bone Joint Surg* 64B:349–356, 1982.

Kavanaugh JH, Brower TD, Mann RV: The Jones fracture revisited. *J Bone Joint Surg* 60A:776–782, 1978.

Wiener BD, Linder JF, Giattini JF: Treatment of fractures of the fifth metatarsal: A prospective study. *Foot Ankle Int* 18:267–269, 1997.

General

Hansen ST Jr: Foot injuries. *In* Browner B (ed): *Skeletal trauma,* 2d ed. Philadelphia, WB Saunders, 1992, pp 1959–1991.

Heckman JD: Fractures and dislocations of the foot. *In Rockwood and Green's fractures in adults.* Hagerstown, JB Lippincott, 1991, pp 2041–2182.

Myerson M: Diagnosis and treatment of compartment syndrome of the foot. *Orthopedics* 13:711–717, 1990.

Glossary

Abduction Motion in the coronal plane; the extremity is moved away from the midline; the opposite of adduction.

Adduction Motion in the coronal plane; the extremity is moved toward the midline (e.g., adduction of the right hip crosses the right leg over the left leg).

Allograft Bone graft from a donor, not the patient.

Ankylosis Fusion of a joint; it may be fibrous or bony.

Arthrodesis Surgical fusion of a joint.

Autograft Bone graft from the patient who is being grafted.

Buddy taping Splinting a finger or toe by taping it to a neighboring finger or toe.

Caudad Toward the foot (e.g., the x-ray beam is angled caudad).

Cephalad Toward the head (e.g., the x-ray beam is angled cephalad).

Comminuted Term applied to fractures indicating that there are several fragments of bone and that the fracture is not simple (i.e., fractured into only two pieces).

Compound Term applied to fractures indicating that the fracture is open.

Contralateral Opposite side (e.g., a femur fracture and contralateral knee dislocation indicates that the fracture and knee dislocation are not in the same leg).

Coronal plane A two-dimensional surface in the frontal plane (e.g., medial and lateral angulation is in the coronal plane).

Coxa The hip and proximal femur (e.g., the coxa magna is the large femoral head).

Cubitus The elbow; cubital pertains to the elbow.

Diastasis Separation of bones attached by fibrous tissue, which is distinct from a dislocation in which the articular surfaces of a diarthrodial joint are separated (e.g., symphysis pubic diastasis or tibiofibular diastasis in a Maisonneuve fracture).

Dislocation Disruption of the joint with complete loss of continuity between the articular surfaces, as opposed to subluxation.

Dorsiflexion Describes motion away from the palmar, plantar, or volar surfaces of the hand or foot (e.g., dorsiflexion of the ankle lifts the forefoot superiorly off the ground).

Eversion Forefoot position in which the sole of the foot faces laterally; opposite of inversion.

Facet   Nearly flat articular surface (e.g., posterior facet of the calcaneus, or facet joint of the spine).

Genu   The knee (e.g., genu valgum, or knock-kneed).

Inversion   Forefoot position in which the sole of the foot faces medially; opposite of eversion.

Ipsilateral   Same side (e.g., ipsilateral femur and tibia fractures indicate that both fractures involve the right or left leg).

Kessler suture   Suture technique used to repair tendons (Fig. G-1).

Lateral   Away from the midline (e.g., apex lateral angulation).

Medial   Toward the midline (e.g., apex medial angulation).

Palmar   Toward or on the palm (e.g., palmar flexion of the wrist or a palmar incision).

Plantar   Toward or on the sole of the foot (e.g., plantar flexion of the ankle or a plantar incision).

Pronation   Forearm rotation resulting in the palm facing down; rotation of the foot and ankle around the axis of the neck of the talus, resulting in the sole facing laterally.

Prone   Describes face-down position of the patient.

Sagittal plane   Two-dimensional surface in the lateral plane (e.g., anterior and posterior angulation is in the sagittal plane).

Spondylolisthesis   Derived from the Greek words *spondylos* meaning "spine" and *olisthanein* meaning "to slip"; denotes foreward subluxation of one vertebral body on the lower vertebral body. May be traumatic or developmental.

Sprain   Denotes an injury of a ligament. Sprains are graded I to III. Grade I is rupture of interligamentous fibers without lengthening of the ligament. Grade II is partial rupture of the ligament with lengthening of the ligament but some interligamentous fibers remaining intact. Grade III is complete rupture of the ligament.

Subluxation   Disruption of a joint with partial loss of continuity between the articular surfaces.

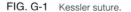

FIG. G-1   Kessler suture.

Supination Forearm rotation resulting in the palm of the hand facing up; rotation of the foot and ankle around the axis of the neck of the talus resulting in the sole of the foot facing medially.

Supine Describes face-up (lying on the back) position of the patient.

Tenodesis Occurs when a tendon is fixed to an underlying bone (i.e., tenodesis of the flexor digitorum profundus by fixing the tendons to the radius results in flexion of the fingers when the wrist is dorsiflexed).

Valgus Term used to describe angulation in the coronal plane. *Varus* and *valgus* are always used in conjunction with a joint; they indicate that the extremity distal to the named joint goes toward the midline (varus) or away from the midline (valgus; e.g., genu varum: the calf, i.e., the extremity distal to the knee, goes toward the midline, resulting in bowing).

Varus Term used to describe angulation in the coronal plane (*see Valgus*).

Volar Refers to the palmar surface of the hand and flexor or anterior surface of the wrist and forearm (e.g., volar flexion of the wrist is the opposite of wrist dorsiflexion).

Index

Page references in *italic* indicate figures; page references followed by the letter *t* indicates tables.

ISBN 0-07-048624-7

90000

9 780070 486249

PERRY/HANDBOOK
FRACTURES